C. Catalano · R. Passariello (Eds.)

Multidetector-Row CT Angiography

With Contributions by

H. Abe · C. Bartolozzi · C. R. Becker · L. Bertoletti · L. Bonomo · A. Caggiati · C. Catalano
D. Caramella · M. D. Dake · M. Danti · R. Ferrari · D. Fleischmann · T. Flohr · F. Fraioli
J. C. Hellinger · T. Hirai · M. Hohn · M. Hori · R. Iannaccone · R. Iezzi · D. S. Katz
A. A. Khankan · T. Kim · Y. Korogi · M. Kuwabara · A. Laghi · J. M. Levin · D. Marin
B. Merlino · T. Murakami · H. Nakamura · A. Napoli · P. Nardis · E. Neri · F. Odoguardi
R. Passariello · F. Pediconi · S. Schaller · U. J. Schoepf · M. Takahashi · J-F. Uhl · P. Vagli
Y. Yamashita

Foreword by

A. L. Baert

With 176 Figures in 345 Separate Illustrations, 85 in Color and 22 Tables

Springer

Carlo Catalano, MD
Associate Professor, Department of Radiological Sciences
University of Rome "La Sapienza"
Policlinico Umberto I
Viale Regina Elena n. 324
00161 Rome
Italy

Roberto Passariello, MD
Professor and Chairman, Department of Radiological Sciences
University of Rome "La Sapienza"
Policlinico Umberto I
Viale Regina Elena n. 324
00161 Rome
Italy

Medical Radiology · Diagnostic Imaging and Radiation Oncology
Series Editors: A. L. Baert · L. W. Brady · H.-P. Heilmann · M. Molls · K. Sartor

Continuation of Handbuch der medizinischen Radiologie
Encyclopedia of Medical Radiology

ISBN 978-3-642-07276-5 e-ISBN 978-3-540-26984-7

Springer is a part of Springer Science+Business Media

http//www.springeronline.com

Softcover reprint of the hardcover 1st edition 2005

Medical Editor: Dr. Ute Heilmann, Heidelberg
Desk Editor: Ursula N. Davis, Heidelberg
Production Editor: Kurt Teichmann, Mauer
Cover-Design and Typesetting: Verlagsservice Teichmann, Mauer

Printed on acid-free paper 21/3150xq – 5 4 3 2 1 0

MEDICAL RADIOLOGY
Diagnostic Imaging

Editors:
A. L. Baert, Leuven
K. Sartor, Heidelberg

Foreword

Intravenous CT angiography (CTA) was first introduced more than 10 years ago following the development of spiral CT. However, considerable technical problems, related to the difficulties in achieving satisfactory spatial resolution of large body volumes or of the extremities, prevented widespread clinical application of this interesting non-invasive diagnostic imaging modality.

The introduction of the multidetector-row technology allowed excellent volume data acquisition and improved considerably the technical quality of CTA imaging while reducing the quantities of iodinated contrast media administered to the patient.

CTA is now a mature and robust technique that increasingly is replacing catheter angiography for diagnostic purposes in daily radiological practice.

This volume covers exhaustively not only the technical and physical bases of multidetector-row CTA but also the correct clinical execution of the study, as well as the new and fascinating applications of this method in all organs of the body as well as in the extremities. The eminently readable text is complemented by numerous superb illustrations.

The editors belong to the department of radiology of the University "La Sapienza", a clinical radiological center with a long-standing interest and competence in new imaging modalities and specifically in angiography and CT. They are widely recognized as experts in the field.

The authors of individual chapters, who come from both sides of the Atlantic and from the Far East, were invited to contribute because of their outstanding personal experience in a specific anatomic area and their major contributions to the radiological literature on the topic.

I would like to thank the editors and the authors and congratulate them sincerely for their superb efforts in writing this excellent volume, which is a much-needed comprehensive update of the considerable diagnostic possibilities of modern CTA.

This book will be of great interest not only for general and vascular radiologists but also for all referring clinical practitioners. I am confident that it will meet the same success with readers as the previous volumes published in this series.

Leuven — Albert L. Baert

Preface

The advent of spiral CT introduced a new era in radiology: three-dimensional acquisition. The possibility to acquire volumes instead of simply bi-dimensional scans allowed to introduce the concept of multiple phases studies after a single intravenous bolus of contrast agent administration and especially to acquire a volume during the passage of the contrast agent in the arteries. The advent of computed tomography angiography (CTA) resulted in a revolution in vascular radiology with more and more pathological entities assessed non invasively, leaving catheter angiography the main and increasing role of treating mini-invasively diseases.

The clinical advantage of CTA appeared immediately clear either in emergency or selected cases. Infact since then the role of CTA is well established in the diagnosis of acute diseases of the aorta (dissection and rupture), pulmonary embolism, thoracic and abdominal aortic aneurysms.

Other applications were also successfully considered, such as the evaluation of the intracranial circulation, the carotid arteries, the renal arteries and the pelvic arteries.

The success of the technique was also related to the development of sophisticated workstations for three-dimensional evaluation and reconstructions of the acquired volume, introducing new algorithms that facilitated the diagnosis and created images analogue or at least similar to those provided by catheter angiography.

As the experience with CTA increased it became evident which were the limitations of spiral CT: the need to reach a compromise between spatial resolution along the *z*-axis and volume coverage and to administer quite large volumes of iodinated contrast agent. In fact if a large volume needed to be acquired a thin slice collimation could not be used; on the contrary a high resolution volume using a thin collimation was possible only for limited volume width. At the same time scan duration was long (considering a minimum gantry rotation time of 0.75 seconds, which nevertheless in most scanners was 1 second) necessitating, in order to achieve a good vascular enhancement, a large amount of contrast agent.

These limitations were then surpassed at the beginning of 1999 when the first multidetector row scanners were introduced and tested clinically, with excellent results. It seems immediately clear that the compromise between volume coverage and spatial resolution had no reason to exist anymore and that the volume of iodinated contrast agent could be reduced.

Since then a large number of articles have demonstrated that computed tomography has entered a new technological era with enormous impact on the routine daily practice; real three-dimensional visualization of all body structures, non invasive assessment of vascular structures, cardiac and coronary imaging, perfusion imaging and more and more screening examinations.

Multidetector row CT technology is under continuous development and at this time we are assisting to decrease of the gantry rotation time, improvement of x-ray tubes performances and increase of number of slices acquired per second.

Computed Tomography Angiography is the application that has most benefited of all these technological improvements opening to non invasive assessment the evaluation of all peripheral vasculature and the coronary arteries with all relative clinical implications.

The aim of this text is therefore to show the potentials and clinical applications of CTA, with its limitations and advantages, also in comparison with other imaging modalities.

Rome

Carlo Catalano
Roberto Passariello

Contents

1 Multidetector-Row CT Angiography: Evolution, Current Usage, Clinical Perspectives and Comparison with Other Imaging Modalities

Douglas S. Katz and Man Hon

CONTENTS

1.1 Evolution of Multidetector-Row CT Angiography

1.1.1 Development of Helical CT Angiography

Helical computed tomography (CT), introduced commercially more than a decade ago, represented a revolutionary advance compared with single-slice "conventional" CT. Shortly after its introduction, Rubin et al. [36, 37], at Stanford University, described CT angiography (CTA) of the abdominal aorta and its branches, utilizing the volumetric data sets which were acquired in a single breath-hold on a helical CT scanner. For CTA, the images were obtained during peak arterial enhancement, using a rapid injection of iodinated contrast, which was given through a large-gauge peripheral IV. The investigators were able to reliably identify up to third-order aortic branches, and they detected pathological conditions such as abdominal aortic aneurysms and dissections, as well as renal artery stenosis, and were able to reformat the data set into various three-dimensional representations, including shaded surface displays and maximum-intensity projections. Rubin and his colleagues [36, 37] noted the significant advantages of CTA compared with traditional catheter angiography: speed, noninvasiveness, need for only a single injection to obtain multiple views, and visualization of the extraluminal as well as intraluminal structures. At the same time, the use of helical CT angiography to noninvasively image the carotid circulation was also reported from Stanford University [45], and Remy-Jardin and her colleagues [34] reported the first prospective evaluation of helical CT for suspected pulmonary embolism. Multiple reports followed, confirming the robustness of CTA for imaging the aorta and other vessels, as well as its many advantages compared with conventional angiography, most significantly that conventional angiography reveals the lumen of an aneurysm, whereas CTA demonstrates the overall aneurysm size and extent, as well as its relationship to adjacent structures. Van Hoe et al. [49], for example, compared CTA with digital subtraction angiography (DSA) in 38 patients with abdominal aortic aneurysms; the proximal extent of the 15 juxta- and suprarenal aneurysms was predicted correctly in 14 cases with CTA but in only 12 cases using DSA, compared with the findings at surgery. Additional reports on the utility of helical CTA emerged, for imaging suspected traumatic aortic injury [8], living renal donors [38], staging

D. S. Katz, MD
Vice Chair and Director of Body CT, Department of Radiology, Winthrop-University Hospital, 259 First Street, Mineola, NY 11501, USA *and* Associate Professor of Clinical Radiology, State University of New York at Stony Brook, Stony Brook, NY, USA
M. Hon, MD
Attending, Department of Radiology, Winthrop-University Hospital, 259 First Street, Mineola, NY 11501, USA *and* Assistant Professor of Clinical Radiology, State University of New York at Stony Brook, Stony Brook, NY, USA

malignancy prior to surgery, and evaluating hepatic transplant recipients before and after surgery [26]. For all of these clinical situations, it was noted that CTA could be combined with additional phases of imaging (unenhanced, portal venous, delayed), e.g., when staging malignancy.

1.1.2 Refinement and Additional Applications of CT Angiography

As helical CT scanners proliferated over the next several years, the utilization of CT angiography increased significantly, as did the number and types of applications. Compared with conventional angiography, CT angiography was more comfortable for patients, faster, and more readily available at most institutions and practices, especially after hours and at weekends. At many institutions, CTA completely or mostly replaced DSA (and other imaging tests) for many applications, including imaging for suspected pulmonary embolism; imaging of aortic aneurysm, dissection, or injury; and imaging of potential living renal donors. The maturation of CTA paralleled the development of commercially available software packages and workstations, which allowed volumetric rendering and other advanced reconstructions of the three-dimensional data set, although the primary method of image interpretation remained review of the axial images.

1.1.3 Development of Multidetector-Row CT Angiography

The introduction of multidetector-row CT (MDCT) scanners further advanced the revolution started by helical CT [4, 39], and has had its greatest impact on CT angiography. The initial MDCT scanners acquired the data for four to eight axial images per second. Current state-of-the-art MDCT scanners can obtain the data for 16 or more slices per second ("16-plus"), further decreasing scan time and routine slice thickness (typically 1 or 1.25 mm), as well as increasing volumetric coverage. Additional advantages of MDCTA compared with single-slice CTA include decreased motion, respiratory, and cardiac artifacts; decrease in contrast volume (if only an arterial phase study is needed); and scanning of isotropic or nearly isotropic voxels, further improving multiplanar and three-dimensional reconstructions [40, 42]. In one early study which showed the superiority of MDCT angiography (MDCTA), 48 patients with aortic aneurysm or dissection were imaged on two separate occasions, once using a single-slice helical CT scanner and the other time using an MDCT scanner. With MDCT, the entire thoracoabdominal aorta was covered in a single 30-s breath-hold, mean contrast volume was decreased by 58%, image quality improved, and aortic enhancement did not decrease [40]. With the advent of MDCT scanners, techniques including lower-extremity CTA and coronary CTA became much more readily performed, especially with the 16-plus per second MDCT units.

1.2 Established Uses of CT Angiography

1.2.1 Thoracic CT Angiography

1.2.1.1 Thoracic Aortic Imaging

Quint et al. [33] demonstrated the high accuracy of CTA of the thoracic aorta in 49 patients with various pathological processes, including dissection and aortic ulcer; there was exact correlation with the findings at surgery in 45 of the patients. CTA has become the test of choice for suspected aortic dissection, as the diagnosis may be excluded or established with an extremely high level of accuracy, the type (Fig. 1.1; including variants such as intramural hematoma; Fig 1.2), extent, and involvement of branch vessels determined, and alternate diagnoses made if dissection is not present. Sommer et al. [46] determined that CTA, magnetic resonance angiography (MRA), and transesophageal echocardiography were all nearly equivalent in a group of symptomatic patients with suspected aortic dissection, but CTA was superior for the evaluation of the arch vessels, and CTA had the advantages of speed and convenience. For imaging suspected thoracic aortic injury, CTA also became established as the initial test of choice, with the additional major advantage (compared with conventional angiography) that the entire body can be scanned if needed, and is globally evaluated, i.e., the lungs, bones, etc., can all be examined (Fig. 1.3). In a series of 1,518 blunt trauma patients, 127 (8%) with apparent aortic injury and/or mediastinal hematoma visible on CT

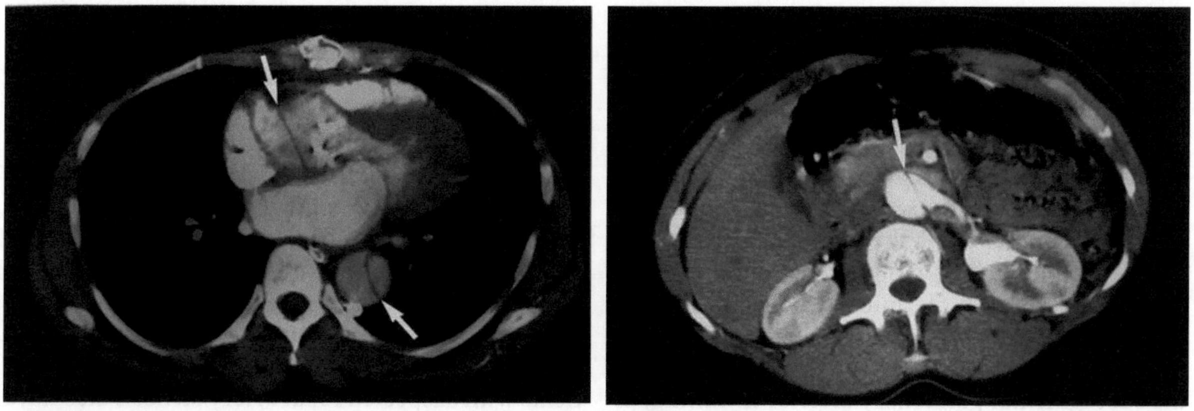

Fig. 1.1a,b. A 45-year-old woman with acute onset of lower back pain and history of aortic valve replacement for rheumatic heart disease. **a** Transverse CT angiography image at the level of the aortic root shows an aortic dissection flap (*arrows*). **b** CT image at the level of the left renal artery shows the dissection flap (*arrow*)

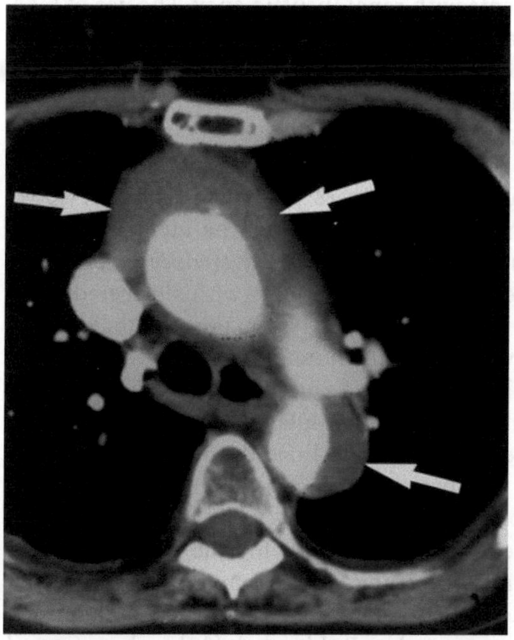

Fig. 1.2. Multidetector-row CT angiography image shows a type A intramural hematoma (*arrows*) in this 77-year-old woman who was imaged for shortness of breath, chest pain, and widening of the mediastinum on plain radiographs

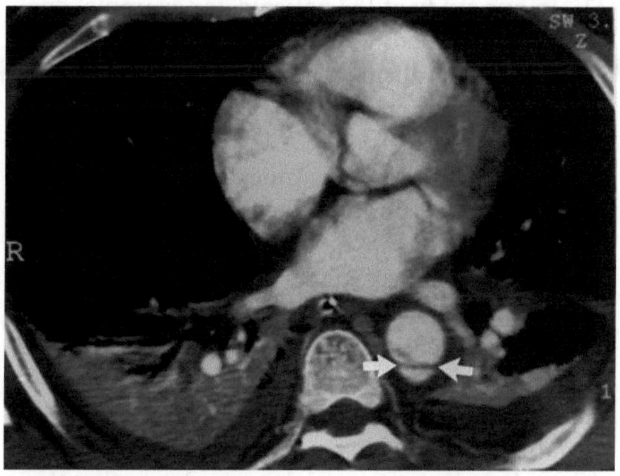

Fig. 1.3. A 59-year-old man underwent multidetector-row CT angiography following a fall from a tree. There is focal disruption of the distal thoracic aorta (*arrows*). CT also revealed pleural effusions, pulmonary contusions and lacerations, and multiple fractures (the latter not shown). The patient was successfully treated with a thoracic aortic stent-graft

angiograms subsequently underwent conventional angiography. In all of these 127 cases, if the aorta itself appeared normal on CT images, it also was normal on angiograms; all aortic injuries were also confirmed, except for two false-positive CT studies, where a ductus diverticulum was shown on conventional angiograms [8]. In another study of 382 patients, all of whom underwent both CTA and DSA, there were ten true-positives, and no false-positive or false-negative CT studies [6].

1.2.1.2
CT Pulmonary Angiography

CT pulmonary angiography (CTPA) for suspected pulmonary embolism, since its introduction by Remy-Jardin and colleagues in 1992 [34], is greatly improved when performed on MDCT scanners, and has correspondingly become a front-line imaging examination at an increasing number of institutions. As a result, at our own institution [25] and at many others, over the past several years, catheter pulmonary angiography has rarely been performed, and the volume of ventilation-perfusion scans has also dramatically decreased. CTPA can be combined with CT venography of the abdomen, pelvis, and lower extremities [17], without the requirement for additional contrast, permitting "one-stop shopping" for pulmonary thromboembolism. The controversy over the reliability of CTPA for imaging the subsegmental pulmonary arteries is waning, as several reports have shown that MDCT is quite accurate for imaging these vessels when thin images are acquired, although the significance of isolated subsegmental emboli – in the absence of residual clot in the lower extremities – remains uncertain [17]. In one study of 157 patients, for example, dual-detector CTPA showed relatively high accuracy for pulmonary embolism, compared with conventional pulmonary angiography [31], and it is assumed that multidetector-row CTA is even more accurate when a state-of-the-art scanner is utilized. For example, a recent study documented the visualization of almost 90% of subsegmental pulmonary arteries using 1.25-mm images and 4-channel MDCT [10]. Very recently, Patel et al. [28] showed that MDCT at 1.25 mm collimation significantly improved visualization of both segmental and subsegmental pulmonary arteries as well as interobserver agreement for pulmonary embolism. Additionally and very significantly, using a pig model, it was shown that there was no difference between CTPA and catheter angiography for the detection of subsegmental emboli, using the gold standard as autopsy of the animals in contrast to catheter angiography itself [2].

1.2.2 Abdominal CT Angiography

1.2.2.1 Renal Artery Imaging

Evaluation of renovascular disease historically involved work-up with systemic renin levels, which was followed with invasive, selective renal vein renin levels for lateralization. Captopril renal scans subsequently improved the diagnostic yield, but the overall sensitivity was suboptimal. Doppler sonography has been used in some centers to screen for renal artery stenosis, but has not gained widespread acceptance due to its relatively high technical failure rate – even in conjunction with IV contrast enhancement – and lower sensitivity compared with other cross-sectional imaging studies. The major advantages of Doppler sonography are lower cost and quicker accessibility [5]. Gadolinium-enhanced magnetic resonance angiography is currently considered by some authorities to be the modality of choice for the routine noninvasive evaluation of suspected renal artery stenosis [23, 32]. Magnetic resonance angiography has the major advantage of not requiring iodinated contrast, since many patients with suspected renal artery stenosis also have a degree of renal insufficiency. Alternative strategies include conventional angiography as an initial examination, although this is obviously an invasive test; conventional angiography can, however, be performed using gadolinium or carbon dioxide in patients with renal insufficiency. The use of CTA for imaging the renal arteries was first reported by Rubin et al. as noted above [36], although subsequent investigations of CTA for renal artery stenosis were somewhat disappointing [7]. By the mid to late 1990s, with use of thinner sections and optimized technique, reports were published of nearly 100% sensitivity and specificity for the identification of greater than 50% renal artery stenoses [3, 14, 29]. For the evaluation of patients with suspected renal artery stenosis, CTA is less expensive than MRA, can reveal flow within metal stents as well as arterial calcification, and can be used to directly plan for renal arterial angioplasty [29]; however, CTA requires the use of iodinated contrast, which requires that patients do not have renal insufficiency. Multiphasic helical CT, including CTA, was also reported as a replacement for the combination of DSA and intravenous urography for the evaluation of patients being considered as living renal donors. As first reported by Rubin et al. [38] and confirmed by multiple investigations (most recently in patients potentially undergoing laparoscopic renal extraction [18]), there was a very high correlation with findings at surgery for the arterial and venous anatomy. Multiphasic CT permitted the identification of calculi, anatomical variations such as multiple renal arteries, early renal branching, and retroaortic/circumaortic renal veins, and renal masses. Similar techniques can also be used for imaging potential living hepatic donors, although in this instance MR is advantageous, because MR cholangiography can easily be performed at the same sitting, and anatomical variants which might preclude donation can therefore be identified.

1.2.2.2
CT Angiography of Aortic Stent-Grafts

CTA has quickly become the test of choice for imaging patients before and after the placement of aortoiliac stent-grafts [1, 43, 44]. The axial CT images, along with maximum-intensity projection and other image reconstructions, can be easily and readily used to plan stent-graft placement and to detect complications after stent-graft placement, most commonly type II endoleaks, where contrast extends into the perigraft sac from patent aortoiliac branches such as the lumbar arteries (Fig. 1.4). The superiority of CTA over DSA for the detection of endoleaks was clearly shown in one study of 46 patients: sensitivities and specificities were 63% and 77% for DSA compared with 92% and 90% for CTA [1].

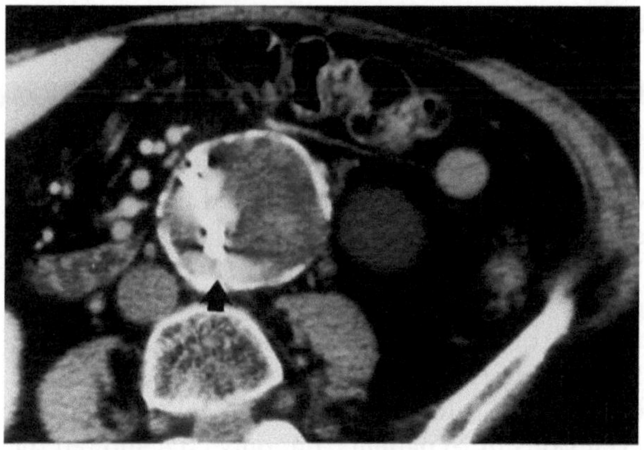

Fig. 1.4. Transverse helical CT angiography image shows a type-II endoleak (*arrow*) in this 81-year-old woman who underwent CT for routine surveillance several months after placement of an aortic stent-graft for an abdominal aortic aneurysm

1.3
Newer and Emerging Uses of Multidetector-Row CT Angiography

1.3.1
CT Angiography of Suspected Mesenteric Ischemia

Mesenteric ischemia is an increasing problem in aging Western populations. Mesenteric ischemia, both acute and chronic, may be multifactorial, is often difficult to correctly diagnose (especially early acute ischemia), and may have devastating effects [52]. Acute mesenteric ischemia is a true medical emergency, with morbidity and mortality related to the time of recognition and treatment. Traditionally, a mesenteric angiogram using conventional catheter technique is performed as soon as the diagnosis is considered [52]. If acute ischemia is diagnosed, intra-arterial infusion of vasodilators will decrease morbidity, even in those patients who require surgery. There is also the rare possibility of treatment with thrombolysis if the acute thrombus is found early enough. If no acute mesenteric ischemia is found, other less urgent imaging can take place. Relatively recently, Horton and Fishman [12] proposed a MDCTA protocol for imaging both suspected acute as well as chronic mesenteric ischemia, which we have adopted at our institution (Fig. 1.5). There are virtually no reports comparing any type of CTA with conventional angiography [52], and there is little published on the accuracy of MDCTA to date, although it is anticipated that with MDCTA the accuracy for acute mesenteric ischemia should improve significantly compared with earlier CT studies. In the only such study we are aware of at this time, Kirkpatrick et al. [19] imaged 47 patients with suspected acute mesenteric ischemia, which was subsequently proven in 21 patients; management was influenced in 4 by the arterial phase images, and an alternate diagnosis was established on CT in 15 of the 26 patients without ischemia. In both acute and chronic mesenteric ischemia, narrowing and calcification of the origins of the celiac and superior mesenteric arteries may be identified on CTA, which are optimally seen on sagittal reformations (Fig. 1.6), although the clinical significance of this finding is not always clear [12]. With

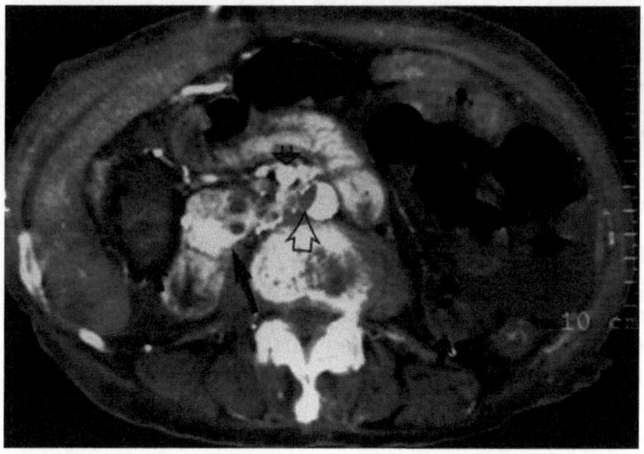

Fig. 1.5. An 82-year-old woman with acute mesenteric ischemia. Transverse multidetector-row CT angiography image shows loops of small bowel with both increased and decreased enhancement. Atherosclerotic changes are noted in the aortic lumen, but the superior mesenteric artery is patent, as is the celiac artery (on other images, not shown)

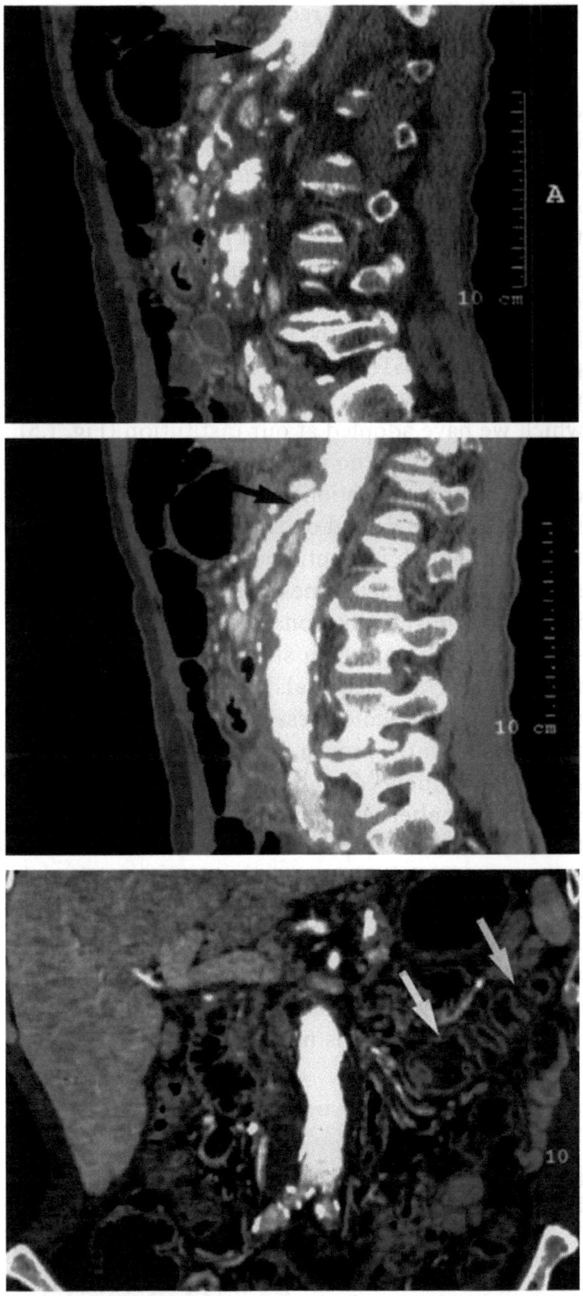

a b c

Fig. 1.6a–c. A 79-year-old man with suspected mesenteric ischemia. **a,b** Sagittal multidetector-row CT angiography reconstructions show patency of the celiac (**a**, *arrow*) and superior mesenteric (**b**, *arrow*) arteries. **c** There is atherosclerosis of the aorta on this coronal reconstruction. Colitis at the splenic flexure is noted, which was believed to be ischemic (*arrows*)

the advent of MDCTA, it is possible to now make the diagnosis of acute mesenteric ischemia in a few minutes, less time than it takes to prepare a patient for catheter angiography, and much less time than it takes to gather the angiography team if the patient presents after hours. In terms of patients with suspected chronic mesenteric ischemia ("intestinal angina"), patients usually present insidiously with classic signs and symptoms of postprandial pain, weight loss, and fear of eating [52]. MDCTA is an ideal imaging modality to evaluate this entity, as the CT is usually performed anyway to evaluate for other causes of the patient's symptomatology. When tailored specifically to evaluate for chronic mesenteric ischemia, the origins and proximal portions of the mesenteric arteries are well visualized on CTA [12]. Treatment of stenoses or occlusions with endovascular angioplasty and/or stent placement, or with surgical therapy, can then be planned using the information from the CTA.

1.3.2
Lower-Extremity CT Angiography

Lower extremity CT angiography, an outgrowth of aortoiliac CTA, is a recent development which can be performed easily and routinely with MDCT [15, 41], but which was first introduced using a single-slice helical CT scanner [3, 22, 35]. Lawrence et al. [22] showed high accuracy of CTA for identifying greater than 75% stenoses, compared with DSA, in the central thigh and calf arteries in 50 patients. Beregi et al. [3] demonstrated 100% concordance of CTA and DSA for revealing popliteal stenoses and occlusions in 26 patients, but only CTA showed the cause of the problem in 10 patients: aneurysm, entrapment syndrome, or cystic adventitial disease. In the first report using MDCTA for imaging the lower extremities, Rubin and colleagues [41] showed 100% concordance for the extent of disease with DSA in 18 patients, and better demonstration of distal runoff vessels on MDCTA in a subset of the patients (Fig. 1.7). The technique worked surprisingly well despite severe asymmetric disease in some patients. Other very recent reports have noted similar findings and equally promising results [24, 27]. MDCTA of the lower extremities, which is performed as a single CTA acquisition of the entire abdomen (and if necessary, chest), pelvis, and legs, has the potential to be cost-effective compared with MRA and other imaging tests [50], and compared with MRA it is much easier to acquire diagnostic images of the calves and feet [15]. Compared with DSA, vascular calcifications are evident, as are soft-tissue abnormalities. Our experience to date is that MDCTA is a robust technique, and surprisingly our vascular surgeons have readily accepted the results of MDCTA

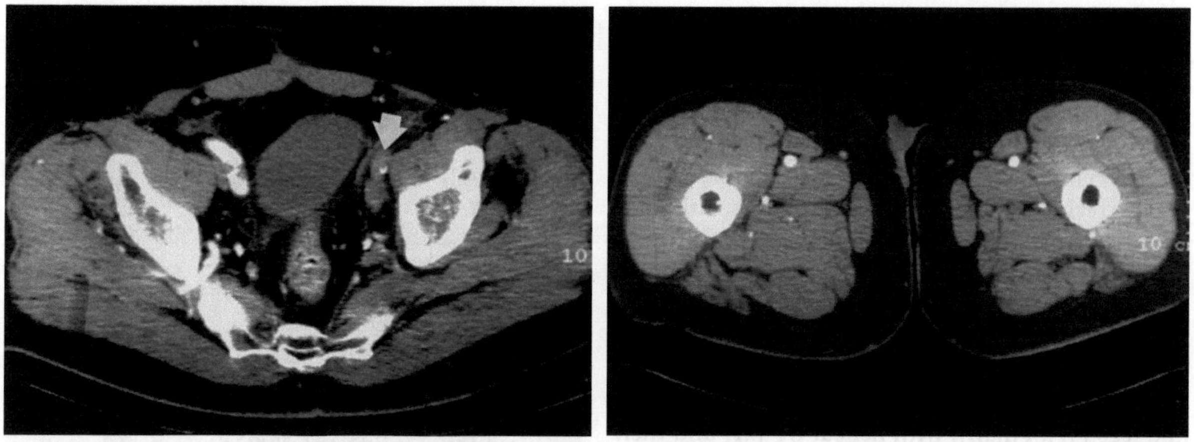

Fig. 1.7a,b. A 60-year-old man with bilateral claudication and an unsuccessful attempt at peripheral arterial access for conventional angiography. **a** Transverse image from a multidetector-row CT angiogram demonstrates no significant flow in the left external iliac artery (*arrow*). **b** Transverse image at the level of the mid thighs reveals patency of both superficial femoral and profunda femoral arteries. The trifurcation vessels in the thighs were also patent bilaterally (not shown)

for a subset of patients with peripheral vascular disease, especially in those patients with limited arterial access for conventional angiography, where reconstitution from distal collaterals gives MDCTA a significant advantage over conventional angiography [15]. There are no studies, to our knowledge, to date which have compared MDCTA of the lower extremities to MRA, and in general larger prospective studies are needed, although determination of a true gold standard, as with many types of MDCTA, is problematic [15].

1.3.3 Cardiac CT Angiography

There has been a recent explosion of interest in cardiac imaging concurrent with the introduction of the latest version of MDCT scanners, although there are few large, prospective peer-reviewed trials by which to judge the true accuracy of MDCTA for coronary arterial imaging, and the current literature is already out of date [9, 13, 20, 48, 51]. Until very recently, temporal resolution was limited to 250 ms, and the previous reports of coronary MDCTA have been somewhat disappointing, as very high accuracy is required if the technique is to compete with conventional coronary angiography. Even with 16-plus MDCT scanners, significant challenges continue, including high radiation doses (primarily related to retrospective cardiac gating), motion artifacts, especially of the right coronary artery, optimization of contrast timing and delivery, problems with patients with high and/or irregular heart rates, optimization of rapid and straightforward yet comprehensive data analysis, and potentially most significantly, "turf" battles with cardiologists. To overcome some of these challenges, CT manufacturers are introducing dedicated software packages, allowing ready performance of ventriculography, quantification of coronary arterial stenoses, and even myocardial perfusion. Additionally, CT has significant potential advantages compared with other modalities: other than the obvious noninvasiveness, compared with echocardiography, the chest wall is not a problem and, compared with MR/MRA, soft versus hard plaque can be distinguished. If these remaining technical challenges are overcome, and the coronary arterial circulation can be routinely imaged with a higher degree of accuracy with improved visualization of the more peripheral coronary arterial circulation, then MDCTA of the heart and coronary arteries may play an important role in the future, including in the comprehensive evaluation of the patient with thoracic pain.

1.3.4 Whole-Body CT Angiography

Whole-body CT angiography is now possible with 16-plus slice MDCT scanners, although the technology must be used judiciously such that all patients do not indiscriminately and unnecessarily receive whole-body radiation. The concept of a single-pass whole-body MDCT protocol for trauma patients, for example, was first proposed by Ptak et al. [30], from the Massachusetts General Hospital. A similar protocol may also be applied when imaging patients with known or suspected atherosclerosis, permitting examination not only for aortic pathology but also for arterial disease in the lower extremities, the carotid arteries, and even the circle of Willis, although at present (in contrast to whole-body MRA [11]), we are not aware of any formal peer-reviewed reports of the utilization of such a protocol. Additionally, CTA has also been shown to be highly accurate as the initial imaging test in patients with suspected injuries to the central arteries of the proximal arms and legs [47]. Finally, with helical CT [21] and then with MDCT [53, 54], active arterial contrast extravasation in the setting of trauma (and to a much lesser extent, in patients without trauma) is being increasingly recognized in the chest, abdomen, and pelvis, even when patients are not being specifically imaged in the arterial phase of contrast administration. The identification of such extravasation strongly suggests the need for immediate surgery or angiographic therapy.

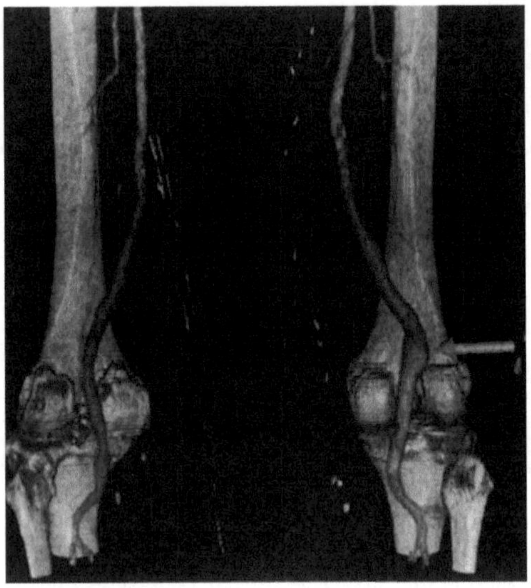

Fig. 1.8. Volumetric reconstruction of a multidetector-row CT angiogram of the lower extremities, performed on a 63-year-old man with suspected atherosclerosis of the aorta and lower extremity arterial circulation, shows patency of the superficial femoral and popliteal arteries, with slight dilatation of the left proximal popliteal artery due to an aneurysm. Bilateral popliteal artery aneurysms were obvious on axial image review (not shown)

1.4 Conclusions

With the continuing advancement of multidetector-row CT technology, the application which has benefited the most, CT angiography, has continued to evolve along with it. Helical CT and now multidetector-row CT have revolutionized noninvasive arterial imaging for an increasing number of examinations and continue to do so to this day. Conventional angiography of course will always play a major role in patient care, because interventional vascular procedures require arterial catheterization, but for diagnostic purposes CT angiography, especially when performed on multidetector-row CT scanners, has become the imaging test of choice for many clinical situations, including suspected aortic dissection or transection, aortic aneurysm imaging, suspected pulmonary artery embolism, tumoral staging, and potential living renal donor evaluation. MR angiography does compete with CT angiography, although, with the increasingly improved spatial resolution of MDCTA and the ease in reformation of the imaging volume, the advantages of MRA have decreased over the past several years for some indications. MRA continues to have a primary role when radiation exposure is a concern (especially in young individuals who may need multiple studies over time or when multiphasic imaging is to be performed) or when iodinated contrast is contraindicated (due to renal dysfunction or allergy). The challenges of viewing, interpreting, and storing increasingly large CT data sets [39] have lessened to some extent as picture-archiving systems and workstations have kept up with these demands. Multiple types of reformations are now available with a click of a button and within a matter of seconds – even volumetric reformations (Fig. 1.8) – although in our opinion review of the images in a cine fashion on a CT monitor or workstation remains the mainstay of initial evaluation, even with CT angiography of the lower extremities or cardiac imaging. Finally, when interpreting CTA studies, attention must always be paid to the extra-arterial structures, since CT is a global examination, and alternative or additional diagnoses may be present [16].

References

1. Armerding MD, Rubin GD, Beaulieu CF et al (2000) Aortic aneurysmal disease: assessment of stent-graft treatment-CT versus conventional angiography. Radiology 215:138–146
2. Baile EM, King GG, Muller NL et al (2000) Spiral computed tomography is comparable to angiography for the

diagnosis of pulmonary embolism. Am J Respir Crit Care Med 161:1010–1015
3. Beregi JP, Djabbari M, Desmoucelle F et al (1997) Popliteal vascular disease: evaluation with spiral CT angiography. Radiology 203:477–483
4. Berland LL, Smith JK (1998) Multidetector-array CT: once again, technology creates new opportunities. Radiology 209:327–329
5. Dowling RJ, House MK, King PM et al (1999) Contrast-enhanced Doppler ultrasound for renal artery stenosis. Australas Radiol 43:206-209
6. Dyer DS, Moore EE, Mestek MF et al (1999) Can chest CT be used to exclude aortic injury? Radiology 213:195–202
7. Galanski M, Prokop M, Chavan A et al (1993) Renal arterial stenoses: spiral CT angiography. Radiology 189:185–192
8. Gavant ML, Manke PG, Fabian T et al (1995) Blunt traumatic aortic rupture: detection with helical CT of the chest. Radiology 197:125–133
9. Gerber TC, Kuzo RS, Karstaedt N et al (2002) Current results and new developments of coronary angiography with use of contrast-enhanced computed tomography of the heart. Mayo Clin Proc 77:55–71
10. Ghaye B, Szapiro D, Mastora I et al (2001) Peripheral pulmonary arteries: how far in the lung does multi-detector row spiral CT allow analysis? Radiology 219:629–636
11. Goyen M, Herborn CU, Kroger K et al (2003) Detection of atherosclerosis: systemic imaging for systemic disease with whole-body three-dimensional MR angiography – initial experience. Radiology 227:277–282
12. Horton KM, Fishman EK (2001) Multi-detector row CT of mesenteric ischemia: can it be done? Radiographics 21:1463–1473
13. Juergens KU, Grude M, Fallenberg EM et al (2002) Using ECG-gated multidetector CT to evaluate global left ventricular myocardial function in patients with coronary artery disease. AJR Am J Roentgenol 179:1545–1550
14. Kaate R, Beek FJ, Lange EE de, et al (1997) Renal artery stenosis: detection and quantification with spiral CT angiography versus optimized digital subtraction angiography. Radiology 205:121–127
15. Katz DS, Hon M (2001) CT angiography of the lower extremities and aortoiliac system with a multi-detector row helical CT scanner: promise of new opportunities fulfilled. Radiology 221:7–10
16. Katz DS, Jorgensen MJ, Rubin GD (1999) Detection and follow-up of important extra-arterial lesions with helical CT angiography. Clin Radiol 54:294–300
17. Katz DS, Loud PA, Bruce D et al (2002) Combined CT venography and pulmonary angiography (CTVPA): a comprehensive review. Radiographics 22:3–20
18. Kawamoto S, Montgomery RA, Lawler LP et al (2003) Multidetector CT angiography for preoperative evaluation of living laparoscopic kidney donors. AJR Am J Roentgenol 180:1633–1638
19. Kirkpatrick ID, Kroeker MA, Greenberg HM (2002) Biphasic CT with CT mesenteric angiography in the evaluation of acute intestinal ischemia. Radiology 225:353–354
20. Kopp AF, Schroeder S, Kuettner A et al (2001) Coronary arteries: retrospectively ECG-gated multi-detector row CT angiography with selective optimization of the image reconstruction window. Radiology 221:683–688
21. Lane MJ, Katz DS, Shah R et al (1998) Active arterial contrast extravasation on helical CT of the abdomen, pelvis, and chest. AJR Am J Roentgenol 171:679–685
22. Lawrence JA, Kim D, Kent KC et al (1995) Lower extremity spiral CT angiography versus catheter angiography. Radiology 194:903–908
23. Leung DA, Hagspiel KD, Angle JF et al (2002) MR angiography of the renal arteries. Radiol Clin North Am 40:847–865
24. Martin ML, Tay KH, Flak B et al (2003) Multidetector CT angiography of the aortoiliac system and lower extremities: a prospective comparison with digital subtraction angiography. AJR Am J Roentgenol 180:1085–1091
25. Mattoo A, Katz DS, Groth ML et al (2003) The search for pulmonary embolism: changing trends in usage of spiral CT and V/Q scan. Scientific poster presentation, American Thoracic Society annual meeting, Seattle, Washington, USA
26. Nghiem HV, Jeffrey RB Jr (1998) CT angiography of the visceral vasculature. Semin US CT MRI 19:439–446
27. Ofer A, Nitecki SS, Linn S et al (2003) Multidetector CT angiography of peripheral vascular disease: a prospective comparison with intraarterial digital subtraction angiography. AJR Am J Roentgenol 180:719–724
28. Patel S, Kazerooni EA, Cascade PN (2003) Pulmonary embolism: optimization of small pulmonary artery visualization at multi-detector row CT. Radiology 227:455–460
29. Prokop M (1999) Protocols and future directions in imaging of renal artery stenosis: CT angiography. J Comput Assist Tomogr 23:S101–S110
30. Ptak T, Rhea JT, Novelline RA (2001) Experience with a continuous, single-pass whole-body multidetector CT protocol for trauma: the three-minute multiple trauma CT scan. Emerg Radiol 8:250–256
31. Qanadli SD, El Hajjam M, Mesurolle B et al (2000) Pulmonary embolism detection: prospective evaluation of dual-section helical CT versus selective pulmonary arteriography in 157 patients. Radiology 217:447–455
32. Qanadli SD, Soulez G, Therasse E et al (2001) Detection of renal artery stenosis: prospective comparison of captopril-enhanced Doppler sonography, captopril-enhanced scintigraphy, and MR angiography. AJR Am J Roentgenol 177:1123–1129
33. Quint L, Francis IR, Williams DM et al (1996) Evaluation of thoracic aortic disease with the use of helical and multiplanar reconstructions: comparison with surgical findings. Radiology 201:37–41
34. Remy-Jardin M, Remy J, Wattinne L et al (1992) Central pulmonary thromboembolism: diagnosis with spiral volumetric CT with the single-breath-hold technique-comparison with pulmonary angiography. Radiology 185:381–387
35. Rieker O, Duber C, Schmiedt W et al (1996) Prospective comparison of CT angiography of the legs with intraaterial digital subtraction angiography. AJR Am J Roentgenol 166:269–276
36. Rubin GD, Dake MD, Napel SA et al (1993a) Three-dimensional spiral CT angiography of the abdomen: initial clinical experience. Radiology 186:147–152
37. Rubin GD, Walker PJ, Dake MJ et al (1993b) Three-dimensional spiral computed tomographic angiogra-

phy: an alternative imaging modality for the abdominal aorta and its branches. J Vasc Surg 18:565–665
38. Rubin GD, Alfrey EJ, Dake MD et al (1995) Spiral CT for the assessment of living renal donors. Radiology 195:457–462
39. Rubin GD, Shiau MC, Schmidt AJ et al (1999) Computed tomographic angiography: historical perspective and new state-of-the-art using multi detector-row helical computed tomography. J Comput Assist Tomogr 23: S83–S90
40. Rubin GD, Shiau MC, Leung AN et al (2000) Aorta and iliac arteries: single versus multiple detector-row helical CT angiography. Radiology 215:670–676
41. Rubin GD, Schmidt AJ, Logan LJ et al (2001) Multidetector row CT angiography of lower extremity arterial inflow and runoff: initial experience. Radiology 221:146–158
42. Rydberg J, Buckwalter KA, Caldemeyer KS et al (2000) Multisection CT: scanning techniques and clinical applications. Radiographics 20:1787–1806
43. Rydberg J, Kopecky KK, Lalka SG et al (2001) Stent grafting of abdominal aortic aneurysms: pre- and postoperative evaluation with multislice helical CT. J Comput Assist Tomogr 25:580–586
44. Sawhney R, Kerlan RK, Wall SD et al (2001) Analysis of initial CT findings after endovascular repair of abdominal aortic aneurysm. Radiology 220:157–160
45. RB, Jones KM, Chernoff DM et al (1992) Common carotid artery bifurcation: evaluation with spiral CT – work in progress. Radiology 185:513–51946.
46. Sommer T, Fehske W, Holzknecht N et al (1996) Aortic dissection: a comparative study of diagnosis with spiral CT, multiplanar transesophageal echocardiography, and MR imaging. Radiology 199:347–352
47. Soto JA, Munera F, Morales C et al (2001) Focal arterial injuries of the proximal extremities: helical CT angiography as the initial method of diagnosis. Radiology 218:188–194
48. Treede H, Becker C, Reichenspurner H et al (2002) Multidetector computed tomography in coronary surgery: first experiences with a new tool for diagnosis of coronary artery disease. Ann Thorac Surg 74:S1398–1402
49. Van Hoe L, Baert AL, Gryspeerdt S et al (1996) Supra- and juxtarenal aneurysms of the abdominal aorta: preoperative assessment with thin-section spiral CT. Radiology 198:443–448
50. Visser K, Kock MCJM, Kuntz KM et al (2003) Cost-effectiveness targets for multi-detector row CT angiography in the work-up of patients with intermittent claudication. Radiology 227:647–656
51. Vogl T, Abolmaali ND, Diebold T et al (2002) Techniques for the detection of coronary atherosclerosis: multi-detector row CT coronary angiography. Radiology 223:2112–2120
52. Wiesner W, Khurana B, Ji H et al (2003) CT of acute bowel ischemia. Radiology 226:635–650
53. Willmann JK, Roos JE, Platz A et al (2002) Multidetector CT: detection of active hemorrhage in patients with blunt abdominal trauma. AJR Am J Roentgenol 179:437–444
54. Yao DC, Jeffrey RB Jr, Mirvis SE et al (2002) Using contrast-enhanced helical CT to visualize arterial extravasation after blunt abdominal trauma: incidence and organ distribution. AJR Am J Roentgenol 178:17–20

2 Multidetector-Row CT: Technical Principles

Thomas Flohr and Stefan Schaller

CONTENTS

2.1 Introduction

Computed tomography has experienced tremendous technological developments since its introduction more than 30 years ago. Acquisition of single images took several minutes on the first scanners in the 1970s. The introduction of spiral CT in the early 1990s was one of the milestones of CT history, resulting in fundamental and far-reaching improvements of CT imaging, and opening a spectrum of entirely new applications, including CT angiography with new visualization techniques such as multiplanar reformation (MPR), maximum-intensity projection (MIP), or even volume-rendering technique (VRT) [1-3]. For the first time, it became possible to perform volumetric imaging of larger scan ranges in a single breath-hold, effectively avoiding misregistration artifacts. However, the goal of isotropic imaging of large scan ranges within one breath-hold could not be reached. As a result, compromises had to be accepted between scan range, longitudinal resolution, and scan time. As an example, to be able to finish a thorax examination within a single breath-hold (i.e., in 20 s) using a 0.75-s rotation time, an 8-mm slice was frequently used. This resulted in table speeds of 16 mm/s at a pitch of 1.5.

Simultaneous acquisition of multiple slices is an effective way of increasing the scan speed at a certain longitudinal resolution or to increase longitudinal resolution at a given scan speed. In 1998, several manufacturers introduced 4-slice scanners with rotation times of 0.5 s, effectively increasing scanning performance by a factor of 6 compared with the previous single-slice scanners rotating at 0.75 s. This allowed for an optimization of protocols in several different respects [4, 5]: the examination time for standard protocols could be significantly reduced, which is clinically important for trauma cases and noncooperative patients. Alternatively, the scan range that could be covered within a certain scan time could be increased by the same factor, relevant for applications such as oncological screening or peripheral CT angiographic examinations (CTAs). The most important clinical benefit, however, turned out to be the possibility to scan a given scan range in a given time at substantially improved longitudinal resolution. However, with four slices, limitations still remained. True isotropic resolution could not be achieved routinely, as the available transverse resolution of around 1 mm did not fully match the in-plane resolution [6–14]. Consequently, more than four simultaneously acquired slices combined with submillimeter collimation for routine clinical applications was the next step on the way toward true isotropic routine CT scanning, leading to the introduction of 16-slice CT systems in 2001 [15, 16]. Figure 2.1 summarizes the development of multislice CT over the past years. It can be observed that, on average, the number of slices in CT doubled approximately every 2.5 years. This is an interesting parallel to Moore's law in the semiconductor industry. Figure 2.2 depicts the decrease in

T. Flohr, PhD; S. Schaller, PhD
Siemens Medical Solutions, CT Concepts, Siemensstrasse 1, 91301 Forchheim, Germany

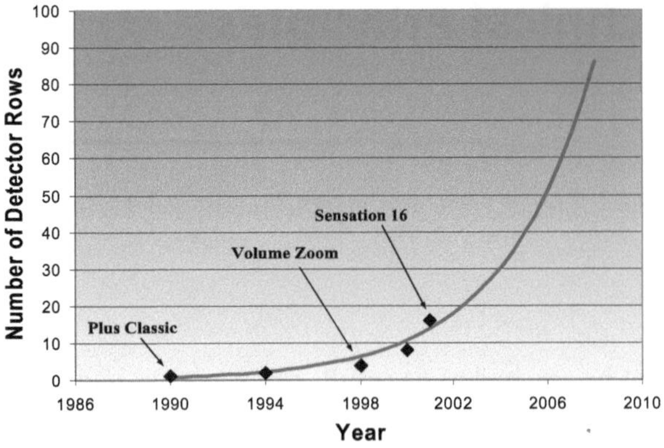

Fig. 2.1. Number of available slices in multislice CT scanners plotted against the year of their market introduction. The number of slices doubles approximately every 2.5 years

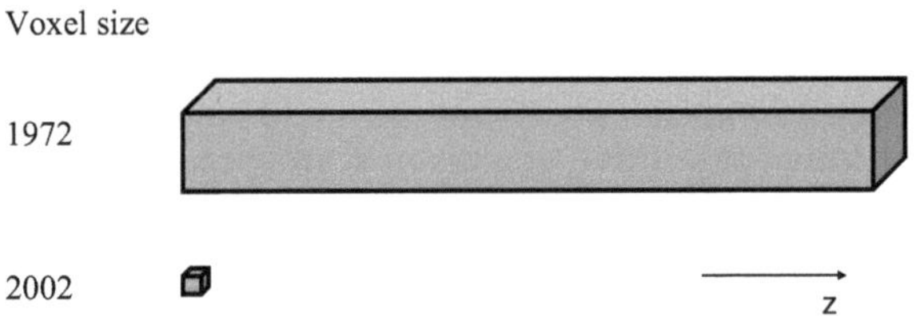

Fig. 2.2. Change in the size of a voxel element over the past 30 years

voxel size corresponding to the increase in spatial resolution. Table 2.1 summarizes the development of the most relevant performance parameters in CT over the past 30 years. Today, a state-of-the-art CT scanner can routinely produce 1,000 images in less than 15 s. This amount of data approximately corresponds to the contents of one CD, i.e., to about 1 h of music in CD quality. While the routine availability of high-quality volume data sets opens the way for new visualization paradigms and novel evaluation techniques, the corresponding large number of images also poses a challenge to the viewing and reading environment of the radiologist. In this chapter, we summarize the technical principles of multidetector-row CT and reflect on some of the new possibilities these developments have opened for volume visualization and evaluation.

2.2 Detector Design, Dose, and Dose Reduction

2.2.1 Detector Design

All recently introduced 16-slice CT systems employ adaptive array detectors. The SOMATOM Sensation 16 (Siemens, Forchheim, Germany) as a representative example uses 24 detector rows [15]. The 16 central rows define 0.75-mm collimated slice width at isocenter; the 4 outer rows on both sides define 1.5-mm collimated slice width. The total coverage in the transverse direction is 24 mm at isocenter. Due to geometric magnification, the actual detector is about twice as wide (see Fig. 2.3). By appropriate combination of the signals of the individual detector rows, either 12 or 16 slices with 0.75-mm or 1.5-mm collimated slice width can be acquired simultaneously. In a "step-and-shoot" sequential mode, any multiple of the collimated width of one detector slice (1.5 mm, 3 mm, 4.5 mm, 6 mm, etc.) can be obtained in principle by adding the corresponding detector signals during image reconstruction. In a spiral mode, the slice width is adjusted in a final *z*-

Table 2.1 Development of characteristic CT performance parameters over time

	1972	1980	1990	1998	2002
Min. scan time (s)	300	5	1	0.5	0.42
Data per 360 scan	58 kB	1 MB	2 MB	12 MB	50 MB
Data per spiral scan	-	-	<50 MB	<500 MB	<1 GB
Image matrix	80×80	256×256	512×512	512×512	512×512
Power (kW)	2	10	40	60	60
Collimation (mm)	13	2–10	1–10	0.5–5	0.75/1.5
Spatial resolution (lp/cm)	3	12	15	24	24
Contrast resolution	5 mm/5 HU/ 50 mGy	3 mm/3 HU/ 30 mGy	3 mm/3 HU/ 30 mGy	3 mm/3 HU/ 30 mGy	3 mm/3 HU/ 30 mGy

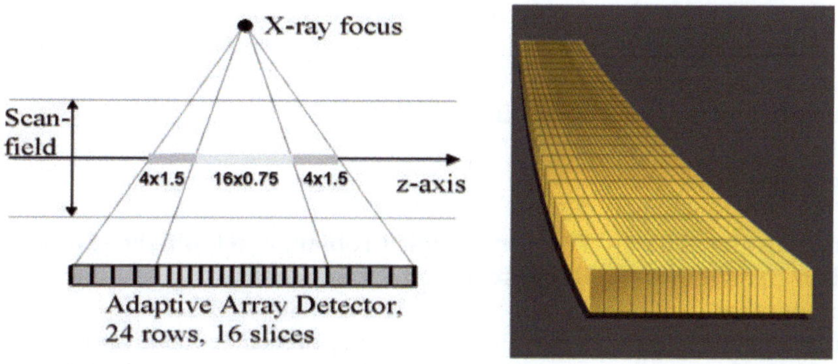

Fig. 2.3. Example of an adaptive array detector used in a commercially available 16-slice CT system (SOMATOM Sensation 16, Siemens, Forchheim, Germany)

filtering step. Therefore, the slice width selection is not restricted to multiples of the collimated width of one detector slice; instead, any slice width equal to or larger than the collimated width of one detector slice (0.75 mm or 1.5 mm) can be realized. Hence, from the same data set, both narrow slices for high-contrast details or as an input to 3D postprocessing and wide slices for low-contrast information and/or overview and filming may be derived.

2.2.2 Dose and Dose Reduction

With multislice CT, a certain dose increase compared with single-slice CT is unavoidable due to the underlying physical principles. The collimated dose profile is a trapezoid in the transverse direction. This is a consequence of the finite length of the focal spot and the prepatient collimation. In the plateau region of the trapezoid, X-rays emitted from the entire area of the focal spot illuminate the detector. In the penumbra regions, only a part of the focal spot illuminates the detector, while other parts are blocked off by the prepatient collimator. With single-slice CT, the entire trapezoidal dose profile can contribute to the detector signal, and the collimated slice width is determined as the full width at half-maximum (FWHM) of this trapezoid. With multislice CT, only the plateau region of the dose profile may be used to ensure equal signal level for all detector slices. The penumbra region has to be discarded, either by a postpatient collimator or by the intrinsic self-collimation of the multislice detector, and represents "wasted" dose. The relative contribution of the penumbra region increases with decreasing slice width, and it decreases with increasing number of simultaneously acquired slices. This is demonstrated by Fig. 2.4, which shows the "minimum width" dose profiles for a 4-slice CT system and a corresponding 16-slice CT system with equal collimated width of one detector slice. Correspondingly, the relative dose utilization of a representative 4-slice CT scanner (SOMATOM Sensation 4, Siemens AG, Forchheim, Germany) is 70% for 4×1 mm collimation and 85% for 4×2.5 mm collimation. A comparable 16-slice CT system (SOMATOM Sensation 16) has an improved dose utilization of 76% (large focal spot) or 82% (small focal spot) for 16×0.75 mm collimation and 85% (large focal spot) or 89% (small focal spot) for 16×1.5 mm collimation.

The most important potential for dose reduction is an adaptation of the dose to the patient size [17, 18]. As a rule of thumb, the dose necessary to maintain constant image noise has to be increased by a factor of 4 if the patient diameter is increased by 8 cm. Correspondingly, for patients 8 cm smaller than the average, a quarter of the standard dose is sufficient for adequate image quality, which is of tremendous importance in pediatric scanning. Most CT manufacturers therefore offer dedicated pediatric protocols, e.g., with dose recommendations according to the weight of the children. In contrast-enhanced studies such as CTAs, the contrast-to-noise ratio for fixed patient dose increases with decreasing X-ray tube volt-

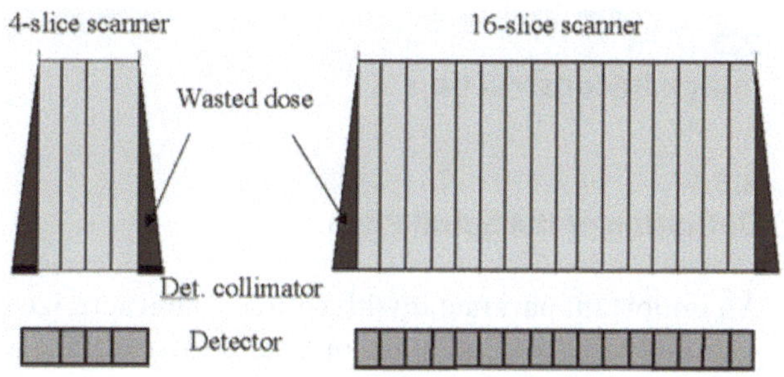

Fig. 2.4. Dose profiles for a 4-slice CT system and a 16-slice CT system with equal collimated width of one detector slice. The relative contribution of the penumbra region, which represents wasted dose, decreases with increasing number of simultaneously acquired slices.

age. As a consequence, to obtain a given contrast-to-noise ratio, patient dose can be reduced by choosing lower kilovolt settings. Compared with a standard scan with 120 kV, the same contrast-to-noise ratio in a 32-cm phantom, corresponding to an average adult, is obtained with 0.49 times the dose for 80 kV (1.3 times the milliampere-seconds) and 0.69 times the dose (1.1 times the milliampere-seconds) for 100 kV [19]. Ideally, 80 kV should be used for CTAs at lowest patient dose. In practice, the maximum tube current available at 80 kV, which is generally not sufficient to scan obese patients, limits the application spectrum. In these patients, 100 kV is a good compromise and the preferable choice for CT angiographic examinations such as thoracic CTAs or cardiac CTAs. In anatomical dose modulation approaches, the tube output is adapted to the patient geometry during each rotation of the scanner to compensate for the varying X-ray attenuation in asymmetrical body regions such as shoulder and pelvis. Depending on the body region, dose can be reduced by 15–35% without degradation of image quality [20]. In more elaborate approaches, the tube output is modified according to the patient geometry in the transverse direction to maintain adequate dose when moving to different body regions, for instance from thorax to abdomen (so-called automatic exposure control). In the special case of electrocardiogram (ECG)-gated spiral scanning for cardiac applications, the output of the X-ray tube can be modulated according to the patient's ECG. It is kept at its nominal value during a user-defined phase of the cardiac cycle, in general the mid- to end-diastolic phase. During the rest of the cardiac cycle, the tube output is reduced to 20% of its nominal value. Depending on the patient's heart rate, dose can be reduced by 30–50% using ECG-controlled dose modulation [21].

2.3 Image Reconstruction

2.3.1 Definition of the Spiral Pitch

An important parameter with which to characterize a spiral scan is the pitch. According to International Electrotechnical Committee (IEC) specifications, the pitch p is given by:

$$p = \frac{\text{table feed per rotation}}{\text{total width of the collimated beam}} \quad (1)$$

This definition holds for single-slice CT as well as for multislice CT. It shows whether data acquisition occurs with gaps (p>1) or with overlap in the transverse direction (p<1).

2.3.2 The Cone-Angle Problem and Multislice Spiral Reconstruction Approaches

Two-dimensional image reconstruction approaches used in commercially available, single-slice CT scanners, such as the convolution-back-projection reconstruction, require all measurement rays contributing to an image to run in a plane perpendicular to the patient's transverse axis (the z-axis). In multislice CT systems, this condition is violated: the measurement rays are tilted by the so-called cone angle relative to a plane perpendicular to the z-axis. The cone angle is largest for the slices at the outer edges of the detector and it increases with increasing number of detector rows. It has been shown [15] that the cone angle can be neglected for multislice CT with up to four slices. As a consequence, all commercially available 4-slice CT scanners rely on image-reconstruction approaches that neglect the cone angle of the measurement rays [22–24]. When a larger number of slices are acquired, however, cone-beam artifacts appear at a level that cannot be tolerated, hence the cone-beam geometry needs to be taken into account. A variety of cone-beam reconstruction algorithms has been published [25–37]. Most of them, however, are not easily applicable to medical CT. Exact spiral reconstruction approaches [34, 35], relying on a 3D Radon inversion, offer a theoretically exact solution of the cone-beam reconstruction problem. They are computationally very expensive and result in image reconstruction times far from being acceptable in a clinical environment. Recently, an exact multislice spiral reconstruction algorithm which does not use 3D Radon inversion has been proposed by A. Katsevich [36]. This approach shows promising properties concerning computational complexity, yet it is still in the research state (as of 2004). In the field of approximate multislice spiral algorithms, approximations are used to handle the cone-beam geometry. Although these algorithms are theoretically not exact, image artifacts may be controlled for a moderate number of simultaneously acquired slices and kept at a level tolerable for medical CT. Two different types of approximate cone-beam reconstruction algorithms are currently implemented in state-of-the art, 16-slice CT systems. The first one uses 3D-back-projection and generalizes the Feldkamp algorithm [32], which was originally introduced for sequential cone-beam scanning, to spiral scanning. Using this approach, the measurement rays are back-projected into a 3D volume along the lines of measurement, in this way accounting for their cone-beam geometry. 3D back-projection is computationally demanding and requires dedicated hardware to achieve acceptable image-reconstruction times. The second reconstruction approach is based on nutating-slice algorithms, which split up the 3D reconstruction into a series of 2D reconstructions on tilted intermediate image planes individually adapted to the local curvature of the spiral path [25–29]. An example is the adaptive multiple-plane reconstruction (AMPR) [30, 31], implemented in the 16-slice scanner SOMATOM Sensation 16 (Siemens, Forchheim, Germany).

2.3.3 Adaptive Multiple-Plane Reconstruction

The AMPR is a generalization of the advanced single-slice rebinning algorithm (ASSR) [28]. In the ASSR, a partial scan interval (~240°) is used for image reconstruction. The image planes are no longer perpendicular to the patient axis; instead, they are tilted to match the spiral path of the focal spot (see Fig. 2.5 for a 16-slice scanner at pitch 1.5). For every view angle in this partial scan interval, the focal spot lies in or nearby the image plane, i.e., measurement rays running in or very close to the image plane are available for image reconstruction. These are the conditions required for a standard 2D convolution-back-projection reconstruction. In a final *z*-reformation step, axial images are calculated by an interpolation between the tilted intermediate image planes. ASSR encounters its limitations when the spiral pitch is reduced to make use of the overlapping spiral acquisition and the resulting dose accumulation. For a 16-slice scanner at pitch 0.5, two full rotations (720°) of multislice spiral data have to be used for every image to ensure complete dose utilization, and there is no way of tilting a single image plane to match the spiral path. A solution for this problem has been found in the AMPR algorithm [30, 31]: instead of using all available data for one single image, it is distributed to several partial images on double oblique image planes, which are individually adapted to the spiral path. These partial images have the same reference projection angle, i.e., they fan out like the pages of a book (see Fig. 2.6a). To ensure full dose utilization, the number of images per reference projection angle (the number of "pages" in the book), as well as the length of the data interval per image, depend on the spiral pitch. The number of images varies from 5, each using 360° of multislice spiral data, at very low pitch values, to 2, each using 240° of multislice spiral data, at high pitch values, greater than 1. The final images with full dose utilization are calculated by a *z*-interpolation between the tilted partial image planes (see Fig. 2.6b). The shape and the width of the interpolation functions are selectable, different slice-sensitivity profiles (SSPs) and different slice widths can therefore be adjusted in this *z*-reformation step. Furthermore, by automatically adapting the functional form of the interpolation functions to the pitch, the spiral concept introduced with Adaptive Axial Interpolation [24] can be maintained with AMPR: the spiral pitch is freely selectable, the slice width is independent of the pitch. As a consequence of the pitch-independent spiral slice width, the image noise for fixed milliamperes (fixed tube-current) would decrease with decreasing pitch due to the increasingly overlapping spiral acquisition. Instead, the tube current (milliamperes) is automatically adapted to the pitch of the spiral scan to compensate for dose accumulation and to maintain constant image noise. The user se-

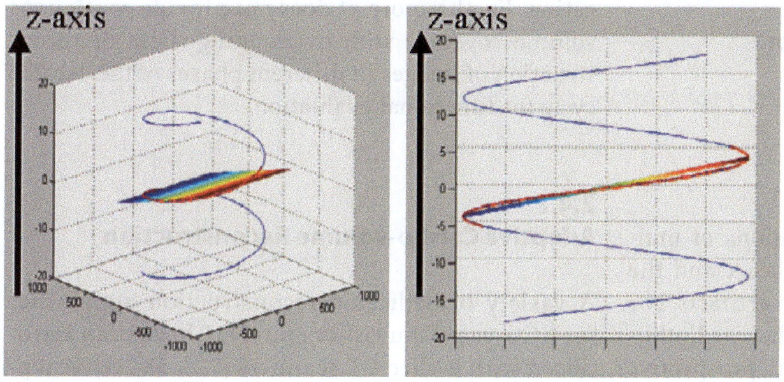

Fig. 2.5. The advanced single-slice rebinning algorithm (ASSR) approach for a 16-slice CT scanner at pitch 1.5. The *blue line* represents the spiral path of the focal spot. On the *right*, a projection into a plane containing the *z*-axis is shown, where the spiral path is represented as a sinusoidal line. A partial scan interval (~240°, marked in *red*) is used for image reconstruction. The intermediate image planes are no longer perpendicular to the patient axis; instead, they are tilted to match the spiral path of the focal spot

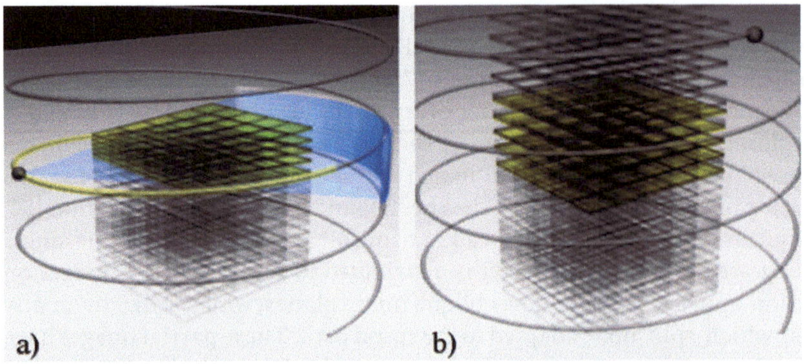

Fig. 2.6a,b. The adaptive multiplane reconstruction (AMPR) approach. As a first step, the multislice spiral data are used to reconstruct several partial images on double oblique image planes, which are individually adapted to the spiral path. Each of these partial images has the same reference projection angle, i.e., they fan out like the pages of a book (**a**). As a second step, the final images with full dose utilization are calculated by a *z*-interpolation between the tilted partial image planes (**b**)

lects an effective milliampere-seconds value, which is also called "volume mAs". The tube current is then automatically adjusted to pitch and rotation time according to:

$$\text{mA} = \text{eff. mAs} \cdot p/T_{\text{rot}} \quad (2)$$

As a consequence of Eq. (2), the patient dose is independent of the pitch p. The weighted CT dose index CTDI_w of an examination is given by:

$$\text{CTDI}_\text{w} = (\text{CTDI}_\text{w})_n \cdot \text{eff. mAs} \quad (3)$$

with $(\text{CTDI}_\text{w})_n$ in milligrays per milliampere-seconds. The subscript n stands for "normalized." The spiral dose is therefore constant and equal to the dose of a sequential scan with the same milliampere-seconds.

2.4 ECG-Synchronized Multislice CT for Cardiothoracic Applications

2.4.1 ECG Triggering and ECG Gating

One of the most exciting new applications of multislice CT is the ability to image the heart and the cardiothoracic anatomy without motion artifacts. For ECG-synchronized examinations of the cardiothoracic anatomy, either axial scanning with prospective ECG-triggering or spiral scanning with retrospective ECG-gating can be used. With prospective ECG-triggering, the heart volume is covered by subsequent axial scans in a step-and-shoot technique. For each axial scan, the number of images corresponds to the number of active detector slices. A partial scan data interval is acquired with a predefined temporal offset relative to the R-waves of the patient's ECG signal which can be either relative (given as a certain percentage of the RR-interval time) or absolute (given in milliseconds) and either forward or reverse [38]. With retrospective ECG-gating, the heart volume is covered continuously by a spiral scan. The patient's ECG signal is recorded simultaneously to allow for a retrospective selection of the data segments used for image reconstruction. Only scan data acquired in a predefined cardiac phase, usually the diastolic phase, is used for image reconstruction [7, 8, 38]. Prospective ECG-triggering has the benefit of a smaller effective patient dose, since scan data is acquired in the previously selected heart phases only. It is, however, more sensitive to arrhythmia than ECG gating. Furthermore, it does not provide continuous volume coverage with overlapping slices or reconstruction of images in different phases of the cardiac cycle for functional evaluation.

2.4.2 Adaptive Cardio-volume Reconstruction

A variety of dedicated reconstruction approaches for ECG-gated multislice spiral CT have been introduced with 4-slice CT scanners [7, 8, 38, 39]. A representative example is the adaptive cardio-volume (ACV) algorithm [38]. An extended and modified version of ACV has been implemented in the 16-slice CT-scanner SOMATOM Sensation 16 (Siemens, Forchheim, Germany). ACV consists of two major steps and combines a partial scan reconstruction optimized for temporal resolution with multislice spiral weighting to compensate for the *z*-movement of the patient table during the spiral scan and to provide a well-defined SSP. During multislice spiral weighting – the first reconstruction step – a "single-slice" partial scan data segment is generated for each image using a partial rotation of the multislice spiral scan data. For each projection angle within the data segment, a linear interpolation is performed between the data of those two detector slices that are in closest proximity to the desired image plane. The cone angle of the measurement rays is neglected; the rays are treated as if they traveled in planes perpendicular to the *z*-axis. Since the heart is usually sufficiently centered and does not contain extended high contrast structures, severe cone artifacts are not expected. Deviating from general-purpose spiral scanning, a cone correction is not necessary for ECG-gated spiral scanning with 16 slices [16].

Depending on the patient's heart rate during the examination, the partial scan data segment is automatically divided into 1 or 2 subsegments (see Fig. 2.7). At heart rates below a certain threshold, one subsegment of consecutive multislice spiral data from the same heart period is used, resulting in a constant temporal resolution of half the gantry rotation time ($T_{rot}/2$) for sufficiently centered objects. At higher heart rates, two subsegments from adjacent heart cycles contribute to the partial scan data segment. In that case, the temporal resolution varies between $T_{rot}/4$ and $T_{rot}/2$ depending on the patient's heart rate, since the heart cycle time and the gantry rotation time have to be desynchronized [38]. The SOMATOM Sensation 16 provides both T_{rot}=0.5 s and T_{rot}=0.42 s for cardiac applications. For T_{rot}=0.5 s, the threshold for two-segment reconstruction is 65 bpm; for T_{rot}=0.42 s, it is 71 bpm. The temporal resolution as a function of the patient's heart rate for both rotation times is indicated in Fig. 2.8. Improved temporal resolution at the expense of reduced transverse resolution by the

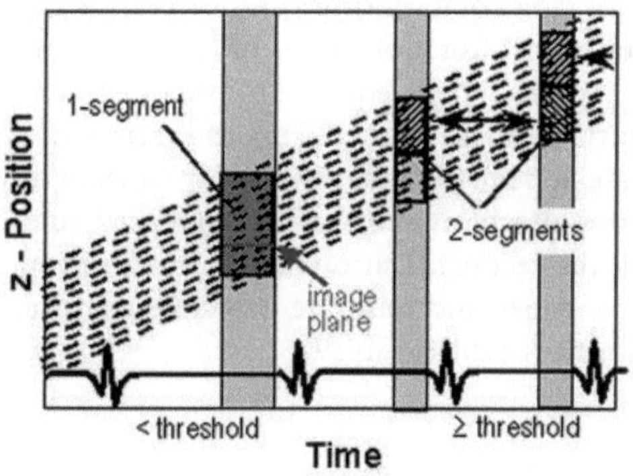

Fig. 2.7. Schematic of the adaptive cardio-volume (ACV) image reconstruction approach for ECG-gated multislice spiral scanning. *Dashed lines* are used to indicate the *z*-positions of the detector slices, which change linearly relative to the patient due to the constant spiral feed. At the *bottom*, the ECG signal is shown schematically. At heart rates below a certain threshold, one segment of consecutive multislice spiral data is used for image reconstruction. At higher heart rates, two subsegments from adjacent heart cycles contribute to the partial scan data segment. For each heart period, a stack of images at different *z*-positions covering a small subvolume of the heart is reconstructed, which is indicated by a *box*

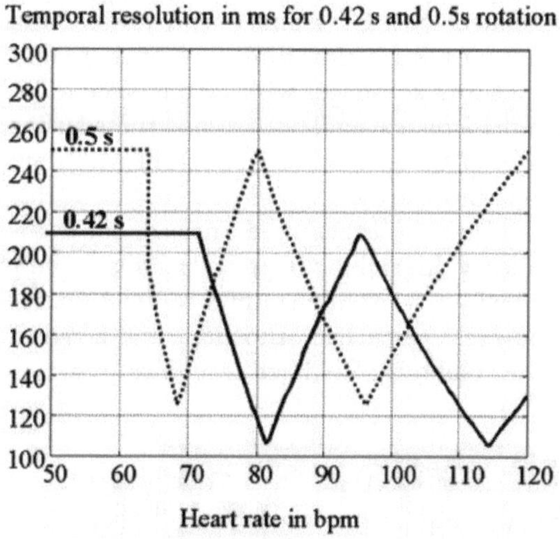

Fig. 2.8. Temporal resolution for sufficiently centered objects as a function of the heart rate for the ACV approach using 0.5-s and 0.42-s gantry rotation time. For 0.42 s rotation time, the temporal resolution reaches its optimum (105 ms) at 81 bpm. This is clinically important, since without administration of beta-blockers the majority of heart rates are in the range 75–85 bpm

use of multisegment reconstruction approaches can degrade the image quality of cardiac examinations by blurring coronary plaques and stenoses [38]. In addition, multisegment approaches encounter their limitations if the patient's heart rate varies during examination, hence the ACV-approach is limited to two segments as a maximum. Similar to the AMPR reconstruction for general purpose spiral scanning, a final *z*-filtering step is applied to the original ACV-images. Shape and width of the filter functions are selectable, different SSPs and different slice widths can therefore be adjusted. The image-quality improvements with 16-slice CT systems compared with established

4-slice scanners can be demonstrated with CT data of a mathematical, anthropomorphic heart phantom. Figure 2.9a shows MPRs along right and left coronary artery (RCA and left anterior descending coronary artery, LAD) of this phantom, which are the result of an ACV reconstruction for a CT scanner with 4×1 mm collimation, 0.5 s rotation time, and pitch p=0.375 (table feed 3 mm/s). Images with 1.3 mm slice width and 0.6 mm increment have been reconstructed using a standard body kernel and an artificial ECG-signal with 55 bpm. The MPRs demonstrate the clinical image quality typical for 4-slice CT-systems and illustrate their performance limits: coronary plaques can be differentiated and classified according to their CT density (Hounsfield units, HU), stents suffer from blooming and artifacts. For the MPRs shown in Fig. 2.9b, the ACV approach has been applied to scan data simulated for a CT scanner with 16×0.75 mm collimation, 0.42 s rotation time, and pitch p=0.28 (table feed 8 mm/s). Images with 1.0 mm slice width and 0.5 mm increment have been reconstructed using an artificial ECG-signal with 55 bpm. The MPRs are free of cone-beam artifacts, thus demonstrating that a cone correction is not required. Instead, due to the smaller slice width and the improved axial sampling compared with a scan with 4×1 mm collimation, the stents show less geometric distortions and a reduction of the "blooming" artifact. In clinical practice,

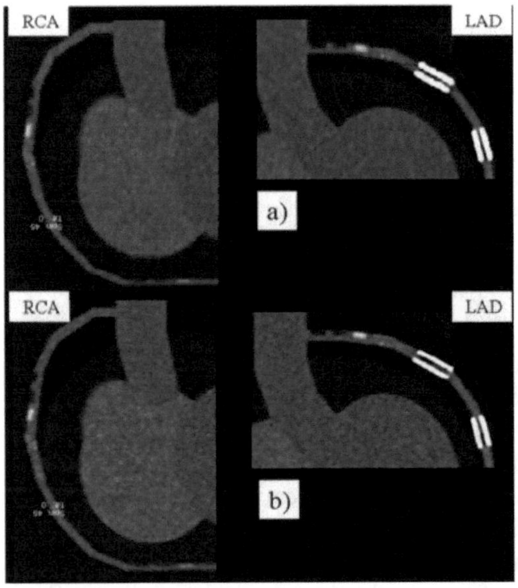

Fig. 2.9a,b. MPRs along the right coronary artery (*RCA*) and left anterior descending coronary artery (*LAD*) of a mathematical heart phantom for virtual CT-scanners with 4×1 mm collimation (**a**) and with 16×0.75 mm collimation (**b**). ACV reconstruction of simulated CT data, neglecting the cone-angle of the measurement rays

the result of the phantom study has been confirmed by patient scans. ECG-gated cardiac scanning benefits from both improved temporal resolution and improved spatial resolution. Characterization and classification of coronary plaques even in the presence of severe calcifications is entering clinical routine as a consequence of the increased clinical robustness of the method. In a recent study, coronary CTA with a 16-slice system was performed on 59 patients. In comparison with conventional catheter angiography, 86% specificity and 95% sensitivity could be demonstrated. None of the patients had to be excluded [40]. Comparable results were obtained by a different group [41].

With a spatial resolution of 0.5×0.5×0.6mm^3, 16-slice CT sets today's benchmark in spatial resolution for noninvasive coronary artery imaging. Motion artifacts in patients with higher heart rates remain the most important challenge for multislice coronary CTA. Although diagnostic image quality can be achieved in most cases by administration of beta-blockers, it is desirable to avoid patient preparation. Further improved temporal resolution will therefore have a much bigger impact on the development of cardiac CT than further increase in the number of simultaneously acquired slices. For robust clinical performance, better temporal resolution has to be achieved by faster gantry rotation rather than by multisegment reconstruction approaches. Obviously, significant improvements will be needed to handle the substantial increase in mechanical forces (~17g for 0.42 s rotation time, >33g for 0.3 s rotation time) and increased data transmission rates. Rotation times of less than 0.2 s (mechanical forces >75g) required to provide a temporal resolution of less than 100 ms independent of the heart rate appear to be beyond today's mechanical limits. An alternative to further increased rotation speed is the reconsideration of a scanner concept with multiple tubes and multiple detectors that was described for the first time in 1975.

2.5 From Slices to Volumes: Impact on Visualization and Postprocessing

The latest generation of 16-slice CT systems allows for truly isotropic imaging in virtually any application. As a consequence, the distinction between transverse and in-plane resolution is gradually becoming a historical remnant, and the traditional axial slice is loosing its clinical predominance. It is replaced by interactive viewing and manipulation of isotropic volume images, with only the key slices or views in arbitrary directions used for filming or stored for a demonstration of the diagnosis. With high-performance visualization software packages, such as the syngo InSpace, one can now interactively inspect large volumes and even navigate through endoscopic visualizations. As an example of the level of image quality available today, Fig. 2.10 shows an endoscopic view into the coronary arteries. At the resolution provided by today's 16-slice scanners, it now becomes possible for the first time to quantitatively evaluate not only calcified but also soft plaques in the coronaries. Figure 2.11 shows an example of the syngo VesselView application, which offers automatic centerline extraction as well as unfolding of the vessel along that central path. Measurement tools provide distance and lumen area measurements. In Fig. 2.12, the syngo Volume package is used to quantitatively evaluate a soft plaque in terms of its volume and average HU-value density.

2.6 Future Perspective for Multislice CT

Improved transverse resolution goes hand in hand with considerably reduced scan times, facilitating the examination of uncooperative patients and reducing the amount of contrast agent needed, but also requiring optimized contrast agent protocols. New clinical applications are evolving as a result of the tremendously increased volume scan speed, such as CTAs in the pure arterial phase. A CTA of the circle of Willis with 16×0.75 mm collimation, 0.5 s rotation time and pitch 1.5 requires only 3.5 s for a scan range of 100 mm (table feed 36 mm/s). A thorax-abdomen CTA with submillimeter collimation takes about 17 s for a scan range of 600 mm. For a CTA of the renal arteries, the table feed can be reduced to 24 mm/s (pitch 1) to make better use of the tube output for obese patients; nevertheless, the total scan time for 250 mm scan range with 16×0.75 mm collimation is not longer than 11 s. An examination of the entire thorax (350 mm) with 16×0.75 mm collimation, 0.5 s rotation time, and pitch 1.375 (table feed 33 mm/s) can be done in 11 s, hence, both a native and a contrast-enhanced scan can be obtained within the same breath-hold period for optimum matching of both image volumes. ECG-gated cardiac scanning also benefits from both improved temporal resolution and improved spatial resolution.

For general purpose CT, we will see a moderate increase in the number of simultaneously acquired slices in the near future; the resulting clinical benefits, however, may not be substantial and have to be care-

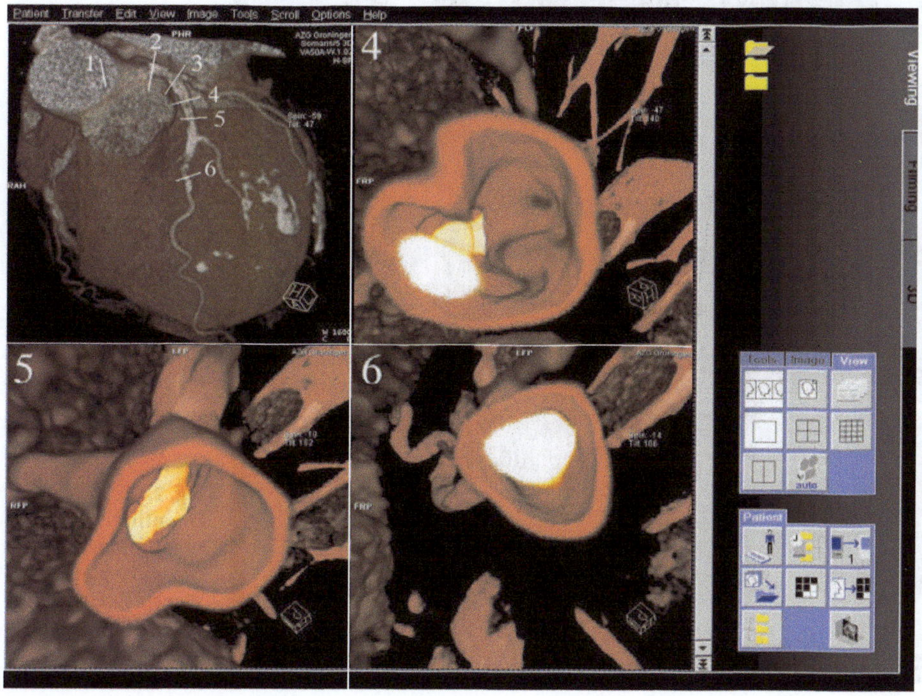

Fig. 2.10 State-of-the-art 16-slice CT: endoscopic view into the coronary arteries. Calcified plaques are visualized as bright lesions

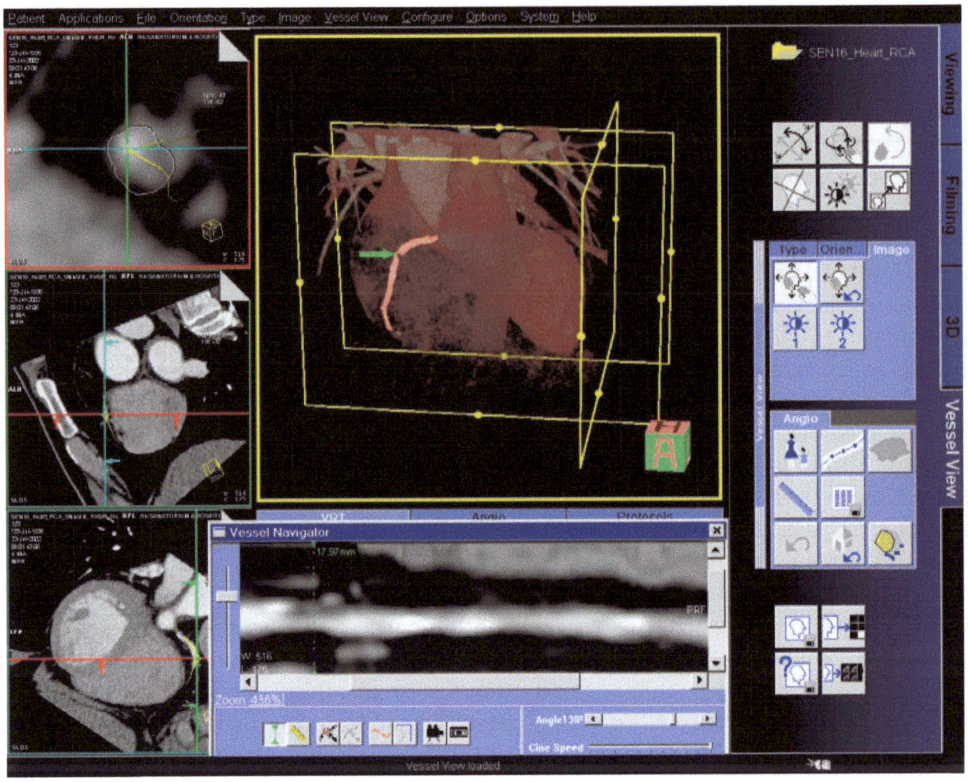

Fig. 2.11. Example of a dedicated software package for vascular applications (syngo VesselView). The software automatically extracts the centerline of the vessels, generates curved reformats, and offers both visual and quantitative assessment of plaque and vessel lumen for grading of stenosis or preoperative planning of endografts

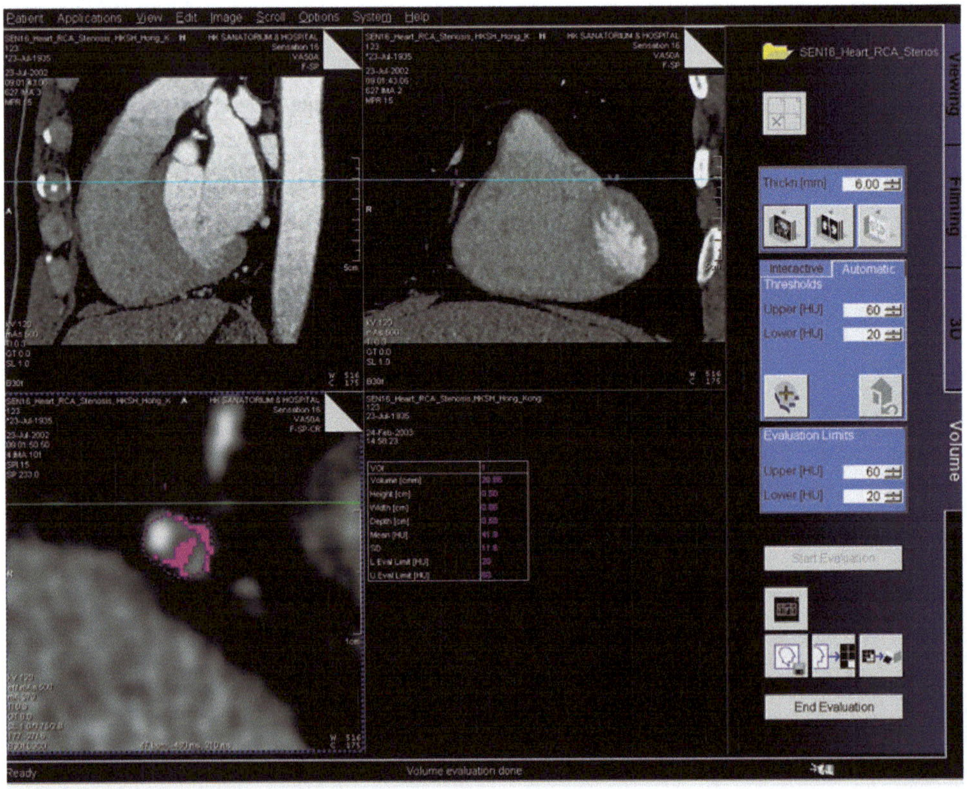

Fig. 2.12. Quantitative evaluation of noncalcified coronary plaque. The software calculates mean density and volume of a selected lesion

fully considered in the light of the necessary technical efforts. As soon as all possible examinations can be performed in a comfortable breath-hold of not more than 10 s, a further increase in the slice number will not give a significant clinical benefit at all. Potential further improvement of the spatial resolution will have to be reserved to special applications due to the inevitable increase in dose that has to be applied for adequate signal-to-noise ratio. It will have to go along with the development of more powerful X-ray tubes and generators. Instead of a mere quantitative enhancement of scan parameters with doubtful clinical relevance, the introduction of area detectors large enough to cover entire organs such as the heart, the kidneys, or the brain in one axial scan (~120 mm scan range) could bring a new quality to medical CT. With these systems dynamic volume scanning would become possible, and a whole spectrum of new applications, such as functional or volume perfusion studies, could arise. Area detector technology is currently under development, yet no commercially available solution so far fulfills the high requirements of medical CT concerning dynamic range of the acquisition system and fast data readout. Initial experience with today's cesium iodide–amorphous silicon (CsI–aSi) flat-panel detector technology originally used for conventional catheter angiography is limited in low contrast resolution and scan speed. Due to the intrinsic slow signal decay of flat-panel detectors, rotation times of at least 20 s are needed to acquire a sufficient number of projections (≥600 per rotation). On the other hand, high contrast resolution is excellent due to the small detector pixel size, yet dose requirements preclude the examination of larger objects. Initial experimental results are limited to small high-contrast objects such as joints, inner ear, or contrast-filled vessel specimens. Figure 2.13 shows a prototype setup incorporating a flat-panel detector into a standard CT gantry (SOMATOM Sensation 16, Forchheim, Germany). The detector covers 25×25×18 cm^3 scan field of view, the pixel size is 0.25×0.25 mm^2, both measured at the center of rotation. Figure 2.14 shows MPRs of a hand specimen, demonstrating excellent spatial resolution. Figure 2.15 shows a VRT of the RCA of a heart specimen, acquired on a flat-panel CT system with 0.25 mm slice width and on a 4-slice CT scanner with 1.3 mm slice width for comparison (courtesy of Klinikum Grosshadern, Munich, Germany). The combination of area detectors of sufficient quality with fast gantry rotation speeds is a promising technical concept for medical CT systems. Due to the present technical restrictions, however, these systems will probably not be available in the near future.

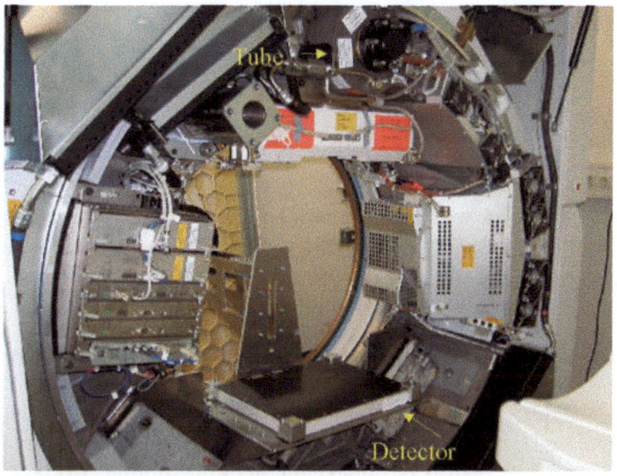

Fig. 2.13. Prototype setup incorporating a flat-panel detector into a standard CT gantry

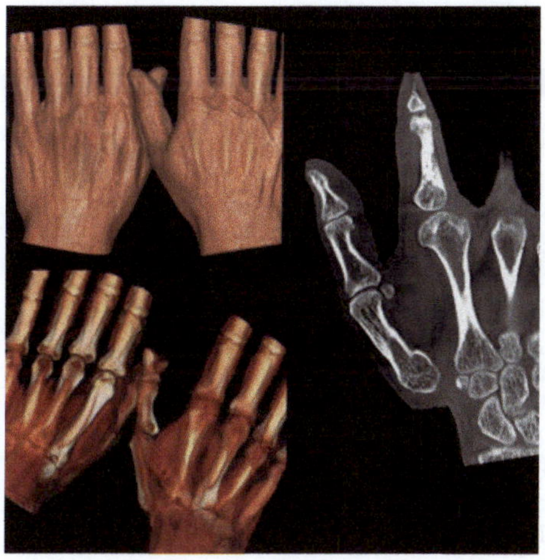

Fig. 2.14. Multiplanar reformation (MPRs) of a hand specimen, scanned with a CT prototype with a flat-panel detector

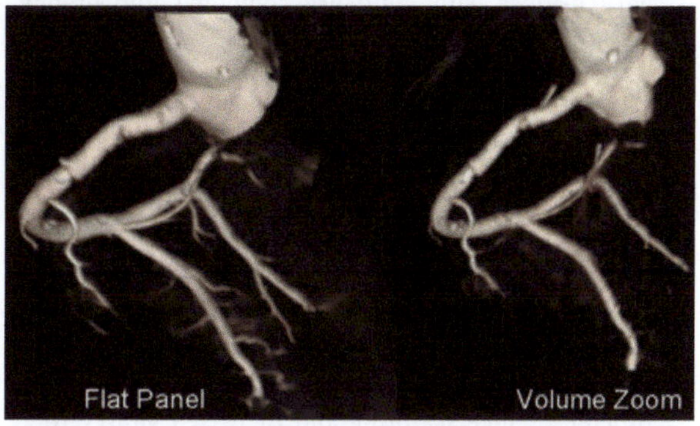

Fig. 2.15. VRT of the RCA of a heart specimen, acquired on a flat-panel CT-system with 0.25 mm slice width and on a 4-slice CT scanner with 1.3 mm slice width for comparison (Courtesy of Klinikum Grosshadern, Munich, Germany)

References

1. Kalender W, Seissler W, Klotz E, Vock P (1990) Spiral volumetric CT with single-breath-hold technique, continuous transport and continuous scanner rotation. Radiology 176:181–183
2. Crawford CR, King KF (1990) Computed tomography scanning with simultaneous patient translation. Med Phys 17:967–982
3. Kalender W (1995) Thin-section three-dimensional spiral CT: is isotropic imaging possible? Radiology 197:578–580
4. Klingenbeck-Regn K, Schaller S, Flohr T, et al. (1999) Subsecond multislice computed tomography: basics and applications. Eur J Radiol 31:110–124
5. Hu H, He HD, Foley WD, Fox SH (2000) Four multidetector-row helical CT: image quality and volume coverage speed. Radiology 215:55–62
6. Ohnesorge B, Flohr T, Schaller S, et al. (1999) Technische Grundlagen und Anwendungen der Mehrschicht-CT. Radiologe 39:923–931
7. Kachelriess M, Ulzheimer S, Kalender W (2000) ECG-correlated image reconstruction from subsecond multislice spiral CT scans of the heart. Med Phys 27:1881–1902
8. Ohnesorge B, Flohr T, Becker C, et al. (2000) Cardiac imaging by means of electro-cardiographically gated multisection spiral CT – initial experience. Radiology 217:564–571
9. Achenbach S, Ulzheimer S, Baum U et al. (2000) Non-invasive coronary angiography by retrospectively ECG-gated multislice spiral CT. Circulation 102:2823–2828
10. Becker C, Knez A, Ohnesorge B, Schöpf U, Reiser M (2000) Imaging of non calcified coronary plaques using helical CT with retrospective EKG gating. AJR Am J Roentgenol 175:423–424
11. Knez A, Becker C, Leber A, et al. (2000) Non-invasive assessment of coronary artery stenoses with multidetector helical computed tomography. Circulation 101: e221–e222
12. Nieman K, Oudkerk M, Rensing B, et al. (2001) Coronary angiography with multislice coputed tomography. Lancet 357:599–603
13. Schroeder S, Kopp A, Baumbach A, et al. (2001) Noninvasive detection and evaluation of atherosclerotic coronary plaques with multislice computed tomography. JACC 37:1430–1435
14. Kopp A, Schröder S, Küttner A et al. (2001) Coronary arteries: retrospectively ECG-gated multidetector row CT angiography with selective optimization of the image reconstruction window. Radiology 221:683–688
15. Flohr T, Stierstorfer K, Bruder H, Simon J, Schaller S (2002) New technical developments in multislice CT. 1. Approaching isotropic resolution with sub-mm 16-slice scanning. Fortschr Rontgenstr 174:839–845
16. Flohr T, Bruder H, Stierstorfer K, et al. (2002) New technical developments in multislice CT. 2. Sub-millimeter 16-slice scanning and increased gantry rotation speed for cardiac imaging. Fortschr Rontgenstr 174:1022–1027
17. Donelly LF, Emery KH, Brody AS et al. (2001) Minimizing radiation dose for pediatric body applications of single-detector helical CT: strategies at a large children's hospital. AJR Am J Roentgenol 176:303–306
18. Frush DP, Soden B, Frush KS, Lowry C (2002) Improved pediatric multidetector body CT using a size-based color-coded format. AJR Am J Roentgenol 178:721–726
19. Schaller S, Niethammer MU, Chen X, et al. (2001) Comparison of signal-to-noise and dose values at different tube voltages for protocol optimization in pediatric CT. Abstracts of the 57th scientific assembly and annual meeting of the RSNA. 366
20. Greess H, Wolf H, Baum U et al. (2000) Dose reduction in computed tomography by attenuation-based on-line modulation of the tube current: evaluation of six anatomical regions. Eur Radiol 10:391–394
21. Jakobs TF, Becker CR, Ohnesorge B, et al. (2002) Multislice helical CT of the heart with retrospective ECG gating: reduction of radiation exposure by ECG-controlled tube current modulation. Eur Radiol 12:1081–1086
22. Taguchi T, Aradate H (1998) Algorithm for image reconstruction in multislice helical CT. Med Phys 25:550–561
23. Hu H (1999) Multislice helical CT: scan and reconstruction. Med Phys 26:5–18
24. Schaller S, Flohr T, Klingenbeck K, et al. (2000) Spiral interpolation algorithm for multislice spiral CT. I. Theory. IEEE Trans Med Imag 19:822–834
25. Larson G, Ruth C, Crawford C (1998) Nutating slice CT image reconstruction. Patent application WO 98/44847, filed 8 April 1998
26. Turbell H, Danielsson PE (1999) An improved PI-method for reconstruction from helical cone beam projections. IEEE medical imaging conference, Seattle
27. Proksa R, Koehler T, Grass M, Timmer J (2000) The n-PI method for helical cone-beam CT. IEEE Trans Med Imag 19:848–863
28. Kachelriess M, Schaller S, Kalender WA (2000) Advanced single-slice rebinning in cone-beam spiral CT. Med Phys 27:754–772
29. Bruder H, Kachelriess M, Schaller S, Stierstorfer K, Flohr T (2000) Single-slice rebinning reconstruction in spiral cone-beam computed tomography. IEEE Trans Med Imag 19:873–887
30. Schaller S, Stierstorfer K, Bruder H, Kachelriess M, Flohr T (2001) Novel approximate approach for high-quality image reconstruction in helical cone beam CT at arbitrary pitch. Proc SPIE Int Symp Med Imag 4322:113–127
31. Flohr T, Stierstorfer K, Bruder H, et al. (2003) Image reconstruction and image quality evaluation for a 16-slice CT scanner. Med Phys 30
32. Feldkamp LA, Davis LC, Kress JW (1984) Practical cone-beam algorithm. J Opt Soc Am A 1:612–619
33. Wang G, Lin T, Cheng P (1993) A general cone-beam reconstruction algorithm. IEEE Trans Med Imaging 12:486–496
34. Kudo H, Noo F, Defrise M (1998) Cone-beam filtered-backprojection algorithm for truncated helical data. Phys Med Biol 43:2885–2909
35. Schaller S, Noo F, Sauer F, et al. (2000) Exact Radon rebinning algorithm for the long object problem in helical cone-beam CT. IEEE Trans Med Imag 19:361–375
36. Katsevich A (2002) Theoretically exact filtered backpro-

jection-type inversion algorithm for spiral CT. SIAM J Appl Math 62:2012–2026
37. Stierstorfer K, Flohr T, Bruder H (2002) Segmented multiple plane reconstruction – a novel approximate reconstruction scheme for multislice spiral CT, Phys Med Biol 47:2571–2581
38. Flohr T, Ohnesorge B (2001) Heart-rate adaptive optimization of spatial and temporal resolution for ECG-gated multislice spiral CT of the heart. JCAT 25:907–923
39. Taguchi K, Anno H (2000) High temporal resolution for multislice helical computed tomography. Med Phys 27:861–872
40. Nieman K, Cademartiri F, Lemos PA, et al. (2002) Reliable noninvasive coronary angiography with fast submillimeter multislice spiral computed tomography. Circulation 106:2051–2054
41. Ropers D, Baum U, Pohle K, et al. (2003) Detection of coronary artery stenoses with thin-slice multidetector row spiral computed tomography and multiplanar reconstruction. Circulation 107:664–666

3 Multidetector-Row CT: Image-Processing Techniques and Clinical Applications

Emanuele Neri, Paola Vagli, Francesco Odoguardi, Davide Caramella, and Carlo Bartolozzi

CONTENTS

3.1 Introduction

Image processing and three-dimensional (3D) reconstruction of diagnostic images represents a necessary tool for depicting complex anatomical structures and understanding pathological changes in terms of both morphology and function.

The importance of 3D reconstructions is evident if we consider that the quantity of native images produced with new-generation cross-sectional techniques has become increasingly large. Volumetric data such as those acquired with multidetector row computed tomography (CT) are particularly well suited to postprocessing. On the other hand the analysis and processing of such data through additional planes over the axial and 3D views is becoming mandatory.

E. Neri, MD; P. Vagli, MD;
F. Odoguardi, MD; D. Caramella, MD;
C. Bartolozzi, MD, Professor and Chairman
Diagnostic and Interventional Radiology, Department of Oncology, Transplants, and Advanced Technologies in Medicine, University of Pisa, Via Roma 67, 56126 Pisa, Italy

Image processing involves operations such as reformatting original CT images and surface and volume rendering. These types of operations are also included in a wide classification which divides the techniques of display of 3D models into projectional and perspective methods.

Projectional methods are those in which a 3D volume is projected into a bidimensional plane; in the perspective methods a 3D virtual world is displayed by means of techniques that aim to reproduce the perspective of the human eye looking at the physical world.

Projectional methods include CT image-reformatting approaches such as multiplanar reformations (MPR) in the sagittal, coronal, oblique, and curved planes. More specific projection techniques include maximum-intensity projection (MIP) and minimum-intensity projection (MinIP). The reformatting process does not modify the CT data but uses them in off-axis views and displays the images in an orientation different from native acquisition.

Surface and volume rendering use algorithms that generate 3D views of sectional two-dimensional data. Surface rendering is based on the extraction of an intermediate surface description of the relevant objects from the volume data, while volume rendering displays the entire volume preserving the whole dynamic range of the image. A more advanced application of surface and volume rendering is represented by virtual endoscopy, which is a simulation of the endoscopic perspective by processing volumetric data sets.

The CT acquisition parameters that have a direct effect on the quality of the image processing are section thickness, reconstruction spacing, and pitch. Thin sections and reconstruction spacing allow better postprocessing results by reducing partial volume averaging effects on the longitudinal plane or *z*-axis (Fig. 3.1). The effect of pitch on 3D imaging of CT data sets is particularly relevant for single-row systems, where the use of high pitch values introduces an increased slice-sensitive profile and consequently determines artifacts on projectional and perspective

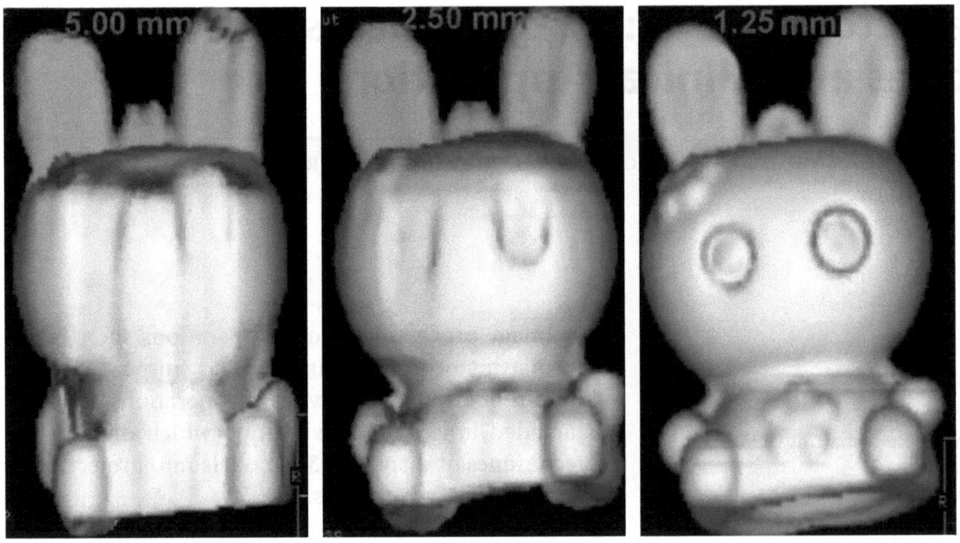

Fig. 3.1 Section thickness influences the diagnostic accuracy of postprocessed images. the morphological detail of the phantom is progressively better depicted by means of thinner sections.

images such as the stair-step artifact. In multirow CT, the effect of pitch on slice-sensitive profiles is less relevant and does not significantly affect 3D imaging.

The acquisition must be performed during one continuous breath-hold to avoid different positions of the scanned organs; movement artifacts, which slightly affect the quality of axial slices, become clearly visible especially in 3D images, where the continuity of the volume acquired is essential to reproduce a reliable 3D model. Isotropic viewing is another factor that can influence the quality of 3D images, in particular MPR; it refers to the situation in which MPR images can be created in any plane with the same spatial resolution as the original sections [25].

In multirow CT, an additional element that influences the quality of 3D images is contrast enhancement, especially in the study of the vascular system. The bright contrast obtained in the vascular system and the absence of background enhancement allow easier application of image-processing algorithms; therefore dedicated CT angiographic protocols are required [2, 13, 17].

3.2 Multiplanar Reformations

Reformatting approaches enable images to be displayed in a different orientation from the original one. The term "reconstruction" is often used instead of "reformations," although it is inaccurate in this context. In fact the reconstruction process, especially in CT, refers to the procedure that converts raw projection data into an axial image.

There are many situations in diagnostic imaging in which identification, generation, and display of the optimal image plane is critical; in the case of CT this issue is even more relevant due to the fixed scanning plane (axial plane for X-ray emission and z-axis for CT table movement to cover the human body). In this setting the use of additional planes, for studying structures of interest which are not oriented along the acquisition plane, is strongly recommended. Therefore, techniques to generate and display optimal 2D views are particularly important.

3.2.1 Sagittal and Coronal Reformatting

Most processing systems allow the selection of series or range of images. The dedicated software "grabs" the highlighted series and begins to load it into a data set to create MPR. Usually processing systems show an axial, a sagittal, and a coronal image. By using appropriate icon-command, it is possible to change any image orientation. At this point the user can select the primary view that acts as the working image (Fig. 3.2). On the basis of the primary view, changes in the other frames can be made. Therefore, the starting point of image reformations includes these "conventional" coronal and sagittal planes for a preliminary view of the 3D data set.

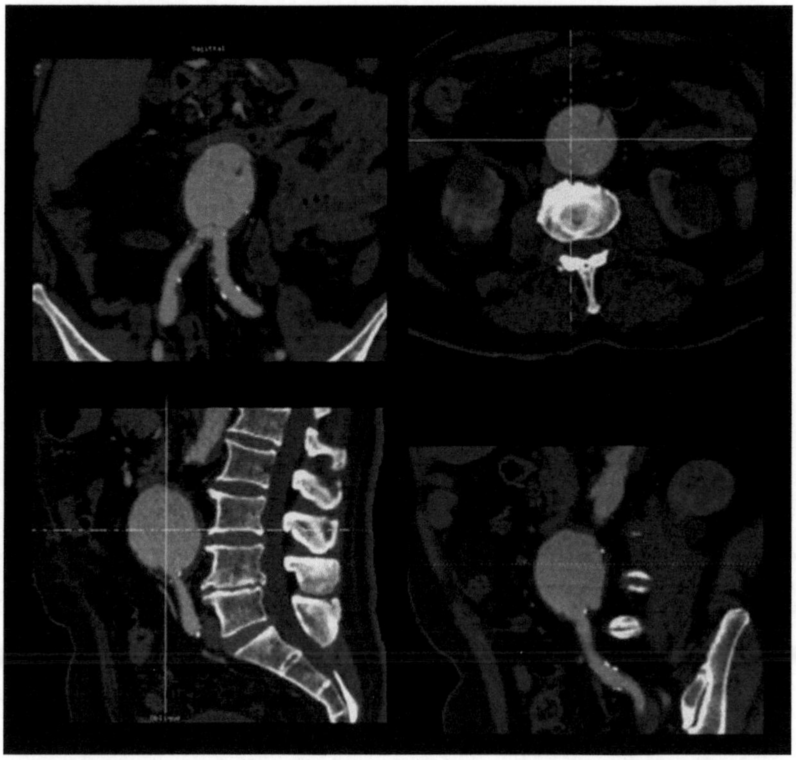

Fig. 3.2 Multiplanar reformation interface shows a four-panel display. In this case an axial image, a coronal image, and two sagittal images are depicted; one of the sagittal images is an oblique image projected in a orthogonal plane. By using appropriate icon-command, it is possible to change any image orientation and to select the primary view. The selected primary view acts as the working image.

3.2.2 Oblique Reformatting

When the user needs additional planes with respect to classic axial, coronal, and sagittal views, oblique reformatting is available. Oblique reformatting is quite similar to sagittal or coronal reformatting, except that the CT voxels in the stack are sampled along an axis that is tilted from either the x- or y-plane. Several organ systems in the human body are not easily visualized with routine sagittal and coronal planes, and oblique reformatting can be useful in these instances (Fig. 3.3a,b). Oblique reformatting is employed when the desired 2D image lies along a plane oriented at an oblique angle to the orthogonal axes of the volume image (Fig. 3.4) [1].

Oblique images are less intuitive and much harder to compute, as simple readdressing of the voxels in a given order will not generate the proper oblique image.

Specification and identification of the oblique image are often done using landmarks in the orthogonal image data. To accomplish this, several images need to be presented to allow unambiguous selection of the landmarks, usually through multiplanar orthogonal images. Two methods can be used for definition of the oblique plane orientation. Selection of three landmarks will uniquely define the orientation of the plane, which may need to be rotated for proper display orientation. Two selected points define an axis along which oblique planes perpendicular to the axis can be generated. This does not uniquely define a single plane, as the oblique image may be generated anywhere along the axis, but this method is often used when a stack of oblique images needs to be generated through a structure. Interactive manipulation of the oblique plane orientation can be achieved if controls for angular rotation maneuvers are provided.

Oblique sectioning, particularly when interactive, requires a visualization method for plane placement and orientation verification. One method uses selected orthogonal images with a line indicating the intersection of the oblique image with the orthogonal images. Another method depicts the intersection of the oblique plane with a rendered surface image, providing direct 3D visual feedback with familiar structural features [23].

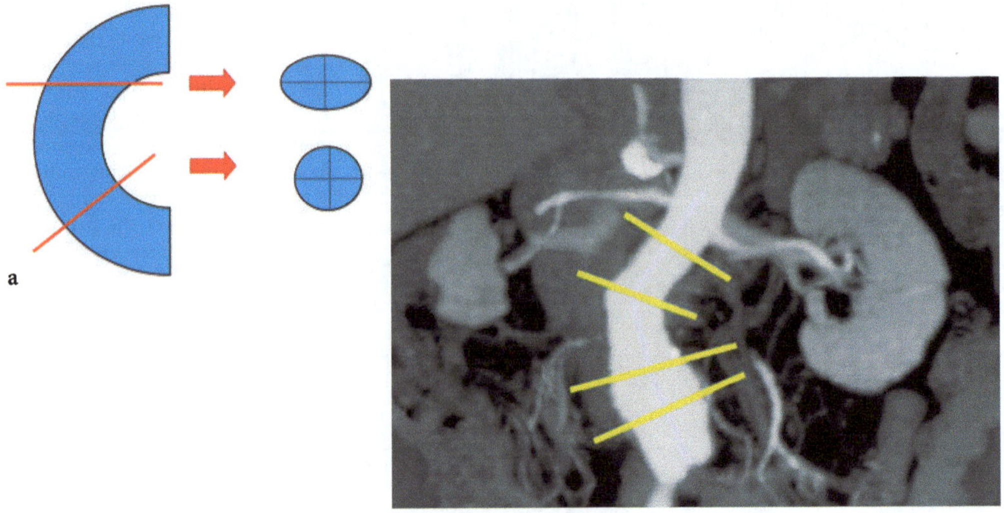

Fig. 3.3. a In some instances (assessment of the diameter of tubular structures) it is crucial to obtain measures from the orthogonal plane, because the employment of other planes may determine overestimation. **b** Abdominal aortic aneurysm: the assessment of the diameters of the aneurismal neck and sac can be obtained only by means of oblique reformatting.

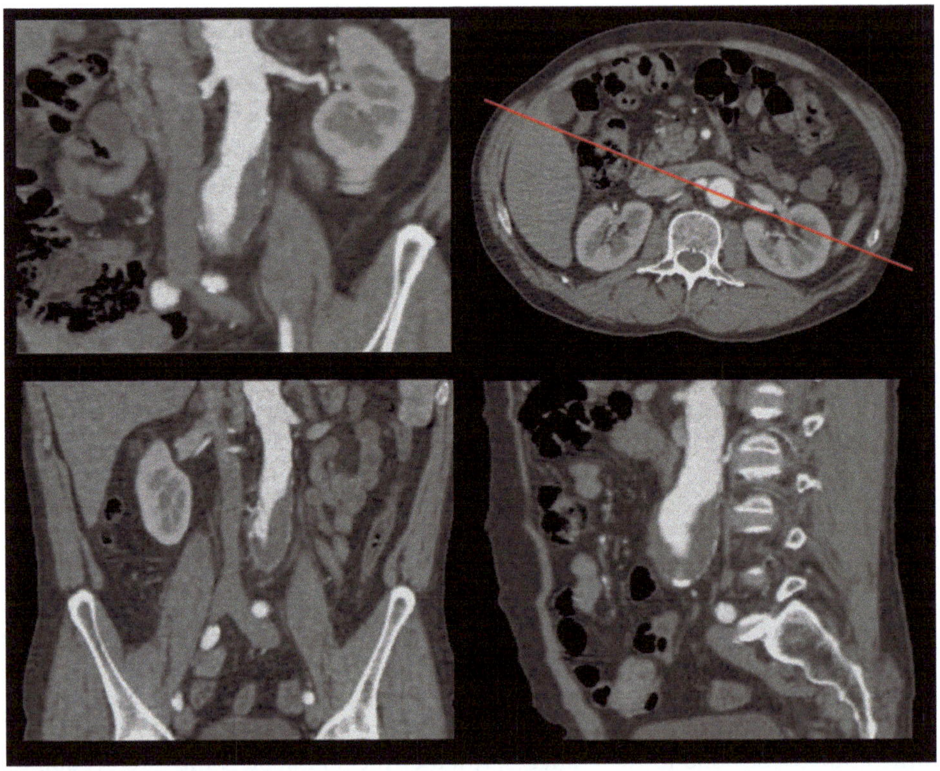

Fig. 3.4 Oblique reformatted images of an abdominal aortic aneurysm were obtained by using thin axial sections. The multiple oblique views show both renal ostia and longitudinal extension of an abdominal aortic aneurysm that could not be directly appreciated in the native axial image.

3.2.3 Curved Reformatting

It is also possible to sample a 3D stack of CT images along a curved plane. Often structures of interest may have curvilinear morphology that orthogonal and oblique reformations cannot capture in a single 2D image. This restriction of planar sections can be overcome using curvilinear reformatting techniques. A trace along an arbitrary path on any orthogonal plane defines a set of pixels in the orthogonal image that have a corresponding row of voxels through the volumetric data set. Each row of voxels for each pixel on the trace can be displayed as a line of a new image, which corresponds to the curved planar structure lying along the trace. Curved planar reformatting represents a variation of MPR.

This technique is useful for curved structures such as the spine, the mandible, and tortuous tubular structures (e.g., blood vessels; Fig. 3.5).

3.3 Maximum-Intensity Projection

Maximum-intensity projection enables the evaluation of each voxel along a line from the viewer's eye through the volume of data and to select the maximum voxel value, which is used as the displayed value.

It represents the simulation of rays that are traced from the operator through the object to the display screen, and only the relative maximum value detected along each ray path into the selected slab (Fig. 3.6a,b) is retained by the computer. This method preferentially displays bone and contrast-filled structures (MIP is largely used for CT angiography; Fig. 3.7).

MIP has a number of related artifacts and shortcomings that must be taken into account to properly interpret the rendered image. The displayed pixel intensity represents only the structure with the highest intensity along the projected ray. A high-density structure such as calcifications (Fig. 3.8) will obscure

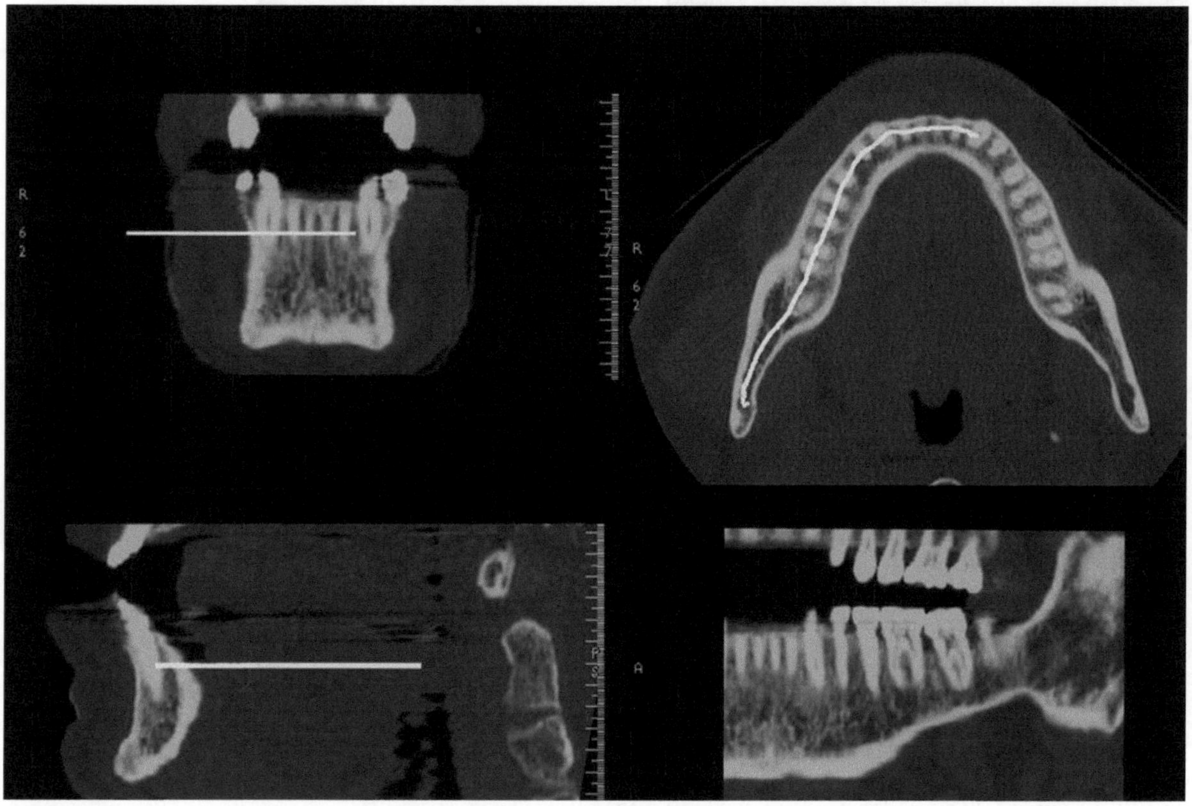

Fig. 3.5 Curved planar reformation enables complete visualization of some curved structures by tracing a cut plane following the anatomical shapes that are confidently represented.

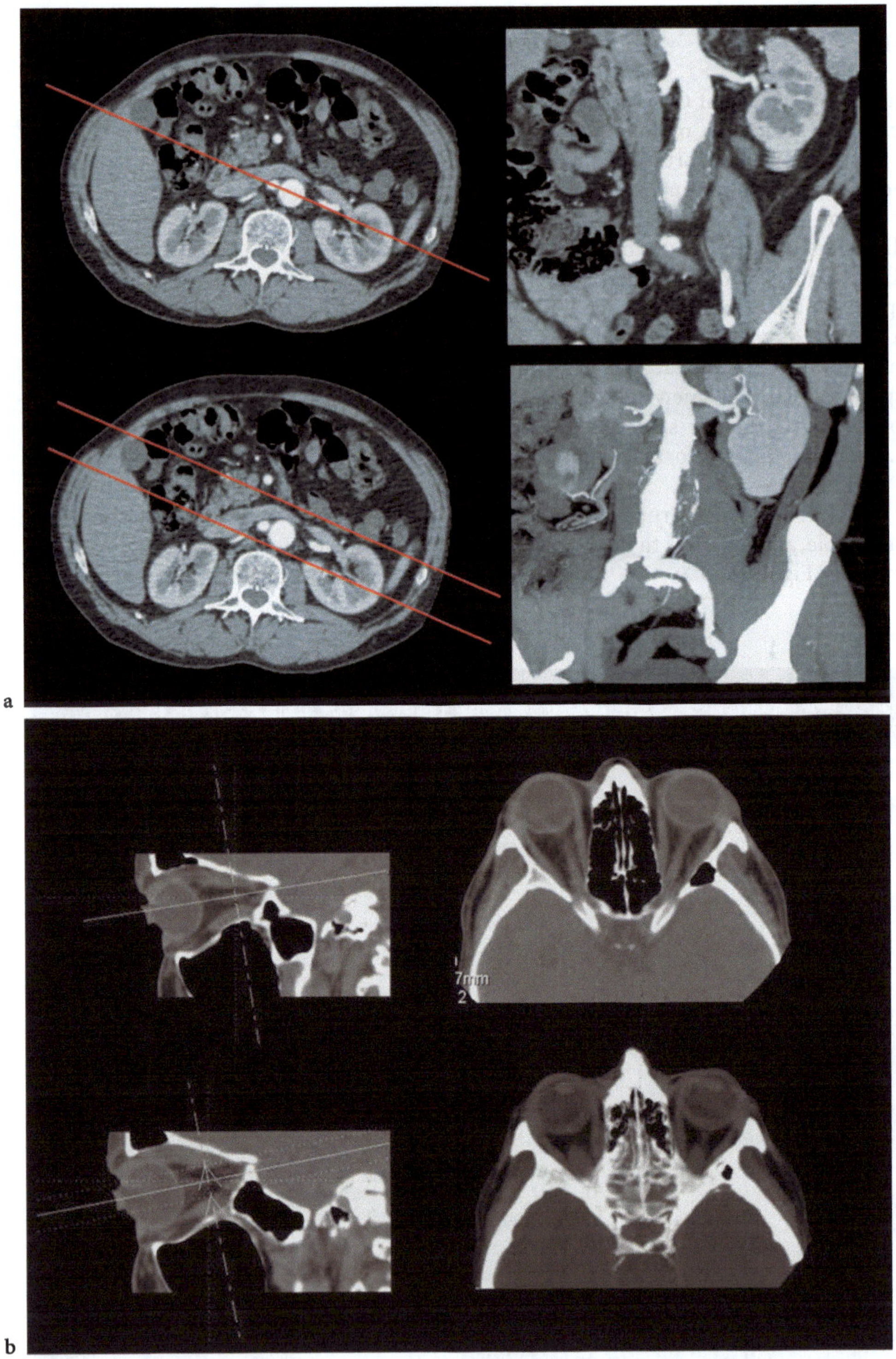

Fig. 3.6a,b A multiplanar approach can be obtained both in maximum-intensity projection (MIP) and multiplanar reformation, although for MIP the thickness of the examined plane should be properly selected.

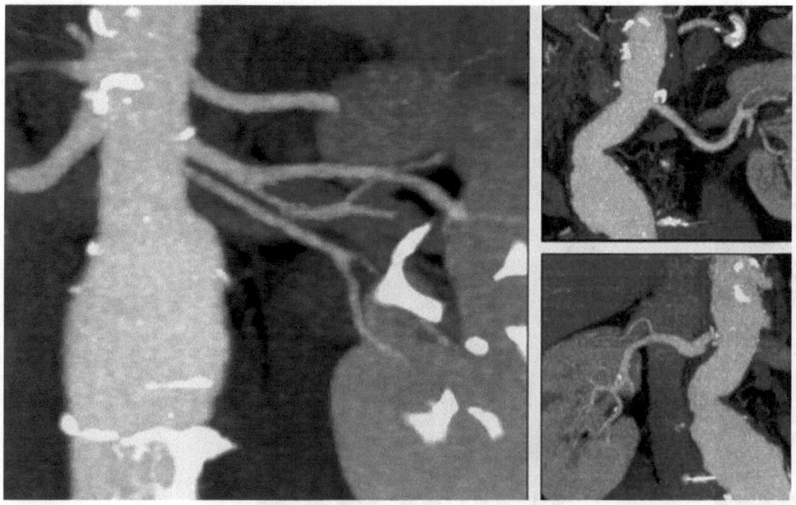

Fig. 3.7 MIP is largely used in CT angiography because the contrast-filled vessels are accurately depicted by this reformation approach. Anatomical details are correctly displayed, showing the patency of the main renal arteries and also the presence of a left accessory.

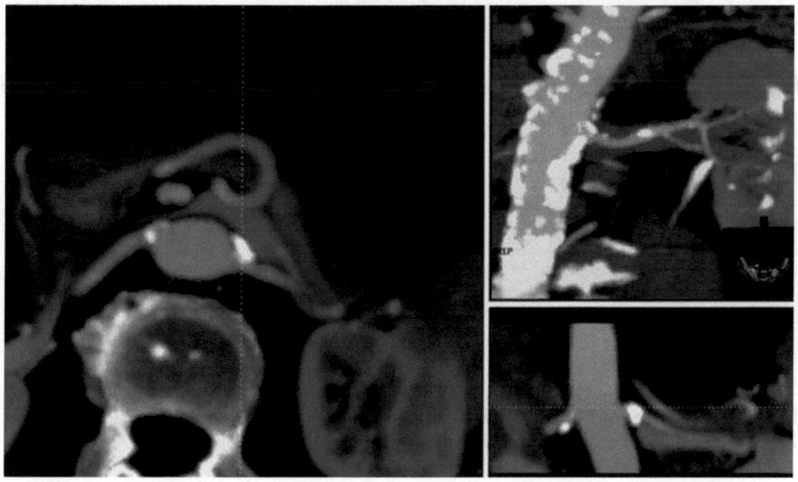

Fig. 3.8 Renal ostia are incompletely visualized for the presence of intimal calcifications.

information from intravascular contrast material. This limitation can be partially overcome with use of nonlinear transfer function or through volume editing to eliminate undesired data [3, 4, 26]. Volume editing can be a preprocessing step (section-by-section "slab" editing) or an interactive process ("sliding-slab" MIP).

The use of the highest intensity value also increases the mean background intensity of the image, effectively selecting the "noisiest" voxels and thereby decreasing the visibility of vessels in enhancing structures such as the kidney and liver. MIP images are typically not displayed with surface shading or other depth cues, which can make assessment of 3D relationships difficult. Also, volume averaging (the effect of finite volume resolution) coupled with the MIP algorithm commonly leads to MIP artifacts. A normal small vessel passing obliquely through a volume may have a "string of beads" appearance, because it is only partially represented by voxels along its length. The impact of these artifacts depends on the resampling filters that are used. Despite its limitations, MIP usually has superior accuracy compared with surface rendering in CT angiography and produces reproducible results with different operators.

Closely related to MIP is the MinIP, which involves detecting the minimum value along the ray paths in each view. This algorithm can be used alternatively to MIP especially in cholangiopancreatographic CT studies [19, 22].

An application defined "variable thickness viewing" enables combining multiple thin sections and visualizing them as slabs, thereby improving noise and coplanar effects. This technique is useful for examinations such as lung studies, because thin sections improve lesion detection (Fig. 3.9) and the accuracy

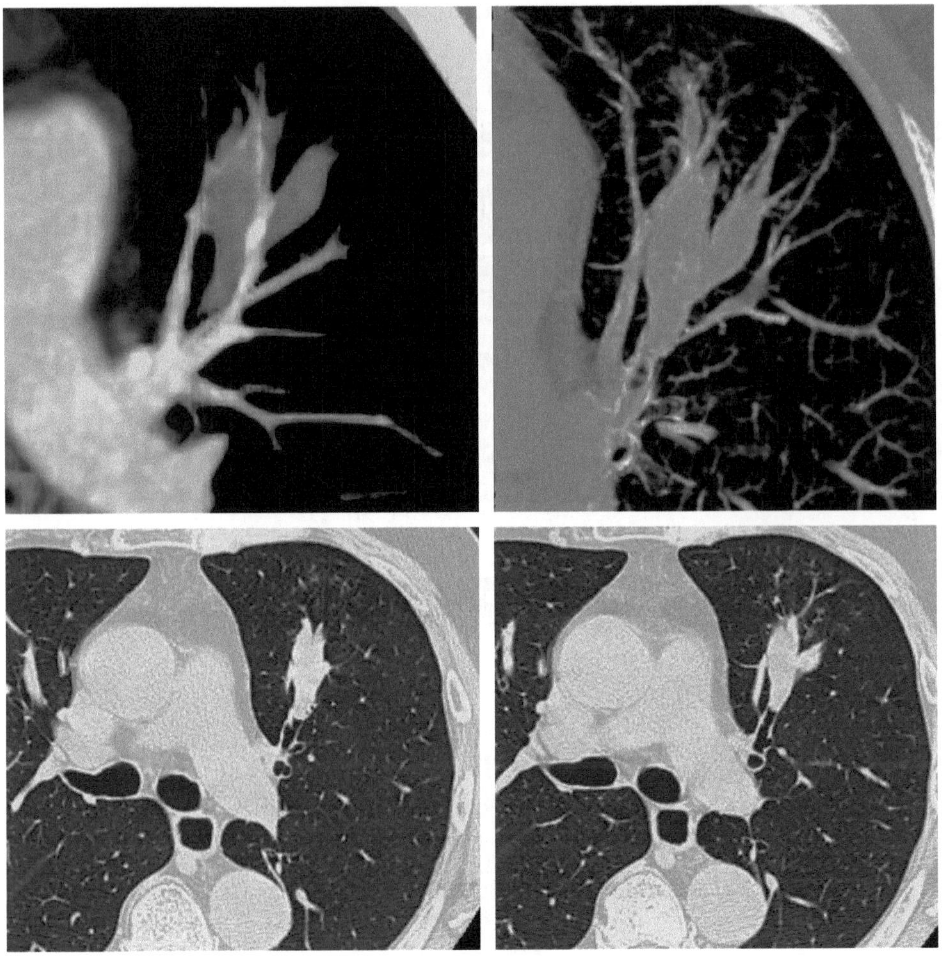

Fig. 3.9 Variable-thickness viewing allows depiction of the topographic relationships of bronchi and pulmonary vessels and also distinguishes them from pathological structures that show the same nodular appearance on the axial image

of lesion volume measurement, while slab mode improves lesion detection [4].

3.4 Volume Visualization

The aim of volume visualization is to realistically represent and analyze volume data by integrating a series of axial CT sections into a form that is easier to interpret than the original images. The medical field was the first to exploit volume visualization, and the first attempts date back to the late 1970s, with clinical applications in craniofacial surgery and orthopedics which required CT visualization of complex bony structures.

There are two basic classes of volume-visualization algorithms in use today: surface and volume rendering. The key idea of surface rendering is to extract an intermediate surface description of the relevant objects from the volume data. Only this information is then used for rendering. In volume rendering, on the contrary, images are created directly from the volume data, and no intermediate geometry is extracted [8].

All 3D rendering techniques represent a 3D volume of data in one or more 2D planes, conveying the spatial relationships inherent in the data with use of visual depth cues. To understand how these techniques work, it may be helpful to think of the volume of data as a cube floating within a computer monitor. The data are organized into a 3D matrix of volume elements (voxels). The screen of the computer monitor is a 2D surface composed of discrete picture elements (pixels). Presenting what is stored in memory on a 2D screen is a challenge, but it is the very problem that 3D reconstruction software has creatively solved.

Each 3D rendering technique relies on mathematic formulas to determine for each pixel what portion of the data in memory should be displayed on the screen and how that portion should be weighted to best represent spatial relationships. Voxel selection is usually accomplished by projecting lines (rays) through the data sets that correspond to the pixel matrix of the desired 2D image. Differences in the images produced with various types of 3D rendering are the result of variations in how voxels are selected and weighted [3]. The different methodological approach of 3D rendering techniques (surface and volume rendering) determines different outcome in practice (Figs. 3.10, 3.11).

Surface-rendering models do not contain any "inside" data and work with the extracted surface, which is manipulated as an empty shell. Volume rendering may display the surface of the superficial voxels of the data set, but it maintains all the data inside the shell as well. The advantage here is that now we can manipulate all the data, and also the dynamic range of the image is preserved generating images with higher flexibility. In volume rendering various parameters such as surface shading and opacity can help reveal both surface and internal detail and the radiologist or clinician is able to clearly distinguish most disease. For this reason a careful selection of these parameters should be performed. The disadvantage is that a volume render takes up more memory and takes longer to build than a surface render.

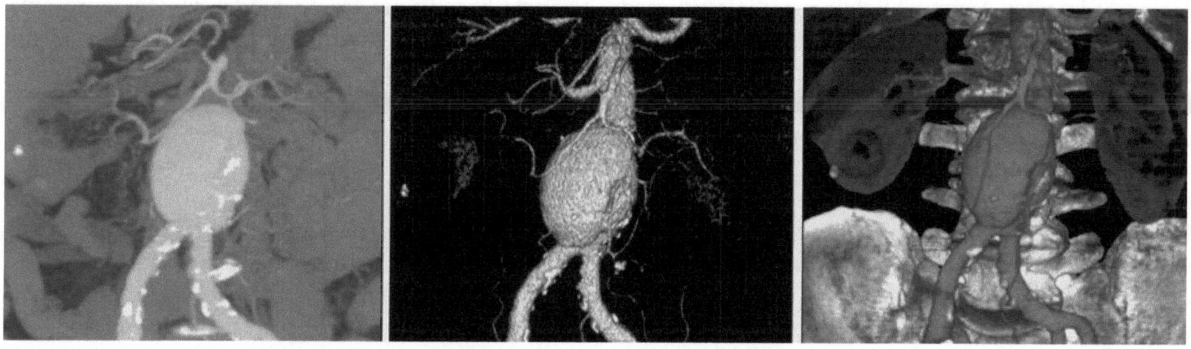

Fig. 3.10 MIP, volume rendering with surface shading and then with a slight transparency applied to the same data set show different aspects of the aortoiliac region. Surface shading and transparent images provides more panoramic views, while MIP allows better depiction of vascular patency and calcification.

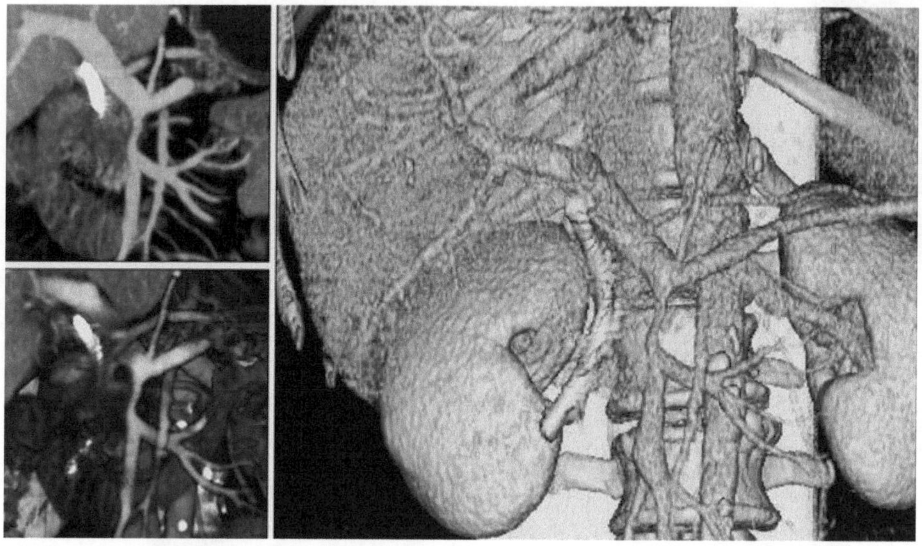

Fig. 3.11 A metallic biliary stent determines many disturbances on MIP images. The correct placement of the device is better appreciated in surface- and volume-rendered images.

3.4.1 Surface Rendering

Surface rendering was the first 3D rendering technique applied to medical data sets. Its early development in the 1970s was a logical extension of new computer graphics and image-processing techniques, and innovations in data segmentation (division of a volume into multiple areas or objects primitives) and display [6, 7].

Surface rendering is a process in which apparent surfaces are determined within the volume of data and an image representing the derived surfaces is displayed. Much of the research in this area has focused on how surfaces are determined. Surface contours are typically modeled as a number of overlapping polygons derived from the boundary of the selected region of interest. A virtual light source is computed for each polygon, and the object is displayed with the resulting surface shading. Multiple overlapping surfaces can be displayed on a single image with the additional implementation of partial opacities.

Simple thresholding is a commonly used technique designed to segment structures of interest for surface rendering. In this technique, each voxel intensity within the data sets is determined to be within some user-specified range of attenuation values (bone attenuation; Fig. 3.12). In surface rendering, the voxels located on the edge of a structure are identified and displayed; the remaining voxels in the image are usually considered invisible. This approach is quite useful for examining the inner surface of hollow structures such as airways (virtual bronchoscopy), colon (virtual colonoscopy), middle ear (virtual otoscopy), etc. The thresholding assignment of the voxels that will be visible is both critical and sometimes difficult to reproducibly define. If the thresholding process is too aggressive, actual protruding structures can be lost from view because of partial volume effects. If the thresholding process is too lax, nondesired voxels (different from the segmented tissue) are included in the 3D model (Fig. 3.13a,b).

After the thresholding process, the surface of the volume data is generated by approximating and connecting the shape of edge voxels of the segmented volume. These visualization pipelines generate a triangle-based wire-frame model, which represents the surface. Most commonly a marching-cubes algorithm [15] is used, which basically decides whether a surface passes through a data element or not. By "marching" through all the cubic cells intersected by the isosurface, the algorithm calculates the intersection points along the edges and produces triangular mesh to fit to these vertices. The wire-frame model can be covered by a virtual surface by assessing surface properties, reflection, and color. In addition a virtual light source can be placed arbitrarily to create shading and depth effects.

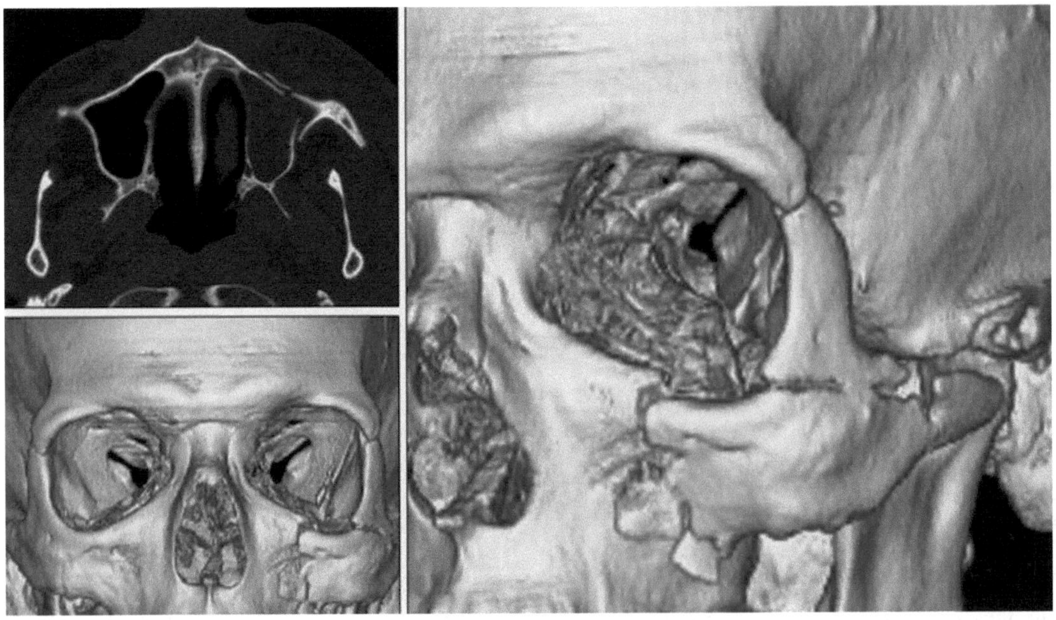

Fig. 3.12 Maxillary and zygomatic bone. Surface rendering clearly depicts the cortical bone and details of fracture lines.

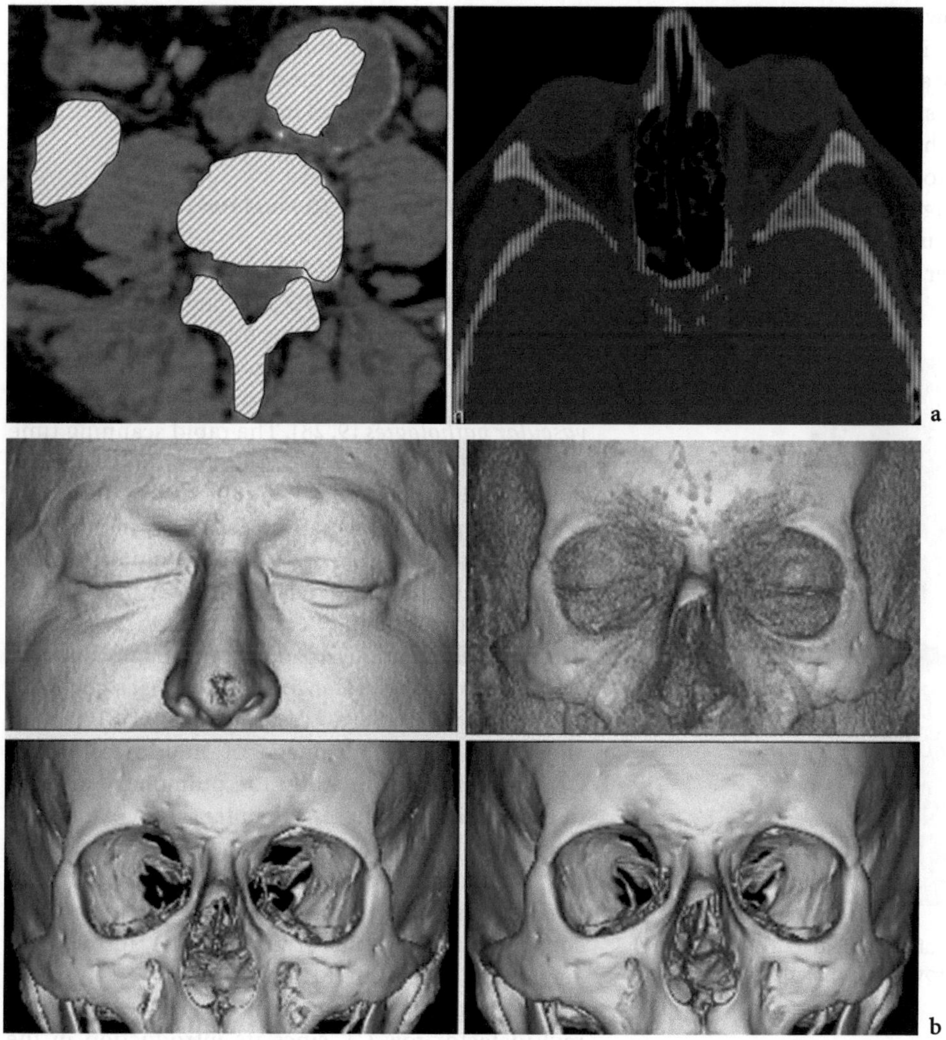

Fig. 3.13a,b Segmentation process eliminates all the structures whose Hounsfield density is lower than a selected value. **a** Segmentation; **b** effects of progressive thresholding values.

3.4.2 Volume Rendering

As mentioned above, volume rendering takes the entire volume of data, sums the contributions of each voxel along a line from the viewer's eye through the data sets, and displays the resulting composite for each pixel of the display.

To optimally display the anatomical structures, volume rendering enables modulation of *window width and level*, *opacity*, and *percentage classification*, and enables also the interactive change of perspective of 3D rendering in real time [3].

Before modulating the visibility of anatomical structures by the mentioned parameters, data resampling and editing can be done, in order to reduce image-processing time, and is applied prior to rendering. Resampling reduces image resolution. Manual or semiautomatic editing is typically performed to "eliminate" an object such as an organ from surrounding structures. One example of editing is represented by clip-plane. This technique defines planes that segment the volume into regions of displayed or suppressed voxels [3].

Rendering parameters are applied to the full-volume data sets and affect the appearance of the image to be displayed. The window width and level functions are similar to windowing parameter settings on standard CT scanners or workstations. Volume rendering typically segments data on the basis of voxel attenuation. The window can be adjusted to standard settings; however, real-time rendering also permits the user to interactively alter the window setting and instantly see the changes.

"Opacity" refers to the degree with which structures that appear close to the user obscure structures that are farther away. High opacity values produce an appearance similar to surface rendering. Low opacity values allow the user to "see through" structures (Fig. 3.14).

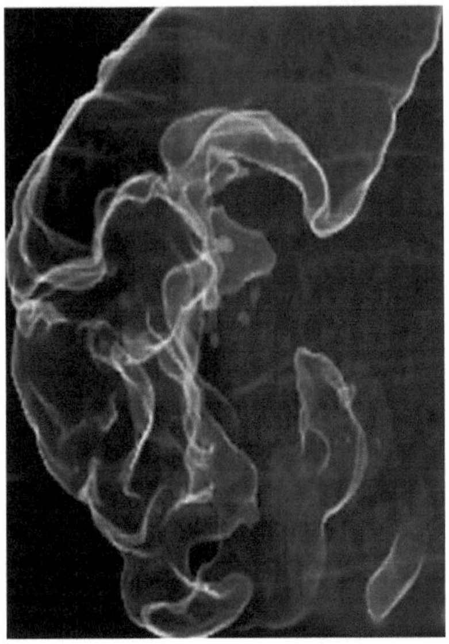

Fig. 3.14 Volume rendering of a polypoid lesion of cecum. The high-transparency mode provides a simulation of double-contrast barium enema.

The use of percentage classification is a more advanced feature of volume rendering which distinguishes between different groups of voxels pertaining to different tissues in an optimal way. Each group is approximated by a trapezoid in the software that can be interactively manipulated to alter the visibility of the tissue, and multiple trapezoidal distributions can be displayed simultaneously [3].

Image display is the final step of image processing and relates to the process by which a "virtual" 3D representation of a volume data set is "flattened" onto one or more 2D planes; this process is required because a 3D model must be represented with a computer monitor, which is a bidimensional device.

The most commonly used display method is *ray-casting*, which is a basic technique for displaying a volume of data in two dimensions. In this technique, an array of parallel lines (rays) are mathematically projected through the volume in alignment with each pixel within a desired 2D plane. A weighted sum of these voxel values encountered by the ray is calculated for each pixel and then scaled to the particular range of gray-scale values in the display.

3.4.2.1 Clinical Applications of 3D Rendering in Multidetector-Row CT

Clinical applications of 3D imaging run parallel to the applications of multidetector-row CT, since both are substantially dependent on each other. The main application of multidetector-row CT is the study of *vascular pathologies* [9, 28]. The rapid scanning time allows a selective and precise evaluation of arterial, portal, and venous phases of the vascular system, even in the peripheral district. Especially in the latter, multidetector-row CT with MIP and volume rendering is valuable. One practical example is the study of patients with pulmonary embolism: in these patients deep venous thrombosis is one of the major causes of embolism and the presence of thrombus is generally evaluated by Doppler ultrasonography (US) or with angiography. The advantage of multidetector-row CT, which is used to study the pulmonary arteries in this clinical setting, is the potential to extend the acquisition caudally, to cover the lower limbs [13]. The accuracy of volume rendering in the study of a variety of applications (thoracic and abdominal aortic aneurysm, renal artery stenosis, intracranial aneurysm) is very high [11, 21, 29].

Due to the fast acquisition and high resolution, multidetector-row CT, since its introduction in the clinical practice, has been found to be effective in the management of *emergency*. In this setting the use of 3D imaging, and especially volume rendering, certainly has been proved useful in musculoskeletal trauma [18, 20]. Volume rendering allows detection of fractures and also characterizes the extent of fracture line as well as the presence of fragments. The provided 3D visualization of the fracture has important surgical outcomes; in fact, on the basis of volume rendering, the correct surgical approach can be easily planned [14].

There are many areas in *oncology* that can benefit from volume rendering, for example to determine tumor resectability and preoperative planning for tumor resection in patients with a variety of neoplasms including pancreatic cancer, primary and metastatic hepatic malignancies, lung cancer, and renal cell carcinoma [3].

A wide variety of applications of 3D image processing can be mentioned for other anatomical areas;

however, among these all the applications in surgical planning will have an impact in clinical practice and in the radiologist's work.

Evaluation of complex craniofacial anomalies played a major role in early clinical applications of 3D reconstruction of CT data [16, 30]. The advantage of 3D reconstruction for surgical treatment of craniofacial malformations was demonstrated in the accurate evaluation of complex spatial relationships, which represented a dramatic improvement over use of axial CT scans alone [3]. Recently, volume rendering has been shown to have advantages over other rendering techniques, particularly in resolving subcortical bone lesions and minimally displaced fractures, and in visualizing hidden areas of interest while creating few artifacts [12].

Postoperative review of patients with *implanted devices* can also be accomplished more effectively, because volume rendering eliminates the vast majority of streak artifact and clearly delineates the anatomical relationship.

3.4.3 Virtual Endoscopy

Virtual endoscopy is a computer-generated simulation of the endoscopic perspective obtained by processing volumetric (CT/MR) data and is one of the applications of virtual reality in medicine [5]. The first presentations of virtual endoscopy in the radiological field were given by Vining in 1993 and 1994 [31, 32], who reported the application in the study of bronchi and colon, respectively. Initial works were oriented to demonstrate the feasibility of the technique in the exploration of the entire human body, but soon focused experiences were carried out for specific clinical problems.

Nowadays virtual endoscopy accounts reports on the study of colon, stomach, bronchial tree, larynx and trachea, middle and inner ear, paranasal sinuses, brain ventricles, vessels, biliary tract, urinary tract, and joints. The terminology used to describe the technique was adapted to the anatomical area under examination: virtual colonoscopy (Fig. 3.15), bronchoscopy (Fig. 3.16), cholangioscopy, ureterorenoscopy, angioscopy, etc.

Most investigators agree that the colon exploration represents the main clinical impact of virtual endoscopy. The unique difference between virtual endoscopy and other 3D imaging methods is the type of perspective. In virtual endoscopy the typical perspective of fiber-optic endoscopes is reproduced by a dedicated computer program; one can freely fly through or around 3D objects that are produced by common 3D processing techniques based on surface or volume rendering. As a consequence the properties of data that are used to generate virtual endoscopy are the same of any data used for other image processing techniques: volumes that respect the spatial relationships of the human body. However, take it for granted, in virtual endoscopy there are specific requirements of image acquisition related to the scope of the virtual endoscopic examination.

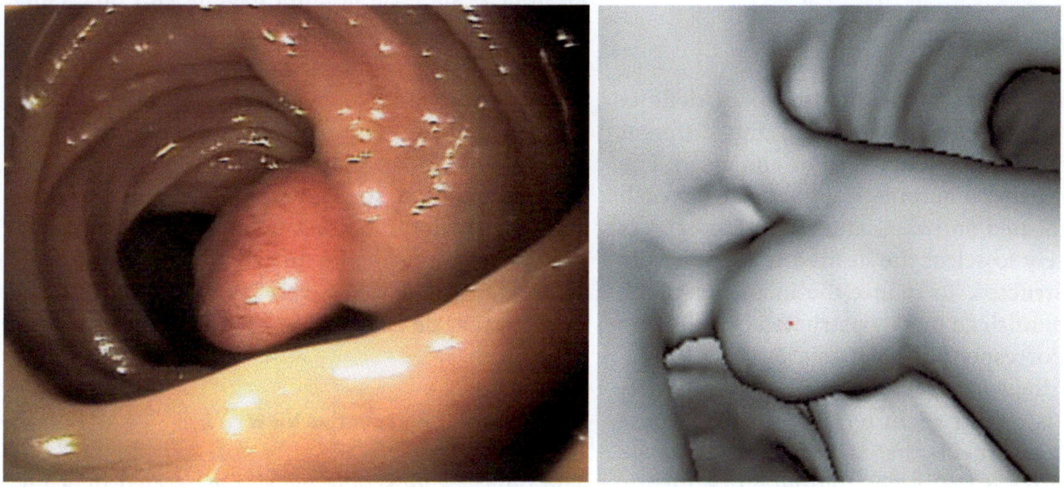

Fig. 3.15 Virtual endoscopy generates endoluminal perspectives similar to conventional endoscopy. A polypoid lesion of the colon is confidently represented by conventional and virtual colonoscopy.

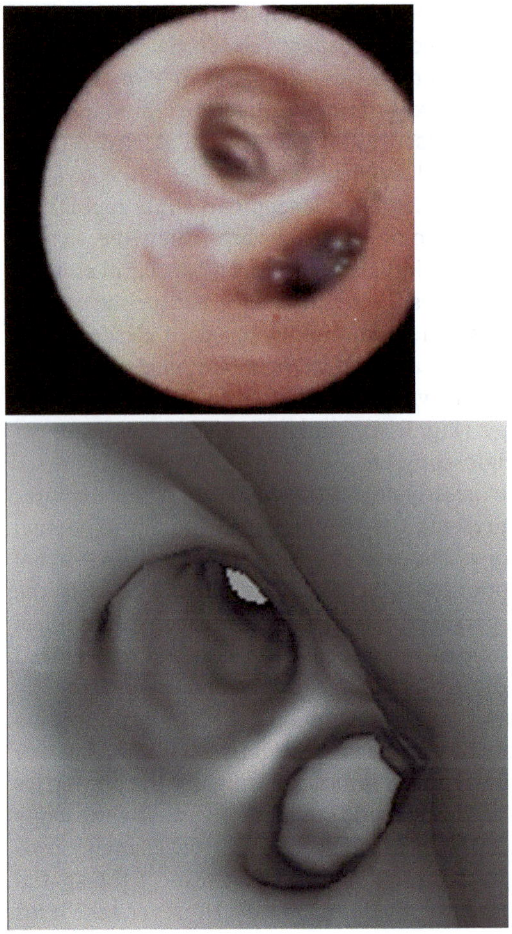

Fig. 3.16 Virtual endoscopy of the main bronchi and conventional bronchoscopy generate similar patterns. The endoscopic view is created by positioning the virtual endoscope within the trachea.

3.4.3.1 Volume Generation

Each patient's data set is composed of a definite number of series corresponding to the different phase of acquisition, unenhanced or enhanced. The volume is in general automatically created by each piece of dedicated software, and the radiologist is asked uniquely to select the desired imaging series to be reconstructed. To reduce the image overload, a reduced volume can be reconstructed by selecting the images corresponding to a selected anatomical area. Within the software architecture, the volumetric data set is organized in terms of voxels. These are near-cubic elements that arise from each image pixel. This latter is the basic building block for the voxel to which a Hounsfield value (in the case of CT) or an intensity value (in the case of MR) is assigned; each voxel has also a defined spatial position and dimension in the volume.

The ideal volumetric data set, which represents precisely the imaged structures, is obtained when all voxels are isotropic and therefore their shape is cubic. Unfortunately conventional CT and spiral CT did not completely fulfill these acquisition requirements. Dedicated MR sequences and multidetector-row CT seem to have overcome these limitations.

3.4.3.2 Volume Segmentation

Surface and volume rendering are the methods used to virtually represent the human body in three dimensions. Each owns a specific principle of dataset segmentation in order to select the anatomical structure to display from the inside. Most available software for virtual endoscopy allows the radiologist to interact with the volumetric sample and segment it in real time. By using surface rendering, the change of visible structure is made by the selection of a threshold which defines the edge line of a surface to display and effectively represents the passage between two different density or intensity values (the colonic mucosa and the colonic lumen filled by air). Thus, before starting the inner visualizations with these methods, the operator should be aware of the different threshold values used. For example the colonic surface in a CT study with pneumocolon can be optimally represented with thresholds ranging from −800 to −700 HU; the middle ear −500 HU and the threshold for displaying aortic lumen depends on the degree of contrast enhancement.

In the volume-rendering technique, the generation of endoscopic view is quite flexible and interactive when the computer used is powerful enough. Almost all commercially available software has been implemented with predefined volume-rendering protocols that produce endoluminal views of specific organs. To simplify the concept, in volume rendering the use of a threshold is strongly smoothed by the use of transfer opacity functions, therefore the passage between structures having different voxel properties is attenuated and progressively increased or decreased by a linear scale of values.

3.4.3.3 Generation of Perspective View

The typical endoscopic view is generated by a ray-casting algorithm [24]. In ray-casting, parallel rays are virtually generated by a source point (the eye of the observer or point in which the endoscope is positioned); the rays transverse the acquired volume along a divergent direction and, applying surface or volume rendering algorithms, the encountered voxels are classified by the attribution of opacity values. In surface rendering the voxels located above or below a specific threshold that are encountered by the rays cast are fixed and transformed in a mesh of polygons reflecting each ray. The algorithm used to perform the surface extraction is called the "marching cube" [15]. It transforms the cubic shape of a voxel into a mesh of triangles (triangulation), and the final composition of the transformed voxels constitutes an isosurface.

In volume rendering the classification of voxels is given by linear opacity functions that attribute different opacity values to particular voxels intensities. The advantages of this approach are the optimization of the dynamic range and the ability to change tissue opacities to produce 3D renderings, which maintain surface details and which represent the entire data set.

The final image of surface- or volume-rendered ray casting will have a conic field of view (as in endoscopy). The field of view can be changed by viewing angle. Many software packages have a large viewing angle, but an increase in this value distorts the surface morphology and alters the potential to recognize pathological findings. This approach seems to have other limitations that are also relevant to real endoscopy.

An exhaustive virtual endoscopic study is time-consuming, especially virtual colonoscopy. To obviate this aspect, new algorithms have been proposed such as virtual dissection of the colon and unfolded cubic rendering of colon [27].

3.4.3.4
Fly-Through Path

Fly-path planning is a critical issue in virtual endoscopy. The navigation through tubular structures is quite difficult, especially if these are tortuous, and presents sharp curves, caliber enlargement, or strong reduction along their path. The calculation of the shorter and central navigation path is required to help the radiologist. The ideal assisted navigation should allow the radiologist to stay comfortably in front of the computer display and take a movie of the complete fly-through of the structure under examination. This is easy to perform in straight structures such as the abdominal aorta or trachea, but become difficult in tortuous structures such as the colon.

The requirements of an assisted navigation are: automatic path-planning, collision detection, and direct interaction with the objects displayed. The last point should consist of the following steps: stop the navigation, look at the object, touch the object, cross correlate with other images (axial, MPR, external 3D models).

Various authors have proposed the calculation of an automatic path. Jolesz [10] proposed a method in which the endoscopic camera is considered as a robot and the walls of the organs as obstacles. However, any given automatic path is not free of errors in calculation, and the collision with the organ's surface is possible. Collision detection algorithms work as in the case of the Jolesz [10] method. The surface is identified as a variation of threshold value and therefore, when the endoscope finds it, performs a change of direction.

The collision detection algorithm is also used in VRML (virtual reality modeling language), where surface-rendered models represent different objects of a virtual world that can be explored through Internet browsers. The direct interaction with the objects displayed in the endoscopic views is an absolute requirement of virtual endoscopy. The main criticism of this technique is that it can wrongly represent objects of the real world. To overcome this problem, most software enables visualization of the target object, pointing to it with the computer mouse, and obtaining the corresponding axial or MPR image crossing through it. On the other hand, we must remember that virtual endoscopy is not a stand-alone technique, but it is one of the possible ways through which volumetric data sets can be represented. Therefore a constant correlation with original data should always be performed, especially to confirm endoscopic findings.

References

1. Baek SY, Sheafor DH, Keogan MT, DeLong DM, Nelson RC (2001) Two-dimensional multiplanar and 3D volume-rendered vascular CT in pancreatic carcinoma: interobserver agreement and comparison with standard helical techniques. AJR Am J Roentgenol 176:1467–1473
2. Batra P, Bigoni B, Manning J (2000) Pitfalls in the diagnosis of thoracic aortic dissection at CT angiography. Radiographics 20:309–320
3. Calhoun PS, Kuszyk BS, Heath DG, Carley JC, Fishman EK (1999) 3D volume rendering of spiral CT data: theory and method. Radiographics 19:745–764
4. Cody DD (2002) AAPM/RSNA physics tutorial for residents: topics in CT. Radiographics 22:1255–1268
5. Geiger B, Kikinis R (1994) Simulation of endoscopy.

AAAI Spring Symposium Series: applications of computer vision in medical images processing. Stanford University, pp 138–140
6. Herman GT, Liu HK (1977) Display of 3D information in computed tomography. J Comput Assist Tomogr 1:155–160
7. Herman GT, Liu HK (1979) 3D display of human organs from computed tomograms. Comput Graph Image Proc 9:1–21
8. John NW (2002) Volume rendering. In: Caramella D, Bartolozzi C (eds) 3D image processing. Springer, Berlin Heidelberg New York, pp 35–41
9. Johnson PT, Heath DG, Kuszyk BS, Fishman EK (1996) CT angiography: thoracic vascular imaging with interactive volume rendering technique. J Comput Assist Tomogr 21:110–111
10. Jolesz FA (1997) Interactive virtual endoscopy. AJR Am J Roentgenol 169:1229-1237
11. Kawamoto S, Montgomery RA, Lawler LP, Horton KM, Fishman EK (2003) Multidetector CT angiography for preoperative evaluation of living laparoscopic kidney donors. AJR Am J Roentgenol 180:1633–1638
12. Kuszyk BS, Johnson PT, Heath DG, Fishman EK (1996) CT angiography with volume rendering: advantages and applications in splanchnic vascular imaging. Radiology 200:564–568
13. Laghi A, Catalano C, Panebianco V (2000) Optimization of the technique of virtual colonoscopy using a multislice spiral computerized tomography. Radiol Med 100:459–464
14. Liener UC, Reinhart C, Kinzl L, Gebhard F (1999) A new approach to computer guidance in orthopedic surgery using real time volume rendering. J Med Syst 23:35–40
15. Lorensen WE, Kline HE (1987) Marching cubes: a high resolution 3D surface reconstruction algorithm. Comput Graph 21:163–169
16. Marsh JL, Vannier MW (1983) Surface imaging from computerized tomographic scans. Surgery 94:159–165
17. Neri E, Vagli P, Picchietti S (2002) Pitfalls and artefacts in virtual endoscopy. In: Caramella D, Bartolozzi C (eds) 3D image processing. Springer, Berlin Heidelberg New York, pp 55–56
18. Pretorius ES, Fishman EK (1999) Volume-rendered three-dimensional spiral CT: musculoskeletal applications. Radiographics 19:1143–1160
19. Park SJ, Han JK, Kim TK, Choi BI (2001) 3D spiral CT cholangiography with minimum intensity projection in patients with suspected obstructive biliary disease: comparison with percutaneous transhepatic cholangiography. Abdom Imaging 26:281–286
20. Philipp MO, Kubin K, Mang T, Hormann M, Metz VM (2003) Three-dimensional volume rendering of multidetector-row CT data: applicable for emergency radiology. Eur J Radiol 48:33-38
21. Portugaller HR, Schoellnast H, Tauss J, Tiesenhausen K, Hausegger KA (2003) Semitransparent volume-rendering CT angiography for lesion display in aortoiliac arteriosclerotic disease. J Vasc Interv Radiol 14:1023–1030
22. Raptopoulos V, Prassopoulos P, Chuttani R (1998) Multiplanar CT pancreatography and distal cholangiography with minimum intensity projections. Radiology 207:317–324
23. Robb RA (1995) Image processing and visualization. In: Robb RA (ed) 3D biomedical imaging: principes and practice. VCH, New York, pp 127–132
24. Roth SD (1982) Ray casting for solid modelling. Comput Graph Image Proc 18:109–144
25. Rydberg J, Buckwalter KA, Caldemeyer KS, et al. (2000) Multisection CT: scanning techniques and clinical applications. Radiographics 20:1787–1806
26. Schreiner S, Paschal CB, Galloway RL (1996) Comparison of projection algorithms used for the construction of maximum intensity projection images. J Comput Assist Tomogr 20:56–67
27. Sorantin E (2002) Technique of virtual dissection of the colon based on spiral CT data. In: Caramella D, Bartolozzi C (eds) 3D image processing. Springer, Berlin Heidelberg New York, pp 197–209
28. Smith PA, Marshall FF, Urban BA, Heath DG, Fishman EK (1997) 3D CT stereoscopic visualization of renal masses: impact on diagnosis and patient management. AJR Am J Roentgenol 169:1331–1334
29. Tomandl BF, Hastreiter P, Iserhardt-Bauer S, et al. (2003) Standardized evaluation of CT angiography with remote generation of 3D video sequences for the detection of intracranial aneurysms. Radiographics 23:e12
30. Vannier MW, Marsh JL, Warren JO (1984) Three dimensional CT reconstruction images for craniofacial surgical planning and evaluation. Radiology 150:179–184
31. Vining DJ (1993) Virtual bronchoscopy: a new perspective for viewing the tracheobronchial tree. Radiology 189:438
32. Vining DJ (1994) Virtual colonoscopy. Radiology 193:446

4 Contrast-Medium Administration

Dominik Fleischmann

CONTENTS

4.1 Introduction

Intravenous contrast-medium (CM) administration remains one of the fundamental components of computed tomography angiography (CTA). The general goal is to achieve adequate opacification of the vascular territory of interest to coincide with the CT acquisition. Many empirical injection protocols have been employed successfully in the past. However, since the introduction of multidetector-row CT (MDCT) – which is a continuously and rapidly evolving technology – scan times have become substantially shorter with each new scanner generation. Injection protocols developed for the early days of CTA are no longer adequate for current MDCT technology, and one may completely miss the bolus if the injection protocol is not adequately adapted to the capabilities of a modern MDCT scanner.

Thus the purpose of this chapter is to provide the reader with the ingredients necessary for the rational design of CM injection protocols for all current and potential future applications of cardiovascular MDCT and CTA. Those ingredients are:

- A basic understanding of the physiological and pharmacokinetic principles guiding arterial enhancement following intravenous CM administration
- Knowledge of the effects of user-selectable injection parameters on vascular enhancement
- Awareness of the technical properties of injection tools (power injectors) and timing devices (bolus tracking) used for CM delivery

Several theoretical and practical examples, as well as suggestions for injection protocols, are provided to illustrate the key points in a logical fashion.

4.2 Contrast Media for CT Angiography

All currently used angiographic X-ray CM are water-soluble derivates of symmetrically iodinated benzene. They are either negatively charged ionic (ionic CM) or nonionic molecules (nonionic CM). The diagnostic use of X-ray CM is exclusively based on the physical ability of iodine to absorb X-rays, not on pharmacological effects – which are generally undesired. The desired effect of CM is thus directly related to the iodine concentration of the agent.

D. Fleischmann, MD
Assistant Professor of Radiology, Department of Radiology, Thoracic and Cardiovascular Imaging Sections, Stanford University Medical Center, 300 Pasteur Drive, Room S-072, Stanford, CA 94305-5105, USA

The selection of intravenous CM for CTA is primarily governed by safety considerations and rate of expected adverse reactions. Nonionic CM are generally safer than ionic CM, with less idiosyncratic (non-dose-dependent, e.g., allergic) adverse reactions [17]. Ionic CM also have a greater potential to cause acute nausea and vomiting, and – as a result – motion, when injection rates greater than 2.0–2.5ml/s are used. Furthermore, extravasation of ionic CM is less well tolerated than nonionic CM. Therefore, nonionic CM are probably the best choice for CTA [14].

4.3 Pharmacokinetic and Physiological Principles

All angiographic X-ray CM are extracellular fluid markers. After intravenous administration they are rapidly distributed between the vascular and interstitial spaces [8]. Pharmacokinetic studies on CM have traditionally concentrated on the phase of elimination (following CM injection) rather than on the very early phase of CM distribution (during CM administration). For the time frame relevant to CTA, however, it is this particularly complex phase of early CM distribution and redistribution that determines vascular enhancement. Early CM dynamics cannot be studied directly (i.e., measuring the rapid changes of the concentration of CM from blood samples). However, as relative CT attenuation values (ΔHU, where HU is Hounsfield units), derived by subtracting background attenuation before administration of CM, are linearly related to the concentration of CM (iodine), CM dynamics may be described and expressed in these units [7, 8].

It is important to recognize at this stage that vascular enhancement (which is the topic of this chapter) and parenchymal organ enhancement are affected by different kinetics. Early vascular enhancement (for CTA and cardiovascular MDCT) is essentially determined by the relationship between iodine administration per unit of time (iodine flux, in milligrams of iodine per second) versus blood flow per unit of time (i.e., cardiac output, in liters per minute). Parenchymal enhancement, on the other hand, is governed by the relationship of total iodine dose (milligrams of iodine) to total volume of distribution (i.e., body weight, BW, in kilograms). Thus, the most important injection parameter to chose in CTA is the injection flow rate, whereas in organ imaging it is the injection volume.

4.3.1 Early Arterial Contrast-Medium Dynamics

Early CM dynamics have gained substantial interest because of their implications for CTA. Whereas time-attenuation responses to intravenously injected CM may vary between vascular territories and across individuals (as discussed below), the basic pattern can be observed in the example in Fig. 4.1.

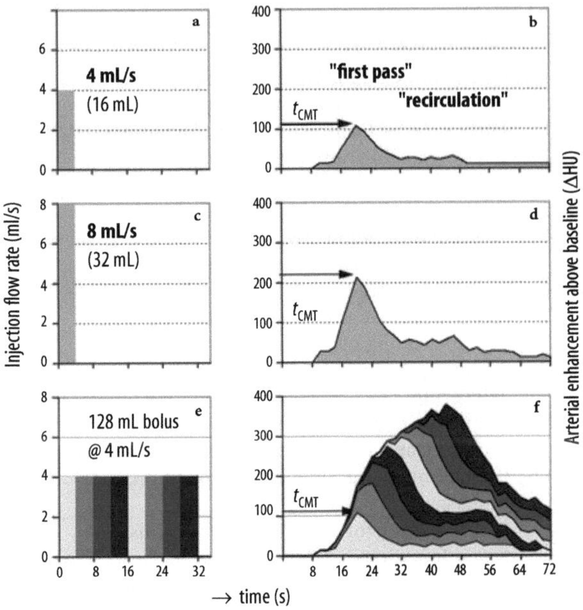

Fig. 4.1a–f. Simple "additive model" illustrates the effects of injection flow rate and injection duration on arterial enhancement. Intravenous contrast medium (CM) injection (**a**) causes an arterial enhancement response (**b**), which consists of an early "first-pass" peak, and a lower "recirculation" effect. Doubling the injection flow rate (doubling the iodine administration rate) (**c**) results in approximately twice the arterial enhancement (**d**). The effect of the injection duration (**e**) can be regarded as the sum (time integral) of several enhancement responses (**f**). Note that due to the asymmetric shape of the test-enhancement curve and due to recirculation effects, arterial enhancement following an injection of 128 ml (the time integral of 8 consecutive 16 ml) increases continuously over time (adapted from [9], with permission)

Figure 4.1 schematically illustrates early arterial CM dynamics as observed in the abdominal aorta: When a 16-ml test-bolus of CM is injected intravenously at a flow rate of 4 ml/s, it causes an arterial enhancement response in the aorta. The time interval needed for the CM to arrive in the arterial territory of interest is referred to as the CM transit time (t_{CMT}). The first peak in the enhancement response is also referred to as the "first-pass" effect. While CM is distributed throughout the vascular and interstitial spaces of the body, a certain proportion of CM-enhanced blood returns rapidly from highly perfused organs, such as the brain and the kidney, to reenter the right heart (*recirculation*). It is important to realize that within the time frame of CTA one will not only observe the first pass of contrast material but also its recirculation effect.

For a given individual and vascular territory, the enhancement response is proportional to the iodine administration rate, or iodine flux (milligrams of iodine per second). Figure 4.1c and d illustrate the effect of doubling the iodine administration rate (by doubling the injection flow rate). One can observe an enhancement response, which is approximately twice as strong. Whereas the effect of the iodine administration rate on arterial enhancement is straightforward and logical, this is not the case for the effect of the injection duration and the shape of the enhancement curve.

A simple additive model – based on the assumption of a time-invariant linear system – may help to explain the effect of prolonged injections on arterial enhancement [9]: As shown in Fig. 4.1e and f, a large (128 ml), prolonged (32 s) bolus of CM can be viewed as the sum of eight subsequent "test boluses" of 16 ml each. Each of these eight test boluses has its own effect (first pass and recirculation) on arterial enhancement. The cumulative enhancement response to the whole 128-ml injection equals the sum (time integral) of enhancement responses to each of the eight test boluses. Note, that the recirculation effects of the earlier test boluses overlap (and thus sum up) with the first-pass effects of later test boluses.

As a result, the general enhancement pattern observed in the arterial system following the intravenous injection of a prolonged bolus (>10 s) of CM can be characterized as follows: After a certain time interval (corresponding to the CM transit time, t_{CMT}), there is a short, steep enhancement increase, which is followed by a continuous increase in arterial opacification as long as CM is injected, which is then followed by a rapid decrease in enhancement after the end of the injection. Note that this enhancement response is delayed in time relative to the beginning of the intravenous injection (t_{CMT}).

4.3.2 Physiological Parameters Affecting Vascular Enhancement

In general, the previously described vascular enhancement response to intravenously injected CM applies to all arterial territories. The specific magnitudes, however, are characteristic for a given vascular territory in a given patient. The exact shape of a time-attenuation curve is determined by individual physiological parameters and beyond the control of the observer.

The *CM transit time* (t_{CMT}) from the injection site to the vascular territory of interest depends on the anatomical distance between them, but also on the encountered physiological flow rates between these landmarks. Injection flow rates hardly affect the arterial t_{CMT}. For systemic arteries, the t_{CMT} is primarily controlled by cardiac output. Cardiac output also accounts for most of the wide interindividual variability of the t_{CMT}. Low cardiac output prolongs, high cardiac output decreases the t_{CMT}. Obviously the t_{CMT} can be substantially delayed in patients with venous obstructions downstream of the injection site.

The *degree of arterial enhancement* following the same intravenous CM injection is also highly variable between individuals. Even in patients considered to have normal cardiac output, mid-aortic enhancement may range from 140 to 440 HU (a factor of 3) between patients [20]. Even if BW is taken into account, the average aortic enhancement ranges from 92 to 196 HU/ml per kilogram (a factor of 2) [13]. Adjusting the CM volume (and injection rates) to BW will therefore reduce interindividual differences of arterial enhancement, but will not completely eliminate them. A reasonable compromise in clinical CTA therefore is to adjust the injection volumes and flow rates for patients with deviations of their BW of more than 20% from an average of 75 kg. The key physiological parameters affecting individual arterial enhancement are cardiac output and the central blood volume.

Cardiac output is inversely related to the degree of arterial enhancement, particularly in first-pass dynamics [1, 2]: if more blood is ejected per unit of time, the CM injected per unit of time will be more diluted. Hence, arterial enhancement is lower in patients with high cardiac output, but it is stronger in patients with low cardiac output (despite the increased t_{CMT} in the latter). This effect is illustrated in two patients with very different physique, in Fig. 4.2. Note that the 51-year-old hypertensive man, with a BW of 88 kg required about 3 times more CM volume to achieve the same degree of arterial enhancement when compared with the 67-year-old woman with 59 kg of body weight.

Central blood volume is also inversely related to arterial enhancement – but presumably affects recirculation and tissue enhancement to a greater extent

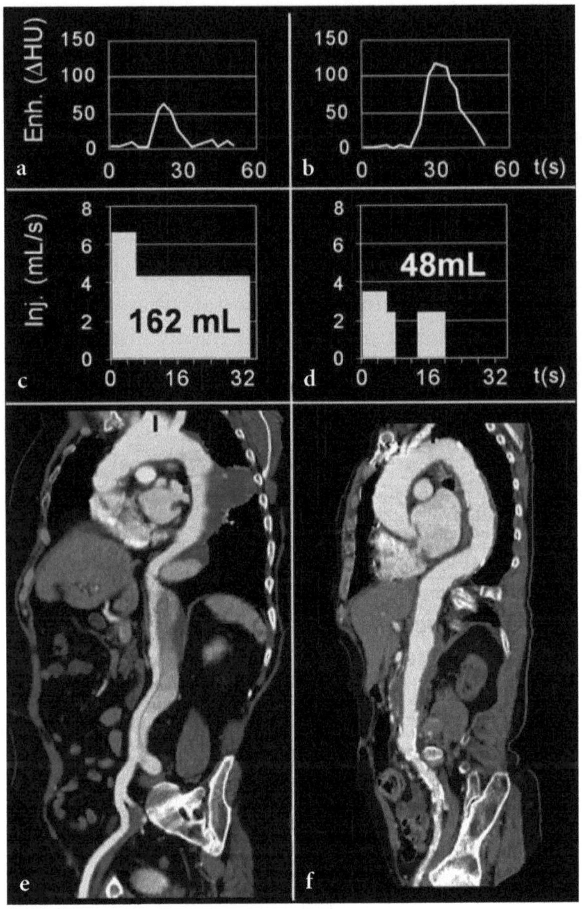

Fig. 4.2a–f. Variability of arterial enhancement between patients of different physique: The aortic enhancement responses (**a**, **b**) to a 16ml test bolus are shown for a 51-year-old hypertensive man with a body weight of 88 kg (**a**), and a 59-year-old woman with 59 kg bodyweight (**b**). Because of a substantially lower enhancement response to the test bolus, the younger, and bigger man required more than 3 times more CM volume (162 ml) than the older and smaller woman (48 ml) (**c**,**d**), to achieve a similar enhancement in the subsequent computed tomography angiogram of the thoracoabdominal aorta (**e**, **f**)

than it affects first-pass dynamics [7]. Central blood volume correlates with BW. If total CM volumes are chosen relative to BW, then 1.5–2.0 ml/kg BW (450–600 mg I/kg BW) are a reasonable quantity for arterial CTA.

Another factor which affects the t_{CMT} but also arterial enhancement is a temporarily diminished venous return caused by a forced Valsalva maneuver of the patient in an attempt to hold his or her breath. In patients but also in previously undiagnosed asymptomatic individuals with a patent foramen ovale, such a maneuver may cause a temporary right-to-left shunt with early arterial enhancement.

4.3.3 Effect of User-Selectable Injection Parameters

With key physiological parameters (such as cardiac output) beyond the control of the observer, it is particularly important to understand the effects of user-controllable injection parameters on arterial enhancement. Traditionally, injection protocols for CTA have been expressed as the volume (milliliters) and flow rate (milliliters per second) of CM. Given the previously described, early arterial CM dynamics, it is more useful, however, to express injection protocols for CTA in terms of iodine administration rate (or its substitute, the injection flow rate, in milliliters per second) and injection duration (seconds). The CM volume is then derived by simple multiplication.

Iodine administration rate (injection flow rate). The number of iodine molecules administered per unit of time (the iodine flux) is proportional to the injection flow rate for a given CM concentration. An iodine flux of 1.0–1.2 g/s (3.5–4 ml/s) is generally considered a minimum injection rate for CTA (15 mg I/s per kilogram of BW). The injection flow rate has a direct, proportional effect on arterial enhancement (Fig. 4.1c,d); e.g., a 50% increase in the injection rate (for a given injection duration) will result in a 50% increase in arterial enhancement (at the cost of 50% more CM volume). Similarly, a 30% increase in the iodine concentration will yield a 30% stronger enhancement. Note that enhancement always refers to increase in attenuation above baseline (nonenhanced) values.

Injection duration. As illustrated in Fig. 4.1, arterial enhancement also increases with the injection duration. This effect is not as straightforward and logical as the effect of the iodine flux; however, it is immediately obvious that very short injection durations – e.g., 5 s – cannot reach an adequate arterial enhancement level (let alone the difficulty of correctly timing a CTA acquisition to such a short enhancement peak). Therefore, the "old rule" of CTA, where the injection duration equals the scanning duration, is no longer applicable to fast acquisitions. There is a minimum injection duration necessary to raise arterial enhancement to an adequate level of opacification, which is probably in the region of about 10 s.

Biphasic or multiphasic injections. As previously noted, the typical arterial enhancement pattern resulting from prolonged (20–40 s) CM injections is a continuous rise of arterial enhancement. Even with correct scan timing, this will result in lower arterial opacification early during the scan, and excessive enhancement later during the data acquisition. A more uniform enhancement can be achieved, however, if the injection rates are varied over time, with high initial flow rates and lower continuing flow rates [3, 11].

4.3.4 Mathematical Modeling

Accurate prediction and controlling of time-dependent arterial enhancement is highly desirable for MDCT, particularly with faster scanners and for CTA. Ideally, one wants to predict and control the time course as well as the degree of vascular enhancement in each individual - independent of an individual's underlying physiology. Two mathematical techniques addressing this issue have been developed.

The first is a sophisticated *compartmental model*, which predicts vascular and parenchymal enhancement using a system of more than 100 differential equations to describe the transport of CM between intravascular and interstitial fluid compartments of the body [1]. For CT angiography, this model suggests multiphasic injections to achieve uniform vascular enhancement. The injection flow rate is maximum at the beginning of the injection followed by a continuous, exponential decrease in the injection rate [1, 3]. The limitation of this approach is, however, that it cannot be individualized, because key physiological parameters are generally unknown in patients with cardiovascular disease.

The second *black-box model* approach is based on the mathematical analysis of a patient's characteristic time-attenuation response to a small test-bolus injection [10]. Assuming a time-invariant linear system, one can mathematically extract and describe each individual's response to intravenously injected CM ("patient factor") and use this information to individually tailor biphasic injection protocols to achieve uniform, prolonged arterial enhancement at a predefined level [11]. The principle of this technique is outlined in Fig. 4.3. The method is robust and has been successfully used in clinical practice, as illustrated in Fig. 4.2.

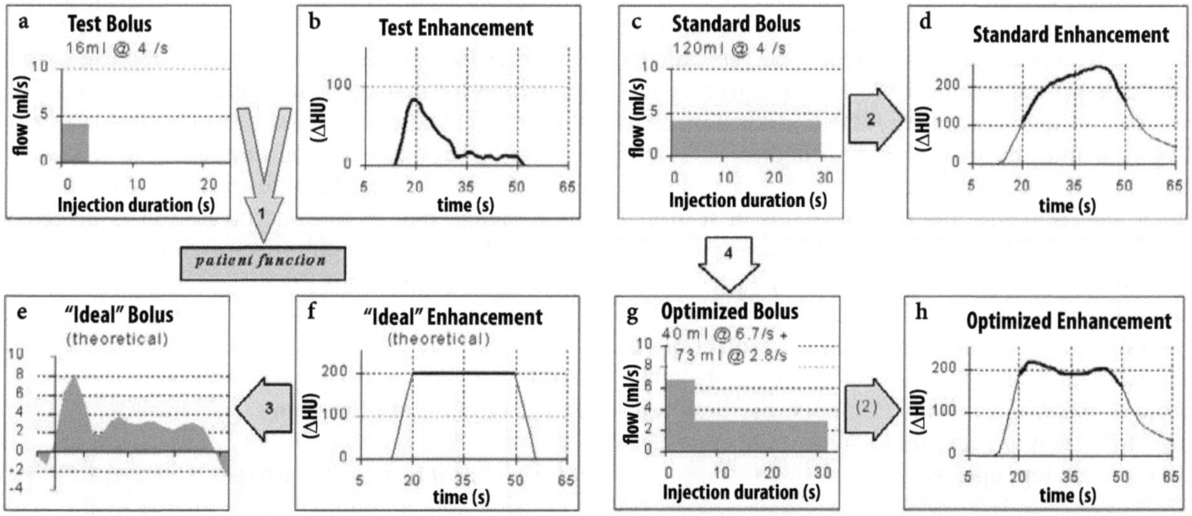

Fig. 4.3a–h Flowchart illustrates the four main steps to characterize, predict, and optimize arterial enhancement in computed tomography angiography of the aorta using the "black-box" model. The calculation of the optimized biphasic bolus for this 65-year-old patients is based on the selection of an "ideal" enhancement of 200 ΔHU for 30 s, with slopes of increase and decrease in 200 HU/6 s:

1. *Step 1:* The patient function is calculated in Fourier space from the relation of a 16 ml test bolus (**a**) to the patient's corresponding aortic time attenuation response, the test enhancement (**b**)

2. *Step 2:* Once the patient function is known, the standard enhancement (**d**) to an orbitrary bolus, e.g., a 120-ml standard bolus (**c**) can be predicted

3. *Step 3:* With the use of the patient function, it is also possible to calculate a theoretically "ideal" bolus (**e**) which is supposed to achieve an "ideal", near rectangular enhancement (**f**)

4. *Step 4:* As the theoretically "ideal bolus" (**e**) contains "unreal" components in the time domain, such as oscillations, or negative flow rates, a fitting algorithm has to be introduced, to approximate the ideal flow rates into a practically applicable "optimized" biphasic (Σ:113 ml) bolus (**g**). The corresponding optimized enhancement (**h**) can be predicted as described in step 2. Despite the pronounced simplification of the optimized bolus (**g**) the resulting optimized enhancement (**h**) does not deviate much from the desired form in the scanning period

Bolus descriptors are given as: total volume (milliliters) at flow rate (milliliters per second). *ΔHU* arterial enhancement over baseline attenuation in Hounsfield units,. (From [10], with permission)

Despite the advantages of mathematically derived injection protocols, both models are not widely used, not being commercially available, because of the additional time needed for calculating individual injection protocols and because of the need for a test-bolus injection. The greatest value of mathematical modeling comes from the gained insights into early CM dynamics for the time frame relevant for current and future CT technology, which allows a more rational design of empirical but routinely applicable injection techniques.

4.4 Instrumentation and Technique

4.4.1 Intravenous Access

A large cubital or antebrachial vein is the most favorable injection site. For a given vein, the largest-diameter peripheral catheter that accommodates the desired injection rate is selected. Whereas cannula lumen diameters as small as 22 g (0.71 mm) may suffice for routine (nonvascular) MDCT, diameters up to 17 g (1.47 mm) have been used for dedicated CTA. If high injection flow rates are desired, a fast manual saline injection with the patient's arms in scanning position (usually above the head) before mechanical CM delivery is recommended to assure correct peripheral catheter position. Injections through a central venous catheter reduce the t_{CMT}, injections in a peripheral vein at the dorsum of the hand slightly prolong the t_{CMT}. In both instances, the flow rates need to be adapted in order to prevent CM extravasation or catheter rupture.

4.4.2 Power Injectors and Safety Issues

Adequate intravenous CM administration for MDCT requires the use of a mechanical, programmable power injector. The general use of CM in MDCT carries the same risk of idiosyncratic (non-dose-dependent) adverse reactions as in other applications. These allergy-like effects are well described [17] and their discussion is beyond the scope of this chapter. Because MDCT requires fast injections, dose-dependent (nonidiosyncratic) adverse effects and the risk of CM extravasation have recently regained interest.

Dose-dependent adverse reactions include nausea, vomiting, arrhythmia, pulmonary edema, and cardiovascular collapse. Based on clinical and experimental evidence for ionic CM, one might naturally assume that rapid injections would be less well tolerated than slower injections [6]. However, at least for injection flow rates up to 4 ml/s, there seems to be no correlation between injection rate and the overall rate of adverse reactions [16].

The rate of CM extravasation during the intravenous administration of CM with power injectors is low, ranging from 0.2 to 0.6% [4]. Whereas this is presumably higher when compared with hand-injection and drip-infusion techniques, no correlation was found between extravasation frequency and injection rates up to 4 ml/s [16]. Most extravasations involve only small volumes and result in minimal to mild symptoms if nonionic CM is used.

Large volumes of CM may be involved, however, in noncommunicative patients such as infants and children, elderly, or unconscious patients. Monitoring of the injection site during CM administration is recommended in this group, because severe extravasation injuries have occasionally been reported, and guidelines for management of extravasation injuries should be at hand [4]. Recently an automated CM extravasation device has been developed, which interrupts the mechanical injection when a skin-impedance change due to fluid extravasation is detected [18]. Such a device might prove useful in high flow-rate MDCT applications [5].

4.4.3 Saline Flushing of the Veins

It is well know from upper-extremity venograms that a considerable amount of CM remains in the arm veins after the end of an injection, from where it is cleared only very slowly. In the setting of CTA, this fraction of CM is not utilized because it does not contribute to arterial enhancement. Flushing the venous system with saline immediately after the CM injection pushes the CM column from the arm veins into the circulation. This has two desirable effects in thoracic MDCT.

First, saline flushing improves arterial opacification. This effect can also be exploited to reduce the total CM volume in routine thoracic MDCT [12, 15]. Second, because saline flushing removes CM from the brachiocephalic veins and the superior vena cava, it reduces perivenous streak artifacts in thoracic and cardiac CT. Precise timing and caudocranial acquisitions allow imaging of upper thorax and thoracic inlet without obscuring artifacts (Fig. 4.4).

Saline flushing has been performed (a) manually – using a three-way valve, (b) by layering saline above contrast in the syringe of a power injector, or (c) by using two interconnected power injectors. The former techniques, however, are impractical for routine CT, because the manual technique may expose the radiologist or technologist to radiation, and the layering technique is time-consuming and poses a risk for contamination. The most convenient technique for routine saline flushing after CM injection involves new, programmable double-piston power injectors (one syringe for contrast material, one for saline) similar to those used in MR angiography. Saline flushing is relatively more important when the total volumes are small and if high-concentration CM is used.

4.4.4 Scanning Delay and Automated Bolus-Triggering

A fixed, empirical injection-to-scan delay may be adequate for many routine thoracic and abdominal CT acquisitions, particularly if maximum vessel opacification is not of critical importance, and in patients without cardiovascular disorders. For dedicated arterial MDCT, however, a fixed scanning delay cannot be recommended, because the arterial t_{CMT} is

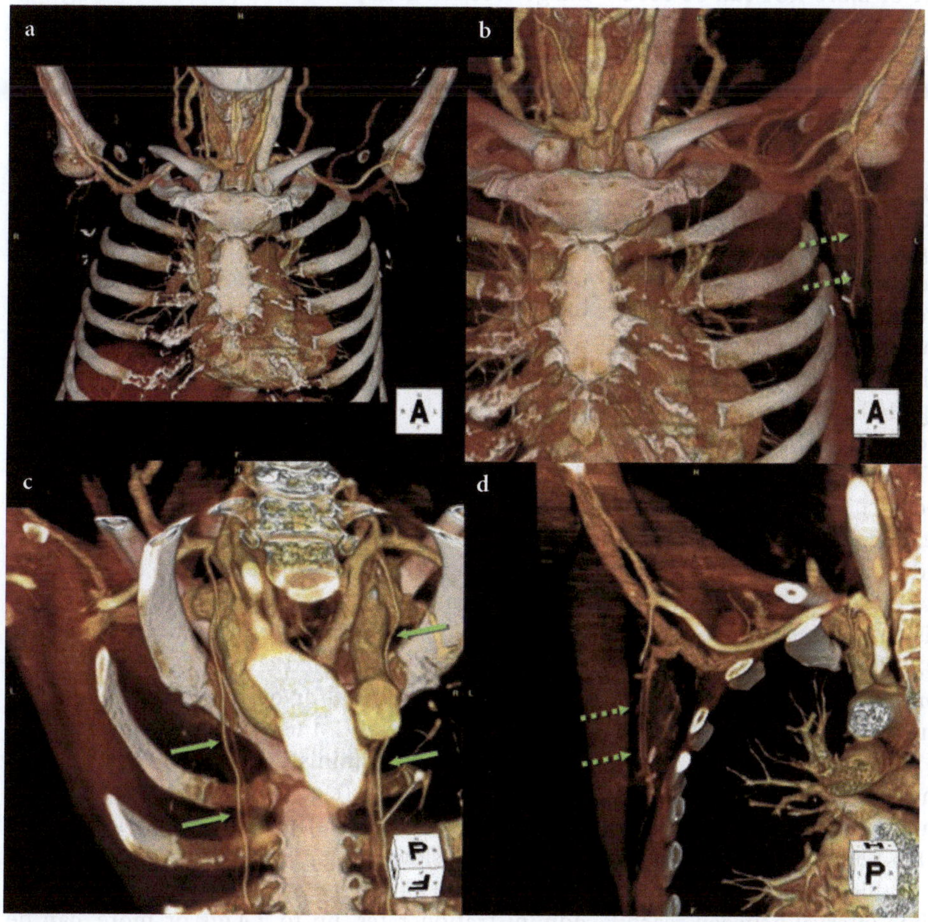

Fig. 4.4a–d. Saline flushing of the veins: CTA of the chest wall in a 57-year-old woman with a history of bilateral breast cancer, referred to evaluate the size and patency of the bilateral internal mammary and thoracodorsal arteries and veins for possible free flap surgical reconstruction. 150 ml of CM were injected biphasically over 55 s, followed by 40 ml of saline using a double-piston power-injector. A fast caudocranial CTA acquisition (16×1.25 mm) was initiated immediately following the end of the CM injection. Volume-rendered images show absence of any streak artifacts at the level of the upper thorax and thoracic inlet (**a**), allowing to assess both internal mammary arteries and veins (*straight arrows* in **c**) and the diminutive thoracodorsal arteries and veins (*dashed arrows* in **b** and **d**)

prohibitively variable between individual patients – ranging from 8 to as long as 40 s in patients with cardiovascular diseases. One might completely miss the bolus with a fast MDCT acquisition if the delay is not properly chosen. In vascular MDCT therefore, the delay needs to be timed relative to the individual t_{CMT}. Transit times can be determined using either a test-bolus injection or an automatic bolus-triggering technique.

Test bolus. The injection of a small test-bolus (15–20 ml) while acquiring a low-dose dynamic (nonincremental) CT acquisition is a reliable means to determine the t_{CMT} from the intravenous injection site to the arterial territory of interest [21]. The t_{CMT} equals the time-to-peak enhancement interval measured in a region-of-interest (ROI) placed within a reference vessel. Furthermore, time-attenuation curves obtained from one or more ROI can be used for individual bolus-shaping techniques using one of the previously described mathematical models (see Sect. 4.3.4). A test bolus is particularly useful to determine the t_{CMT} if unusual CM injection sites need to be used (e.g., lower-extremity veins).

Bolus triggering. Many CT scanners have this feature built into their system. In principle, a circular ROI is placed into the target vessel on a nonenhanced image. While CM is injected, a series of low-dose, nonincremental scans are obtained, and the attenuation within a ROI is monitored or inspected visually. The CT acquisition is initiated when the desired enhancement threshold (e.g., 100 ΔHU) is reached.

Four specific parameters need to be selected when bolus triggering is used. The details as well as the terminology are scanner specific:

- Monitoring delay determines when the first monitoring slice is acquired after the beginning of the injection, usually between 5 and 10 s
- Monitoring interval is the sampling interval for the monitoring slices. While some vendors (e.g., Toshiba) provide continuous monitoring (and radiation), others acquire the monitoring slices at predefined intervals (1–3 s)
- Trigger threshold is the enhancement value within the ROI which, when reached, initiates the CTA acquisition. Values of 80–120 HU (above baseline) are reasonable values in this context
- Trigger delay is the time interval between reaching the trigger threshold (or CM arrival) and the beginning of the actual CTA data acquisition. The minimum trigger delay depends on the scanner (see below). The trigger delay can and should be increased with short acquisition times (see Sect. 4.5)

While bolus triggering is a very effective and robust means for individualizing the scanning delay, it is important to be aware of the fact that it inherently results in longer scanning delays compared with the test-bolus technique. This is because the scanner needs a minimum of 2–3 s to begin data acquisition after the trigger threshold is reached (or more if the starting position of the scan is not identical to the table position of the monitoring series). In addition to this, one has to add the time for image reconstruction and the sampling interval of the monitoring images, which may substantially differ between manufacturers and between scanner models. Notably in early models of General Electric MDCT scanners, this image reconstruction time is 3 s ("what you see is 3 s old"). In these particular scanners, the actual scan is initiated approximately 8 s after the true t_{CMT} (3 s image reconstruction time, 3 s minimum "diagnostic delay", 2 s potential sampling error). While this is not necessarily a disadvantage – because arterial enhancement only gets better with a longer delay – it has to be taken into account for by also increasing the injection duration accordingly – in order to not run out of CM at the end of the acquisition (see also Sect. 4.5).

When the specific details of the bolus-triggering technique of a given scanner are known and taken into account, bolus triggering is a very robust and efficient method, which does not require an additional test-bolus injection.

4.4.5 Contrast-Medium Concentration

Vascular enhancement is proportional to the number of iodine molecules administered per unit of time. This *iodine administration rate* (iodine flux) can therefore be increased either by increasing the injection flow rate and/or by increasing the iodine concentration of the CM used. Thus, if one aims for a certain iodine administration rate (e.g., 1.2 g/s), this requires a faster (e.g., 4 ml/s) injection flow rate with standard-concentration CM (300 mg I/ml) compared with a slower (e.g., 3 ml/s) flow rate with high-concentration (400 mg I/ml) CM. Very high iodine administration rates, up to 2.4 g/s or more, can be safely injected with a 400 mg I/ml solution at 6 ml/s, whereas an injection flow rate of 8 ml/s would be required using a standard (300 mg I/ml) solution. High iodine administration rates are useful in CTA, notably in patients with a shallow enhancement response due to underlying cardiocirculatory disease. Figure 4.5

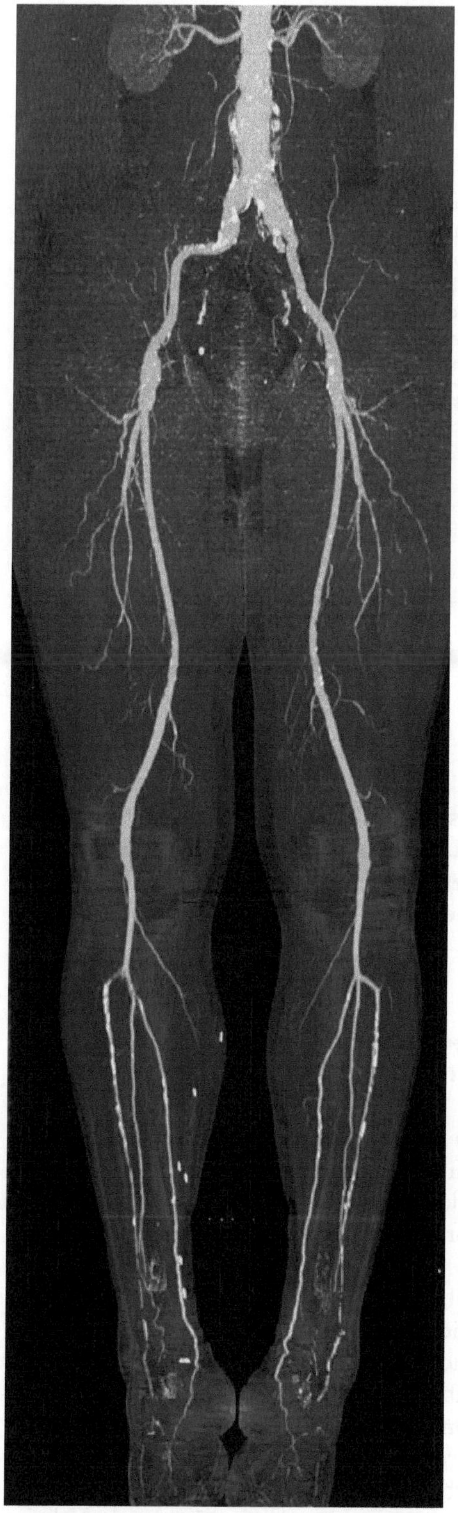

Fig. 4.5. Peripheral CTA in a 62-year-old man. Note the bright arterial opacification in the abdominal aorta, and the entire peripheral arterial tree achieved with a biphasic injection using high-concentration CM (400 mg I/ml). The first 36 ml were injected at 6 ml/s, the following 90 ml were injected at 2.5 ml/s

shows excellent arterial enhancement of the entire peripheral arterial tree using such high-concentration CM and high initial iodine administration rates (2.4 g/s). Furthermore, high iodine administration rates are particularly desirable for nonvascular imaging purposes, e.g., for detecting hypervascular liver lesions or in organ perfusion studies.

Low-concentration CM, on the other hand, have the advantage that they cause less perivenous artifacts at the level of the brachiocephalic veins and the superior vena cava in thoracic MDCT, particularly if saline flushing of the veins is not employed [19].

4.5 Clinical Contrast-Medium Injection Protocols

The most crucial parameter to be considered for designing rational injection protocols is the CT acquisition time. Scanning times have become substantially shorter with latest scanner technology, and further technical developments can be expected in the near future. When bearing in mind that the acquisition times for current CTA applications may range from more than 30 s (e.g., thoracoabdominal CTA with a 4-channel MDCT) to as short as 5 s (abdominal CTA with a 16-channel MDCT), it becomes obvious that the widely followed rule of thumb – where the injection duration equals the scanning duration – is not universally applicable. This is illustrated by the following example: Assume that the same patient who underwent a prior CTA with a slow scanner and a scan time of 32 s (Fig. 4.1f) is rescanned with a new faster scanner, with a scan time of 16 s (Fig. 4.6). It is readily apparent that if the original injection flow rate of 4 ml/s would have been used for the shorter injection duration of only 16 s(compared with 32 s), the arterial enhancement with the faster scanner would be less than with the slower scanner. To compensate for that, arterial enhancement needs to be increased, either by increasing the iodine flux (e.g., by increasing the injection flow rate from 4 to 5 ml/s; but also by increasing the iodine concentration of the CM) and/or by increasing the injection duration and scanning delay (e.g., for 8 s), respectively.

The following two basic injection strategies (for slow and for fast acquisitions) serve as templates for various clinical CTA applications and vascular territories. The suggested protocols are based on pharmacokinetic considerations, published clinical and experimental data, mathematical approximations, and practical experience. The protocols are targeted

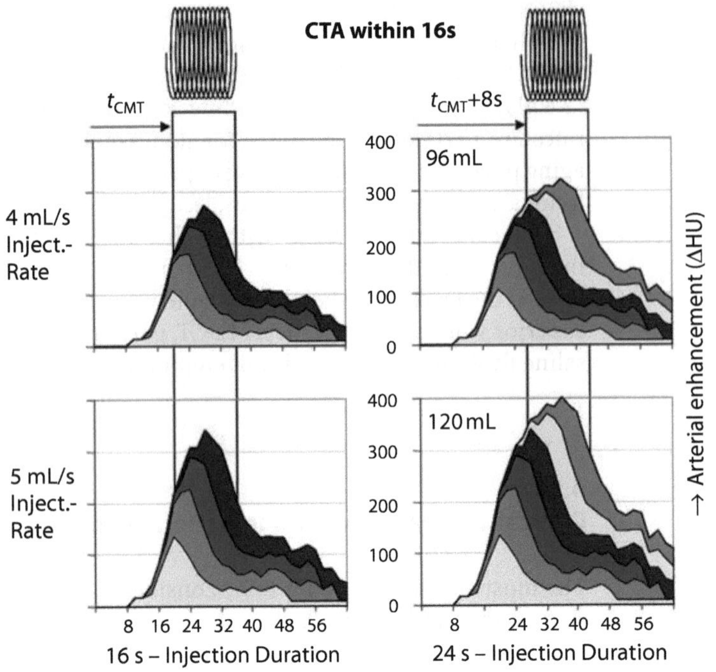

Fig. 4.6. Two strategies to increase arterial enhancement when compared with a 16-s injection at 4 ml/s (upper left panel) can be employed – either alone or in combination: Increasing the injection rate from 4 to 5 ml/s increases the enhancement approximately 20% (lower left panel). Alternatively, one can also increase the injection duration and the scanning delay – taking advantage of the fact that enhancement increases with longer injection durations (right upper panel). Maximum enhancement can be achieved when both – the injection rate (and or the iodine concentration), as well as the injection duration are increased (right lower panel) simultaneously. tCMT Contrast medium transit time

at average patients with a BW of 75 kg. CM injection protocols are tabulated as their iodine dose and administration rates, together with injection volumes and rates for 300, 350, and 400 mg I/ml concentration CM. Adjusting both the total iodine dose and the iodine administration rate to BW is recommended for patients with a BW less than 60 kg and more than 90 kg (e.g., by subtracting or adding 20% of the injected volume and flow rate, respectively).

4.5.1 Basic Strategy for Slow CTA Acquisitions: Biphasic Injections

Biphasic (or multiphasic) injections are ideal for prolonged injections (20–40 s) (Table 4.1), because they provide a more uniform enhancement in the vascular territory of interest [11] (Fig. 4.3). In general, the injection duration is chosen equal to the scanning duration. The initial iodine administration rate should be 1.8g/s for 5 s. The second, maintaining injection phase should be in the order of ≥1.0 g/s (iodine administration rate). The scanning delay should be short (equal to the t_{CMT} or only slightly longer, up to t_{CMT} +2 s; see also Figs. 4.2 and 4.3).

Biphasic injections are less useful for short acquisition times (because enhancement is uniform enough during fast scan times), and particularly when the scanning delay is longer than the t_{CMT} +2 s, because the initial peak caused by the initially high injection rate would be missed.

4.5.2 Basic Strategy for Fast CTA Acquisitions: Rapid Injections

As shown in Fig. 4.6, fast acquisitions require higher iodine administration rates and require that the scanning delay be increased relative to the t_{CMT}. This is shown for scan times in the range of 25–5 s in Table 4.2.

In general, the injection durations are longer than the acquisition times in this setting, and the iodine administration rates are high. High-concentration CM is favorable in this setting, because it avoids excessive injection flow rates. Saline flushing of the veins is generally recommended, notably when short scan-times and when high-concentration CM is used.

For routine CTA applications with 8- and 16-channel GE scanners (models prior to the Xtreme console), and with scan times in the range of 10–20 s, the following ball-park rule can be applied: Select an injection rate between 4 and 5 or 6 ml/s (≥350 mg I/ml concentration). Inject at the selected injection rate for

Table 4.1.

		Iodine		300 mg I/ml CM		350 mg I/ml CM		400 mg I/ml CM	
Acquisition time (s)	Scanning delay (s)	Total dose (g)	Biphasic iodine-flux (g @ g/s)	Total volume (ml)[a]	Biphasic injections (ml @ ml/s)[a]	Total volume (ml)[b]	Biphasic injections (ml @ ml/s)[b]	Total volume (ml)[c]	Biphasic injections (ml @ ml/s)[c]
40	t_{CMT}+2	42	9 @ 1.8 + 33 @ 0.95	140	30 @ 6 + 110 @ 3.1	120	25 @ 5.1 + 95 @ 2.7	105	23 @ 4.5 + 82 @ 2.4
35	t_{CMT}+2	39	9 @ 1.8 + 30 @ 1.0	130	30 @ 6 + 100 @ 3.3	110	25 @ 5.1 + 85 @ 2.9	100	23 @ 4.5 + 77 @ 2.5
30	t_{CMT}+2	36	9 @ 1.8 + 27 @ 1.1	120	30 @ 6 + 90 @ 3.6	105	25 @ 5.1 + 80 @ 3.1	90	23 @ 4.5 + 67 @ 2.7
25	t_{CMT}+2	33	9 @ 1.8 + 24 @ 1.2	110	30 @ 6 + 80 @ 4.0	95	25 @ 5.1 + 70@ 3.4	85	23 @ 4.5 + 62 @ 3.0
20	t_{CMT}+2	30	9 @ 1.8 + 21 @ 1.25	100	30 @ 6 + 70 @ 4.2	85	25 @ 5.1 + 60 @ 3.6	75	23 @ 4.5 + 52 @ 3.1
15	t_{CMT}+2	27	9 @ 1.8 + 18 @ 1.35	90	30 @ 6 + 60 @ 4.5	80	25 @ 5.1 + 55 @ 3.8	70	23 @ 4.5 + 47 @ 3.4

CM, contrast medium; t_{CMT}, CM transit time, as established with a test bolus or bolus-triggering technique
[a] Volume and flow rate calculated for 300 mg I/ml concentration CM
[b] Volume and flow rate calculated for 350 mg I/ml concentration CM
[c] Volume and flow rate calculated for 400 mg I/ml concentration CM

Table 4.2. Injection protocols for fast CTA acquisitions

		Iodine		300 mg I/ml CM	350 mg I/ml CM	400 mg I /ml CM
Acquisition time (s)	Scanning delay (s)	Dose (g)	Iodine flux (g/s)	CM volume @ inj. rate (ml @ ml/s)[a]	CM volume @ inj. rate (ml @ ml/s)[b]	CM volume @ inj. rate (ml @ ml/s)[c]
25	t_{CMT}+8	42	1.2	135 @ 4.0	115 @ 3.5	100 @ 3.0
20	t_{CMT}+8	39	1.35	125 @ 4.5	110 @ 4	95 @ 3.4
15	t_{CMT}+8	36	1.5	115 @ 5	100 @ 4.5	90 @ 3.8
10	t_{CMT}+8	33	1.8	110 @ 6	90 @ 5	85 @ 4.5
5	t_{CMT}+10	27	1.8	90 @ 6	80 @ 5	70 @ 4.5
1	t_{CMT}+10	23	1.8	75 @ 6	65 @ 5	60 @ 4.5

t_{CMT}, contrast-medium transit time, as established with a test bolus or bolus-triggering technique
[a] Volume and flow rate calculated for 300 mg I/ml concentration CM
[b] Volume and flow rate calculated for 350 mg I/ml concentration CM
[c] Volume and flow rate calculated for 400 mg I/ml concentration CM

8 s longer than the scan time (e.g., for a 10-s acquisition, inject 5 ml/s for 18 s, resulting in 90 ml total volume). Use SmartPrep for scan timing, with its default minimum diagnostic delay of 3 s (the actual acquisition will start approximately 8 s after the t_{CMT}, in this setting; for details, see Sect. 4.4.4). The same approach can be chosen with other scanners; however, the diagnostic delay should be slightly longer (5–8 s).

4.5.3 Modifications of Basic Injection Strategies

Adaptations of the basic injection strategies may be necessary for specific vascular territories and certain patient conditions. Also, as mentioned earlier, injection volumes and flow rates should be adapted to a patient's weight.

4.5.3.1
Suboptimal Intravenous Access

Occasionally small-bore cannulas and/or small veins (e.g., on the dorsum of the hand) have to be used for CTA. Because of the cumulative enhancement effect of prolonged injections, it is still possible to achieve bright arterial enhancement even with low (3 ml/s) injection rates. The total amount, however, has to be increased when compared with a standard CTA acquisition, and the delay has to be increased also. Careful monitoring of the injection site is recommended in this setting.

4.5.3.2
Lower-Extremity Injection Site

Arterial enhancement is more difficult to predict from lower-extremity (e.g., femoral line or peripheral) venous injections, particularly in patients with congestive heart failure. Bolus-triggering can be used; however, a test bolus may be more reliable to determine the CM transit time.

4.5.3.3
Pregnancy

If CTA is carried out in a pregnant patient – e.g., to rule out pulmonary embolism – one has to keep in mind that the cardiac output may be substantially increased during late pregnancy, which, in turn, reduces vascular opacification. This is particularly relevant when low-dose CT acquisition parameters are chosen to reduce the radiation dose, because the resulting images tend to be noisy. To avoid the diagnostic dilemma of insufficient opacification of the pulmonary arteries (which would require repeat scanning), large amounts of CM and high injection rates (5 ml/s) are recommended.

4.5.3.4
Pulmonary CT Angiography

In general, it is easier to opacify the pulmonary vasculature than the systemic arteries, because the bolus is less broadened in the pulmonary circulation. Furthermore, the interindividual variation of the t_{CMT} is not as marked as in the systemic circulation (except in patients with chronic thromboembolic pulmonary hypertension, CTEPH).

Moderate amounts of iodine and flow rates (1 g/s) are required to allow a distinction between opacified blood and intraluminal abnormalities. Large amounts of iodine are necessary, however, if an additional, delayed (approx. 2–3 min) acquisition of the lower-extremity veins is desired. A fixed delay is adequate in the majority of patients and should be chosen so that the injection ends 3 s earlier than the end of MDCT acquisition. Saline-flushing is always recommended. For patients with severely compromised cardiocirculatory disease (CTEPH), slower injection rates suffice (because diminished cardiac output leads to brighter enhancement). Image quality is more consistent if the delay is timed relative to the CM transit time in this setting.

4.5.3.5
Coronary CT Angiography

Depending on the scanner capability, either the slow (biphasic) or the rapid injection protocol can be used to opacify the coronary arteries. Particularly with fast acquisitions, saline flushing is recommended, because it reduces the otherwise bright opacification and artifacts in the right atrium and ventricle, which may obscure the right coronary artery. Ideally, all the CM is flushed out of the right side of the heart, to result in a "laevocardiogram."

4.5.3.6
Thoracic Outlet

For the assessment of the structures of the thoracic inlet and the costoclavicular space, it is necessary to inject into the contralateral arm or/and use saline-flushing to remove excess CM from the central veins. With saline-flushing, a caudocranial scanning direction is used, and the acquisition is initiated immediately after the CM is delivered. Large amounts of contrast with prolonged injections allow simultaneous venous opacification during a single CTA acquisition (Fig. 4.4).

4.5.3.7
Abdominal CTA Combined with Abdominal MDCT

If an abdominal CTA acquisition is part of a multiphasic abdominal MDCT study, the injection protocol needs to be adapted to achieve both excellent arterial and parenchymal enhancement. Thus, high iodine administration rates (for arterial enhancement) are combined with high total iodine dose (for parenchymal opacification). Scan timing is chosen according to the clinical question: If pure arterial imaging is desired (e.g., in the assessment of living related kidney or liver donors), the CTA acquisition is obtained at an "early arterial phase" (t_{CMT} + 2–8 s). If hypervascular liver lesions are also sought after (e.g., in patients before and after transarterial embolization), the CTA acquisition is obtained during a "late arterial phase" (t_{CMT} + 10–15 s). The parenchymal acquisitions are usually obtained after approximately 60 s (or t_{CMT} + 40 s).

4.5.3.8 Peripheral CT Angiography

In patients with peripheral arterial occlusive disease, the blood flow from the aorta down to the crural and pedal arteries may be substantially diminished. With table speeds greater than 30 mm/s, it is possible to outrace the bolus in patients with severe disease.

Two injection strategies are possible to guarantee excellent opacification of the entire peripheral arterial tree: (a) For slow scanning speeds (with scan times in the range of 30–40 s), biphasic injections are most favorable, with an initial iodine administration rate of 1.8 g/s for 6 s, followed by a second injection phase at 1.0 g/s for a duration of the scan-time minus 10 s (Fig. 4.5); (b) alternatively, with fast acquisitions (≤30 s), one can inject at a constant rate for 35 s and then choose a delay of 40 s minus the scan time. In patients without peripheral arterial occlusive disease (e.g., in lower-extremity trauma), the standard injection strategies can be used.

4.6 Conclusion

CM delivery remains an integral part of cardiovascular MDCT and CTA. While CT technology continues to evolve, the physiological and pharmacokinetic principles of arterial enhancement will remain unchanged in the foreseeable future. A basic understanding of early CM dynamics thus provides the foundation for the design of current and future CM injection protocols. With these tools at hand, CM utilization can be optimized for various clinical applications of CTA and optimized for each patient. This ensures optimal CM utilization while exploiting the full capabilities of continuously evolving MDCT technology.

References

1. Bae KT, Heiken JP, Brink JA (1998) Aortic and hepatic contrast medium enhancement at CT. I. Prediction with a computer model. Radiology 207:647–655
2. Bae KT, Heiken JP, Brink JA (1998) Aortic and hepatic contrast medium enhancement at CT. II. Effect of reduced cardiac output in a porcine model. Radiology 207:657–662
3. Bae KT, Tran HQ, Heiken JP (2000) Multiphasic injection method for uniform prolonged vascular enhancement at CT angiography: pharmacokinetic analysis and experimental porcine model. Radiology 216:872–880
4. Bellin MF, Jakobsen JA, Tomassin I, Thomsen HS, Morcos SK (2002) Contrast medium extravasation injury: guidelines for prevention and management. Eur Radiol 12:2807–2812
5. Birnbaum BA, Nelson RC, Chezmar JL, Glick SN (1999) Extravasation detection accessory: clinical evaluation in 500 patients. Radiology 212:431-438
6. Dawson P (1998) Does injection rate affect the tolerance? In: Dawson PH, Clauss W (eds) Contrast media in practice: questions and answers. Springer, Berlin Heidelberg New York, pp 135–136
7. Dawson P, Blomley MJ (1996) Contrast agent pharmacokinetics revisited. I. Reformulation. Acad Radiol [Suppl 2] 3:261–263
8. Dawson P, Blomley MJ (1996) Contrast media as extracellular fluid space markers: adaptation of the central volume theorem. Br J Radiol 69:717–722
9. Fleischmann D (2002) Present and future trends in multiple detector-row CT applications: CT angiography. Eur Radiol 12:11–16
10. Fleischmann D, Hittmair K (1999) Mathematical analysis of arterial enhancement and optimization of bolus geometry for CT angiography using the discrete fourier transform. J Comput Assist Tomogr 23:474–484
11. Fleischmann D, Rubin GD, Bankier AA, Hittmair K (2000) Improved uniformity of aortic enhancement with customized contrast medium injection protocols at CT angiography. Radiology 214:363–371
12. Haage P, Schmitz-Rode T, Hubner D, Piroth W, Gunther RW (2000) Reduction of contrast material dose and artifacts by a saline flush using a double power injector in helical CT of the thorax. AJR Am J Roentgenol 174:1049–1053
13. Hittmair K, Fleischmann D (2001) Accuracy of predicting and controlling time-dependent aortic enhancement from a test bolus injection. J Comput Assist Tomogr 25:287–294
14. Hopper KD (1996) With helical CT, is nonionic contrast a better choice than ionic contrast for rapid and large IV bolus injections? AJR Am J Roentgenol 166:715
15. Hopper KD, Mosher TJ, Kasales CJ, et al. (1997) Thoracic spiral CT: delivery of contrast material pushed with injectable saline solution in a power injector. Radiology 205:269–271
16. Jacobs JE, Birnbaum BA, Langlotz CP (1998) Contrast media reactions and extravasation: relationship to intravenous injection rates. Radiology 209:411–416
17. Katayama H, Yamaguchi K, Kozuka T, et al. (1990) Adverse reactions to ionic and nonionic CM. A report from the Japanese Committee on the Safety of Contrast Media. Radiology 175:621–628

18. Nelson RC, Anderson FA Jr, Birnbaum BA, Chezmar JL, Glick SN (1998) Contrast media extravasation during dynamic CT: detection with an extravasation detection accessory. Radiology 209:837–843
19. Rubin GD, Lane MJ, Bloch DA, Leung AN, Stark P (1996) Optimization of thoracic spiral CT: effects of iodinated contrast medium concentration. Radiology 201:785–791
20. Sheiman RG, Raptopoulos V, Caruso P, Vrachliotis T, Pearlman J (1996) Comparison of tailored and empirical scan delays for CT angiography of the abdomen. AJR Am J Roentgenol 167:725–729
21. Van Hoe L, Marchal G, Baert AL, Gryspeerdt S, Mertens L (1995) Determination of scan delay-time in spiral CT-angiography: utility of a test bolus injection. J Comput Assist Tomogr 19:216–220

5 CT Angiography in the Assessment of Intracranial Vessels

Toshinori Hirai, Yukunori Korogi, Mutsumasa Takahashi, and Yasuyuki Yamashita

CONTENTS

5.1 Introduction

Computed tomographic angiography (CTA), a rapidly evolving field in CT imaging, is a noninvasive tool for visualizing blood vessels. The acquisition of thin-slice continuous images of the blood vessels, in which contrast material is used, is necessary to create three-dimensional (3D) reformations of the intracranial vessels. This technique offers a greater capability for identification and characterization of intracranial vascular diseases. While magnetic resonance angiography (MRA) also allows accurate depiction of intracranial vascular diseases and may be used as a screening method, CTA may be used as a further definitive evaluation or preoperative evaluation. Compared with single-detector helical CT, multidetector-row CT improves temporal and spatial resolutions, allowing nearly isotropic images with large volumes such as the entire bed of intracranial vascular structures. Since CTA has some limitations such as inferior spatial and temporal resolutions to digital subtraction angiography (DSA), this technique may not be able to replace DSA in general.

This article aims to illustrate the state-of-the-art techniques of CTA and three-dimensional reconstruction, as well as their application in the evaluation of intracranial lesions.

5.2 Data Acquisition Techniques

3D CTA of the intracranial vessels can be performed with conventional single-detector helical CT or multidetector-row CT scanners. Multidetector-row CT scanners have several advantages over single-detector helical CT in general. These include improved temporal resolution, improved spatial resolution in the *z*-axis, decreased image noise, and longer anatomical coverage [1]. Multidetector-row CT scanners acquire data more quickly, allowing isotropic or nearly isotropic images with large volumes such as the entire vascular structures of the head. When the vascular diseases are in a limited region such as the circle of Willis, the advantages of multidetector-row CT may be small because the image quality of the vessels in a limited area is usually sufficient even by single-detector helical CT.

According to the location of the vascular lesions or suspected vascular lesions on CT, MRI, or MRA, the scanning volume of CTA is usually determined in each case. When the location of lesions is at the circle of Willis or supratentorial region, the volume scanning usually begins at the level of the sellar floor

T. Hirai, MD; Y. Korogi, MD; Y. Yamashita, MD
Department of Radiology, Kumamoto University School of Medicine, 1-1-1 Honjo, Kumamoto 860-8556, Japan
M. Takahashi, MD
Kumamoto University School of Medicine, International Imaging Center, 1-2-23 Kuhonji, Kumamoto 862-0976, Japan

and is continued cranially. When the lesions are multiple or unknown, the volume scanning may begin at the level of the foramen magnum and be continued cranially. Multidetector-row CT scanners are preferable for wider anatomical coverage such as the entire vascular structures from the aortic arch to the intracranial vessels.

In four-detector-row multisection helical CT for the head region, volume data may be acquired in 10–20 s using a slice thickness of 1.0–1.25 mm and a table speed of 3.0–3.75 mm/s (200 mAs; 120 kV); the scanning volume may be 30–60 mm with a 512×512 matrix (Table 5.1). The actual acquired voxel size was 0.47×0.47×0.5 mm. With 16-detector-row multisection helical CT, the scanning speed is 4 times faster than that of four-detector-row multisection helical CT.

5.3 Methods of Contrast-Agent Administration

In order to obtain high-quality CTA images, high concentration of contrast material in the vessels is necessary. Technique-related factors such as contrast material volume and concentration, rate of injection, and type of injection and patient-related factors such as body weight may affect CT contrast enhancement [2, 3]. When the attenuation of the intracranial vessels is usually more than or nearly 300 HU, the image quality of 3D or multiplanar reformations (MPR) are usually satisfactory. Intravenous contrast-agent administration is generally performed in conventional intravenous CTA, while contrast agent is intraarterially administrated in intraarterial CTA

In intravenous contrast-agent administration, there are three methods available: a fixed scan delay technique, a test bolus injection technique, and an automated bolus-tracking technique (Table 5.2). A total of 100–150 ml of nonionic contrast material (300 mg I/ml) is usually injected into the antecubital vein with a flow rate of 2.0–4.0 ml/s by using a power injector.

A fixed scan delay (15–45 s) after the initiation of intravenous contrast injection has been used commonly to obtain the intracranial arterial phase, without taking into account differences in transit time of contrast material [4–7]. This technique has a potential of missing the optimal timing of intracranial arterial phase. To avoid the situation, a larger volume of contrast material may be needed.

A test bolus injection technique is a method to measure the time between the initiation of intravenous contrast injection and the arrival of contrast material in the vessels interested [8, 9]. This technique requires additional volume of contrast material and monitoring the arterial enhancement by periodical CT scanning. Based on this result, a scan delay is determined.

An automated bolus-tracking technique is another method to obtain the optimal arterial phase [10, 11]. Placement of region of interest (ROI) and choice of a threshold of arterial enhancement are needed for radiologists or technologists. The ROI may be placed in the carotid artery near the skull base. Then this technique consists of automated ROI measurement in the selected artery during low-dose scans obtained every few seconds after contrast medium injection. When arterial enhancement reaches the threshold, the spiral scan is initiated.

Table 5.1 Acquisition parameters for intracranial CTA

Detectors of CT	Collimation (mm)	Table speed (mm/s)	Slice thickness/ reconstruction interval (mm)	Scanning time (s)
Single detector	1	1–1.5	1/0.5–1	30–40
Four-detector	1–1.25×4	3–3.75	1–1.25/0.5–0.8	10–20

Table 5.2 Intravenous contrast-agent administration for intracranial CTA

Techniques of contrast-agent administration	Volume of contrast agent (ml)	Monitoring arterial enhancement	Placement of region of interest	Reliability
Fixed scan delay	100–200	No	No	Relatively low
Test bolus injection	100–150	Yes	No	High
Automated bolus tracking	100	Yes	Yes	High

The technique of contrast-agent administration may be determined by the capability of CT unit and radiologist's preference. Unlike intravenous contrast-material injection in conventional CTA, intraarterial CTA is a relatively invasive examination and is performed with a combined angiography and CT unit [12]. This method has theoretical advantages compared with intravenous contrast-agent administration, because a higher concentration of contrast material can be obtained in the intracranial artery without considering the appropriate timing of injection, and a smaller amount of contrast material can be used. When evaluating intracranial aneurysms, a total of 16–24 ml of diluted contrast agent, 4–6 ml of nonionic contrast material (300 mg I/ml) diluted with triple volume of saline (12–18 ml), is injected into the carotid artery at a flow rate of 0.6–0.8 ml/s by using a power injector [12].

5.4 Postprocessing and Display Techniques

There are various display techniques in CTA. They include axial, MPR, maximum-intensity projection (MIP), surface rendering, volume rendering, and virtual endoscopy methods. Although all these techniques are valuable in displaying CTA data, it has not been established which technique or which combination of the techniques is the best or better method for identification and characterization of intracranial vascular diseases.

Axial and MPR images have basic information from the volume data for the intracranial vessels. They enable the evaluation of relationship between calcification or bony structure and intracranial vessel lumens. The assessment of the intracranial vessels is not able to perform with 3D reformatted images alone [11]. In the evaluation of the vessels in the skull base, axial and MPR images are essential (Fig. 5.1). The curved MPR method may be useful for the assessment of the tortuous vessels and the vessels surrounded by bony structures [13].

MIP is a widely used method for CTA and MRA (Fig. 5.2b). The single layer of the brightest voxels is displayed without use of attenuation threshold. When arterial luminal attenuation is smaller than calcification, calcification can often be differentiated from arterial lumens. Although the attenuation information is maintained, the depth information is lost. Therefore, intracranial vessel structures are superimposed as two-dimensional projection angiograms.

The surface rendering method shows the first layer of voxels within defined thresholds, that is, the visualization of the surface of all structures. The caliber of the intracranial artery varies depending on the thresholds selected. This may lead to a slight overestimation of the vessel structures. Unlike MIP, the attenuation information is lost but the depth information is preserved. Calcification cannot be separated from arterial lumens but the spatial relationship between the vessels is understood.

3D images with volume rendering have a number of theoretical advantages over MIP and surface rendering [14, 15] (Figs. 5.1, 5.2, 5.3). Groups of voxels within defined attenuation thresholds are chosen and relative

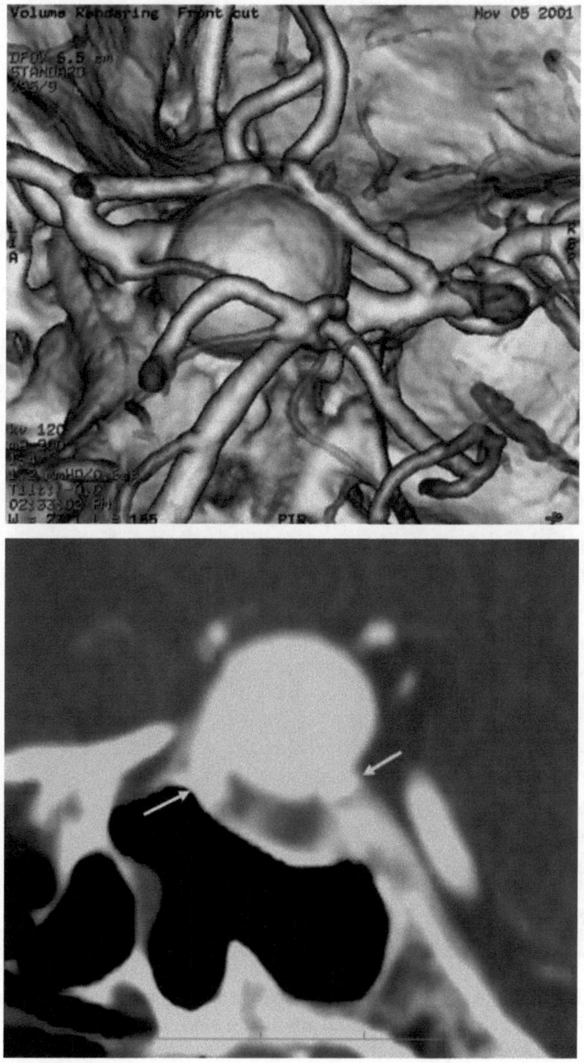

a

b

Fig. 5.1a,b A 60-year-old woman with an unruptured giant aneurysm of the left internal carotid-ophthalmic artery. **a** Volume-rendered computed tomography angiogram (CTA) from behind and above demonstrates a giant aneurysm extending to the anterior communicating artery. **b** Multiplanar reconstruction image of CTA shows the relationship between the giant aneurysm and the left internal carotid artery (arrows).

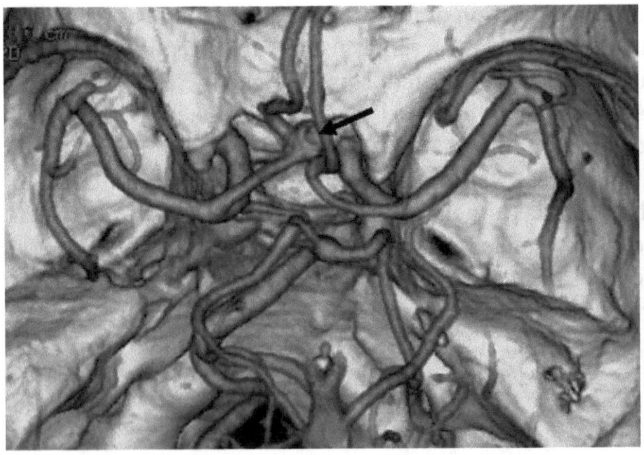

a

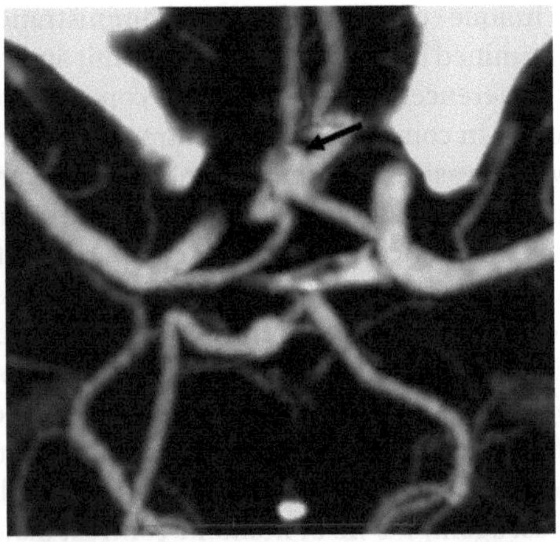

b

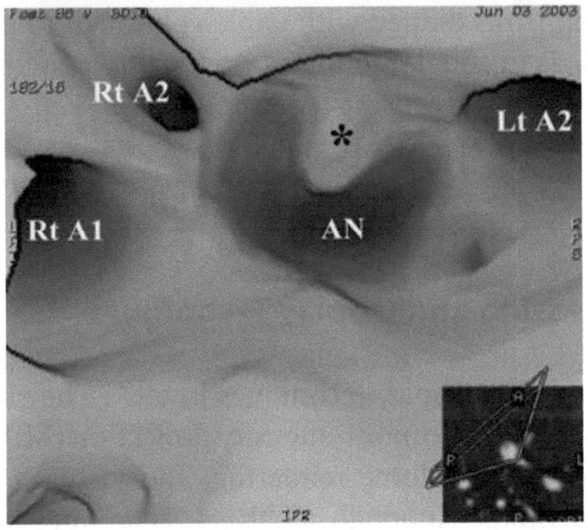

c

Fig. 5.2a-c A 61-year-old man with an unruptured aneurysm of the anterior communicating artery. **a** Volume-rendered CTA from above shows an aneurysm at the anterior communicating artery (*arrow*). **b** Maximum-intensity projection image of CTA from above depicts an aneurysm at the anterior communicating artery, but the relationship between the aneurysm (*arrow*) and the adjacent arteries is not clearly understood. **c** Virtual endoscopy from the left A1 segment shows thrombus (*star*) within the aneurysm (*AN*) and the adjacent arteries. *Rt A1*, right A1 segment; *Rt A2* right A2 segment; *Lt A2*, left A2 segment

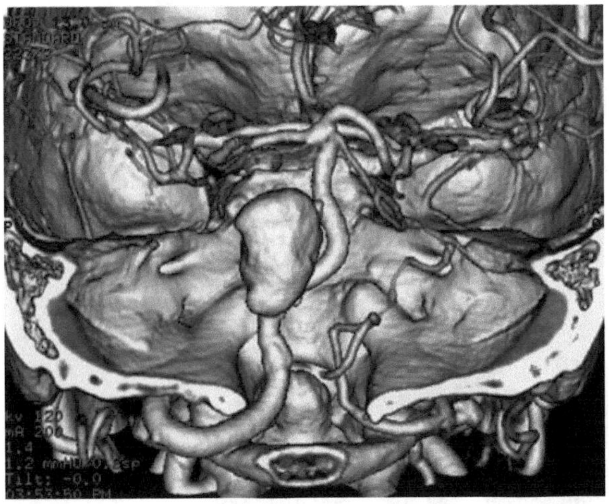

a

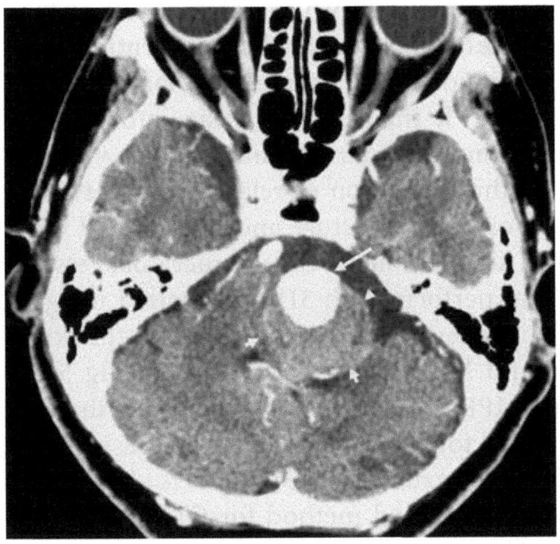

b

Fig. 5.3a,b A 67-year-old woman with an unruptured giant aneurysm of the left vertebral artery. **a** Volume-rendered CTA from behind and above shows a giant aneurysm of the left vertebral artery. Thrombus in the aneurysm is not depicted. **b** Axial source image of CTA shows partial thrombus (*arrowheads*) within the aneurysm. The lumen of the aneurysm is located anteriorly (*arrow*).

Fig. 5.4a–d A 76-year-old man with severe stenoses of the left vertebral artery. **a** Anteroposterior digital subtraction angiogram of the left vertebral artery shows severe stenoses and segmental dilatation in the intracranial segment of the left vertebral artery (*arrows*). **b** MRA image also depicts severe stenoses and dilatation in the left vertebral artery (*arrows*). **c** Volume-rendered CTA image from behind shows aneurysm-like dilatation of both vertebral arteries (*arrows*), which correspond to the calcification of the vessel wall. **d** Axial source image of CTA demonstrates no apparent lumen in the stenotic artery because of circumferential calcification. (Adapted from [11]) voxel attenuation is conveyed by means of a gray scale, which yields images that are more accurate than those with surface rendering [15]. The volume-rendered images maintain the original anatomical spatial relationships of the 3D angiography data set and have a 3D appearance, facilitating interpretation of vascular interrelationships, which is limited with MIP images [15]. The quality of volume-rendered 3D angiography is essential in the imaging of the intracranial vasculature, especially vascular lesions such as aneurysms. Although the volume-rendering technique has much larger data volume than MIP and surface-rendering techniques, new computer processing and display systems do not limit its practical and versatile use.

Virtual endoscopic images can be obtained by a perspective volume-rendering method [16, 17] (Fig. 5.2c). With this method, the volume data are rendered from a point source at finite distance to approximate the human visual system.

5.5 How to Analyze Images

The axial or MPR images are always analyzed in conjunction with the corresponding 3D images because of the potential for misinterpretation inherent in the evaluation of 3D images alone.

Calcifications in the arterial wall are the limiting factor of 3D images owing to the inability to separate mural calcification and intramural contrast material (Fig. 5.4). MIP may allow the visualization of both calcification and arterial lumen. To minimize this limi-

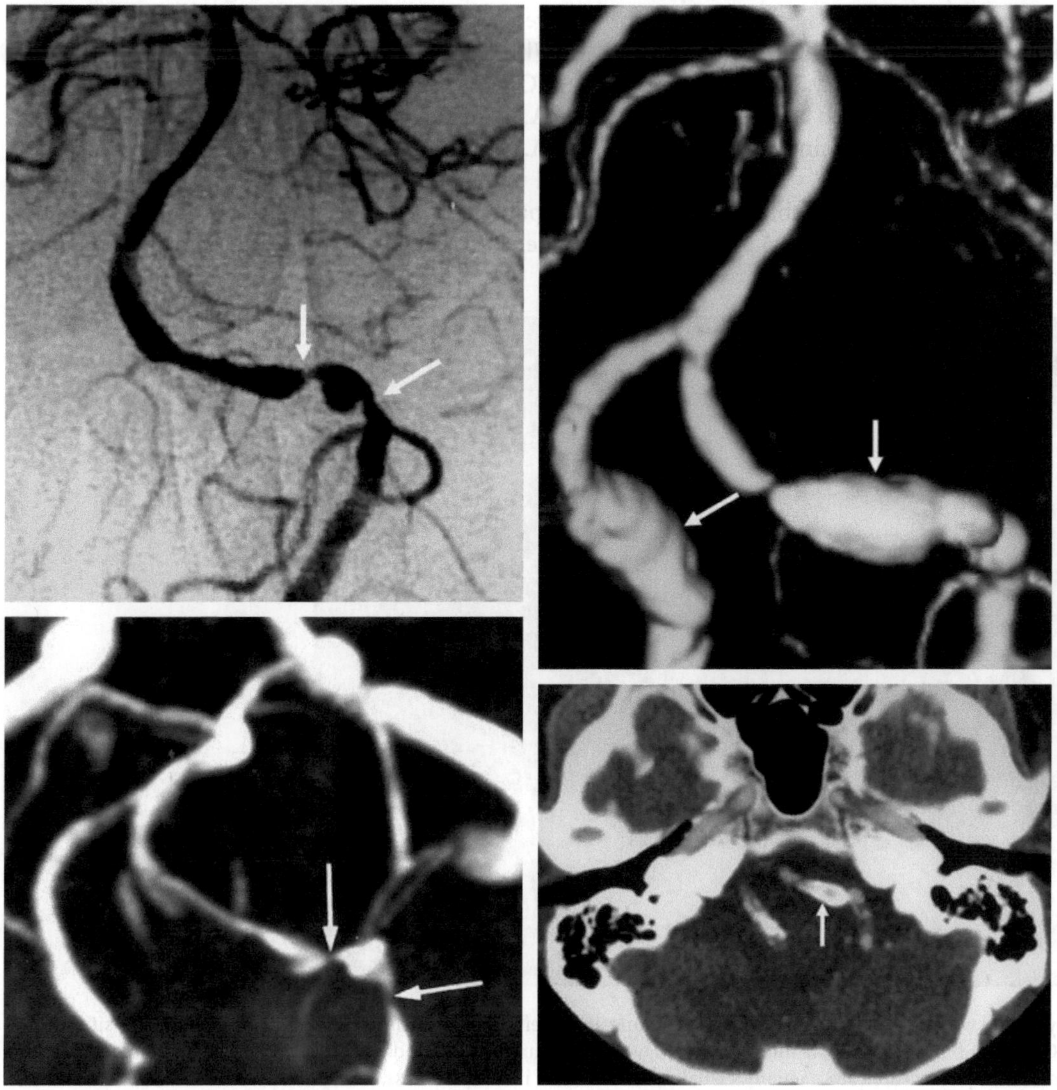
a b c d

tation, analysis in conjunction with the axial source or MPR images is necessary. Dense circumferential calcification of the arterial wall may cause artifacts that interfere with the evaluation of the arterial lumen on axial or MPR images of CTA [11].

In the skull base region, CTA often fails to identify the lumen of the internal carotid artery within the cavernous sinus, because the cavernous sinus is enhanced [11]. When the density of the arterial segment is greater than that of the cavernous sinuses, the MPR or curved MPR images can usually assess the lumen of the arterial segment. However, when the cavernous sinuses are equally enhanced relative to the carotid artery, this arterial segment cannot be differentiated from the venous structure.

Careful evaluation for the superimposition of the bone and venous structures is needed when the intracranial arteries are assessed. The basal vein of Rosenthal may overlap with the middle and posterior cerebral arteries. The skull base structures such as the anterior and posterior clinoid processes contact with the internal carotid artery. This overlapping of the structure is usually resolved by careful evaluation of continuity of the vessels using MPR and axial source images.

To eliminate the skull base bone, subtraction methods have been developed [18–20] (Fig. 5.5). Although the techniques allow the visualization of the internal carotid artery without bony structures, this issue has not been completely resolved.

5.6 Comparison with Other Modalities

MRA is another noninvasive imaging modality. This technique includes time-of-flight (TOF) and phase-contrast methods. In the evaluation of intracranial vessels, TOF MRA is widely used because of its better spatial resolution and shorter examination time. On TOF MRA, 3D images are preferable for intracranial arteries and 2D images are often used for intracranial venous structures. In the assessment of the cervical carotid arteries, contrast-enhanced MRA has become a more accurate diagnostic method than conventional MRA [21].

With regard to depiction of the intracranial vessels, CTA has several advantages compared with TOF MRA. Acquisition time for CTA is faster than for TOF MRA. Since patients may have claustrophobia and need patience for longer examination time for MRI, the patient acceptance of the examination is much higher for CTA. CTA provides the information about

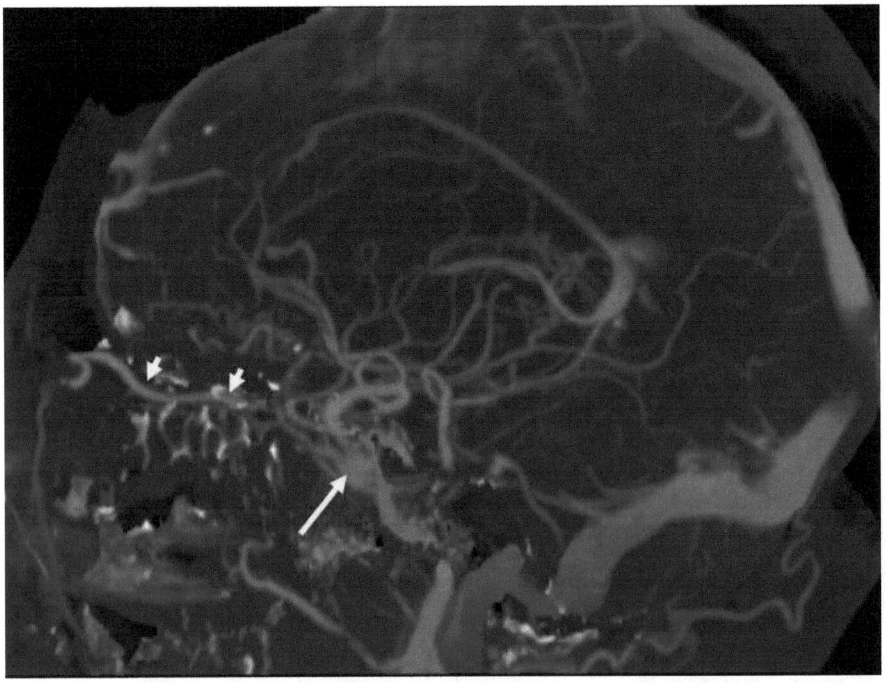

Fig. 5.5 An 81-year-old woman with dural arteriovenous fistula at the left cavernous sinus. Selective maximum-intensity projection image of CTA with bone subtraction shows the left cavernous sinus (*arrow*) and the dilatation of the left superior orbital vein (*arrowheads*). Bony structures are partially visualized because of incompleteness of subtraction.

the relationship between the vessels and the bony structure, while TOF MRA does not.

TOF MRA has several limitations in identifying and grading stenoses. First, the vessels that lie near the sphenoid sinus are subject to artifactual narrowing or nonvisualization owing to the large susceptibility gradient present in this area [22], although this issue is not so problematic with recent MRI units, resulting in a superiority of MRA over CTA in this region [11]. The artifacts may be minimized with the development of MRA sequences. Second, acceleration of flow in the carotid siphon and loss of laminar flow and resultant intravoxel dephasing can also contribute to artifactual signal loss in the C2 and C3 portions of the internal carotid artery, making it difficult to evaluate narrowing of this segment of the vessel [22] (Fig. 5.6). Third, MR angiograms of severely stenotic vessels often show an apparent discontinuity in a vessel. The flow void results from intravoxel spin dephasing and the acceleration of spins through the area of stenosis [23]. These artifacts may result in overestimation of stenosis on MRA alone. These disadvantages are not seen on CTA, because CTA shows the vessel lumen filled with contrast material such as DSA.

Disadvantages of CTA include the need for exposure to ionizing radiation, injection of iodinated contrast material, optimization of imaging delay time, and careful evaluation for superimposition of the bone and venous structures. Since CTA has inferior spatial resolution to DSA and does not provide information about intracranial hemodynamics, CTA cannot replace DSA in general. The amount of radiation exposure during CTA is without doubt greater than that during conventional CT but is significantly less than that during DSA [7]. The amount of ionizing radiation may not be an important concern in the predominantly older patient population. Iodinated contrast agents must be used with caution in patients with serious risk factors, such as renal insufficiency, congestive heart failure, or hypersensitivity to contrast material.

5.7 Clinical Application

The most useful application of CTA among intracranial diseases is diagnosis of aneurysms. CTA for intracranial aneurysms is widely used and established. CTA for steno-occlusive diseases is also useful, but it has some limitations. In other vascular diseases such as arteriovenous malformations, dural arteriovenous fistulas, and brain tumors, CTA may be applied as an alternative to MRI/MRA or limited purposes. According to each vascular disease, advantages and limitations of CTA need to be understood.

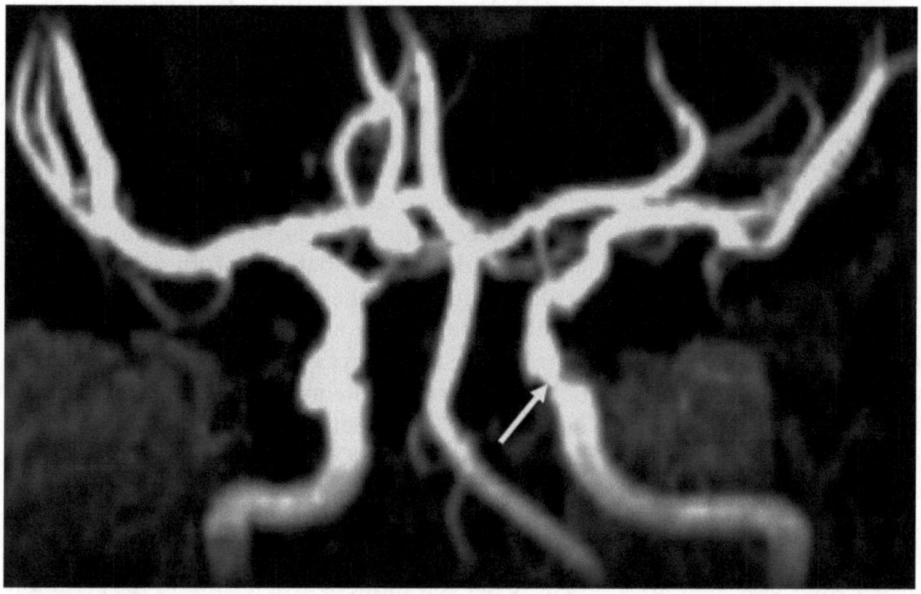

Fig. 5.6 A 48-year-old man with psychiatric problems. Maximum-intensity projection image of MRA from the front shows a stenosis-like area (*arrow*) in the left carotid siphon. The stenosis-like area is caused by artifactual signal loss due to turbulent flow in the carotid siphon.

5.8 Intracranial Aneurysms

5.8.1 Diagnosis and Preoperative Evaluation

Conventional angiography has been considered to be the gold standard for diagnosis and preoperative evaluation of intracranial aneurysms. However, there are several limitations to obtain sufficient information prior to treatment. Superimposition of vessel loops, tortuosity of vessels, small aneurysm size, or complicated aneurysm shape may cause an erroneous detection of an aneurysm or insufficient delineation of the aneurysm and adjacent vessels. To avoid these situations on conventional angiography, different projections, stereoviews, increased magnification, and high frame-rate acquisition may be needed [24]. Also, the limitation of conventional angiography for diagnosis and preoperative study of intracranial aneurysms has been recognized by studies with CTA [4, 5, 25–30] and 3D angiography [31, 32].

The usefulness of CTA for the diagnosis and preoperative evaluation of intracranial aneurysms has been advocated [4, 5, 25–30]. Diagnostic accuracy of CTA is greater for detection of aneurysms larger than 3 mm than for detection of aneurysms 3 mm or smaller [28, 29]. According to previous studies with single-detector helical CT [4, 5, 25–29], the sensitivity and specificity of CTA for intracranial aneurysms larger than 3 mm are 83–100% and 79–100%, and those for intracranial aneurysms 3 mm or less are 51–98% and 79–100%, respectively.

Some authors have suggested that CTA may replace the use of conventional angiography in assessment of acute subarachnoid hemorrhage [25, 26, 30]. In the future, surgery would be performed on the basis of CTA findings alone; however, some limitations in current CTA are considered as follows [27, 28]. First, it requires relatively large amounts of contrast materials and proper timing of the scanning. Second, patient movement due to poor patient condition causes unsatisfactory CT angiographic quality. Third, CTA cannot always be repeated because of risk factors such as renal insufficiency or heart failure. Intravenous injection site and heart function may affect CT angiographic results.

Aneurysms adjacent to the skull base may not always be depicted on CTA. Several authors have described that aneurysms at the skull base that arise from the intracavernous or paraclinoid carotid artery may be obscured by the bone, calcium, or venous blood in CTA studies [25, 26, 28]. The axial source and MPR images of CTA may play an important role in assessing the aneurysms at the intracavernous or paraclinoid carotid artery (Fig. 5.1).

CTA is especially useful for the following conditions: complex-shaped aneurysms, aneurysms with large diameter, thrombosed aneurysms, and complex-overlapping vessels such as the anterior communicating artery aneurysm. Even if carotid angiograms with manual compression of the carotid artery during arteriography are used, DSA does not always clearly depict its presence and the relationship to the anterior communicating artery and bilateral A1 and A2 segments of the anterior cerebral artery in the anterior communicating aneurysm. In thrombosed aneurysm, axial source and MPR images of CTA are useful for assessing the relationship between aneurysm lumen and thrombus within the aneurysm [25] (Fig. 5.3).

Although intraarterial CTA using a combined CT and angiographic unit is a limited method to use, it may be useful for preoperative evaluation of intracranial aneurysms as a supplement to DSA [12]. The additional findings of intraarterial CTA to DSA may affect the following treatment.

5.8.2 Postoperative Follow-up Study

After surgical treatment of an intracranial aneurysm, posttreatment evaluation may be necessary for assessing clipping status. Potential problems include partial clipping of the neck, inadvertent occlusion of vessels after improper clip placement, and migration of the clip. The dome and the neck of the aneurysm after clipping can be evaluated with CTA [33, 34]. CTA is not severely degraded by the presence of nearby aneurysm clips (Fig. 5.7). The very thin collimation of 1 mm or less reduces the severe beam-hardening artifacts seen on routine head studies [33]. CT artifacts may depend on material of the clip [34]. The artifacts caused by the titanium clips are relatively small compared with artifacts from other clips [34].

In the posttreatment evaluation of aneurysm embolization using Guglielmi detachable coils, MRA is a noninvasive useful tool [35–37]. Several reports have described that 3D TOF MRA had high sensitivity with few coil-induced artifacts in detecting residual necks of aneurysms treated with Guglielmi detachable coils. Embolic materials made of platinum seem to have few coil-induced artifacts. Since the platinum coils cause remarkable artifacts on CT, MR studies are more preferable for patients treated with platinum coils than CT studies.

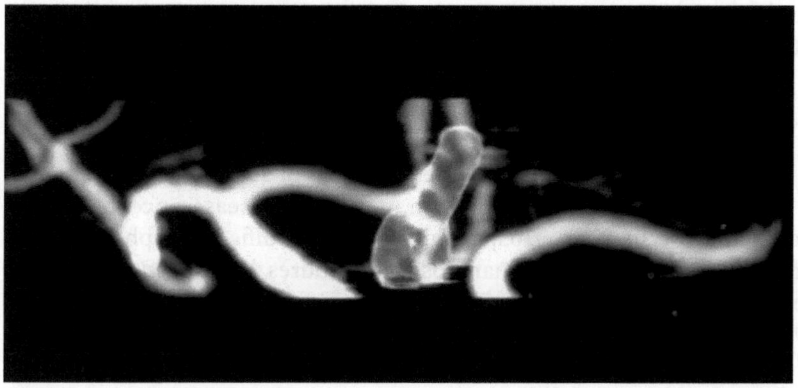

Fig. 5.7 A 52-year-old man with post-surgical clipping of ruptured anterior communicating aneurysm. Volume-rendered CTA image reveals the clip and the adjacent arterial structures. Residual lumen of the aneurysm is not depicted. Contrast angiography also shows no residual lumen of the aneurysm.

5.9 Steno-occlusive Diseases

5.9.1 Atherosclerotic Narrowing

Atherosclerotic narrowing of the major intracranial arteries is associated with the risk of stroke [38]. A warfarin–aspirin symptomatic intracranial disease study showed that symptomatic patients with 50–99% stenosis of an intracranial artery benefited from anticoagulation therapy [39]. Although conventional angiography is a gold standard for evaluating intracranial steno-occlusive diseases, cerebral angiographic complications still remain. Among noninvasive imaging modalities, MRA allows accurate discovery of intracranial steno-occlusive diseases and is widely used as a screening method [40–42]. However, MRA has a potential for consistent overestimation of stenosis. The clinical efficacy of CTA in the evaluation of narrowing of the lumen of the intracranial artery has already been shown to be sensitive and specific [6, 7, 43]. Skutta et al. [44] retrospectively studied the usefulness of CTA for evaluating the intracranial steno-occlusive diseases in 112 patients. They concluded that CTA was a reliable method for grading intracranial steno-occlusive lesions, with the exception of the petrous segment of the carotid artery. Hirai et al. [11] prospectively studied intracranial steno-occlusive diseases with MRA, CTA, and DSA. MRA had a sensitivity of 92%, a specificity of 91%, and an accuracy of 91% for the identification of stenosis of 50% or greater, while additional use of CTA yielded a sensitivity of 100%, a specificity of 99%, and an accuracy of 99% [11]. The combined MRA and CTA provided significantly higher diagnostic accuracy than did MRA alone. The combined evaluation reduced the tendency to overestimate stenosis seen with MRA and improved the specificity for detecting stenosis of 50% or greater. The combined MRA and CTA could achieve equal accuracy to DSA in measuring stenosis and detecting occlusion of the major intracranial arteries in most patients with suspected steno-occlusive diseases [11]. However, CTA may not always correctly delineate the lumen of the artery with circumferential calcification and the cavernous portion of the internal carotid artery [11] (Fig. 5.4).

5.9.2 Acute Embolic Stroke

In patients with large-vessel embolic stroke, intraarterial thrombolytic treatment performed within 6 h of stroke onset can reduce the incidence of disability [45, 46]. Large-vessel stroke may be difficult to distinguish from transient ischemic attacks, lacunar infarctions, postseizure states, peripheral neuropathies, complex migraine, and toxic metabolic encephalopathies [47]. In order to perform effective treatment, it is important to accurately and rapidly detect intracranial steno-occlusive diseases. Knauth et al. [11] prospectively evaluated the usefulness of CTA of the intracranial vessels compared with conventional angiography in 21 patients with acute ischemic stroke. In this study, CTA correctly demonstrated all trunk occlusions of the basilar artery, the internal carotid artery, and the middle cerebral artery. Lev et al. [48] studied 44 consecutive intraarterial candidates who were examined with CTA. Sensitivity and specificity for the detection of large-vessel occlusion were 98.4% and 98.1%, respectively. They concluded that CTA is highly accurate for the detection and exclusion of large-vessel intracranial occlusion and may be valuable in the triage of hyperacute stroke patients to intraarterial thrombolytic treatment.

5.9.3 Moyamoya Disease

Moyamoya disease is a rare cerebrovascular occlusive disease of unknown cause that occurs predominantly in the Japanese, although cases in other ethnic groups have also been described [49, 50]. The angiographic features of this disease include (a) bilateral stenosis or occlusion of the supraclinoid portion of the internal carotid artery (ICA) that extends to the proximal portions of the anterior cerebral artery and the middle cerebral artery, and (b) the presence of parenchymal, leptomeningeal, or transdural collateral vessels that supply the ischemic brain [51, 52]. Although conventional angiography remains the principal imaging technique for demonstrating anatomical changes in detail, less invasive CTA provides an accurate means of diagnosing moyamoya disease when it is suspected on CT, MRI, or clinical grounds [53].

5.9.4 Arterial Dissection

Dissections of the intracranial artery are relatively uncommon vascular diseases that usually affect the supraclinoid carotid, middle cerebral, or vertebrobasilar arteries [54–57]. These lesions have been recognized as a cause of stroke in young and middle-aged adults [54–57].

The accurate diagnosis of intracranial dissections is important for appropriate management of patients. Although conventional angiography is the classic gold standard for the diagnosis of intracranial artery dissection, it rarely demonstrates specific angiographic signs such as a double lumen or intimal flap. Noninvasive imaging techniques including MRI, MRA, and CTA have been reported to be valuable methods for establishing the initial diagnosis and for follow-up studies [58–61].

5.10 Extracranial–Intracranial Bypass

In patients with ischemic cerebrovascular disease, extracranial–intracranial (EC-IC) bypass can be used to improve cerebral blood flow and halt the extension of affected areas or reduce the risk of future strokes, although the effectiveness of this technique remains controversial [62]. The superficial temporal artery–middle cerebral artery anastomosis is frequently performed for the treatment of supratentorial ischemia. In patients with moyamoya disease, encephaloduroarteriosynangiosis and modified encephaloduroarteriosynangiosis procedures have been performed. To examine the patency of EC-IC anastomosis after surgery, conventional cerebral angiography has been the most reliable imaging method among several modalities [63].

CTA using a multidetector CT unit is useful for assessing EC-IC bypass routes [64]. The wide scanning range is valuable for demonstrating the donor and recipient arteries on a single image.

5.11 Arteriovenous Malformation

Intracranial arteriovenous malformations (AVMs) are a complex network of abnormal vascular channels that consists of arterial feeders, the AVM nidus, and venous drainage channels. Cerebral angiography is a gold standard of this disease and can provide the hemodynamic information and the angioarchitecture.

Three-dimensional reconstruction of CTA is very helpful in demonstrating the nidi, drainers, and 3D structure of AVMs [65] (Fig. 5.8). Demonstrations of feeders are not remarkable. CTA of cerebral AVMs could be performed routinely, and 3D imaging is helpful in demonstrating the complex anatomy of cerebral AVMs. This technique may be helpful in planning gamma-knife radiosurgery.

5.12 Carotid-Cavernous Sinus Fistulas

Carotid-cavernous sinus fistulas (CCFs) are classified into dural and direct types. CCFs usually appear as neuro-ophthalmologic symptoms that include proptosis, chemosis, cranial nerve palsies, and dilated episcleral veins.

Although DSA is currently the standard of reference for the diagnosis of dural and direct CCFs, CTA can provide noninvasive diagnosis of these diseases [66]. CTA depicts an enlarged enhancing cavernous sinus and venous drainage channels such as the superior ophthalmic vein, petrosal sinus, sphenoparietal sinus, and intercavernous sinus [66] (Fig. 5.5).

5.13 Brain Tumors

CTA is an alternative method to evaluate extra-axial brain tumors. However, it is not usually applied to intra-axial brain tumors. In large skull base tumors such as meningiomas and pituitary adenomas, CTA may be useful for preoperative evaluation.

5.13.1 Meningiomas

Skull-base meningiomas often involve intracranial vessels. Preoperative evaluation of the tumor is essential for successful surgical removal. Although DSA clearly demonstrates the vascular structure of meningiomas, it does not show the relationship between tumors and bony structures and has a risk of neurological complication. MRA is a noninvasive method that is widely used in the evaluation of patients with meningiomas.

CTA depicts the relationship between skull-base meningiomas and neighboring bony and vascular structures clearly, with minimal risk to the patients [67] (Fig. 5.9).

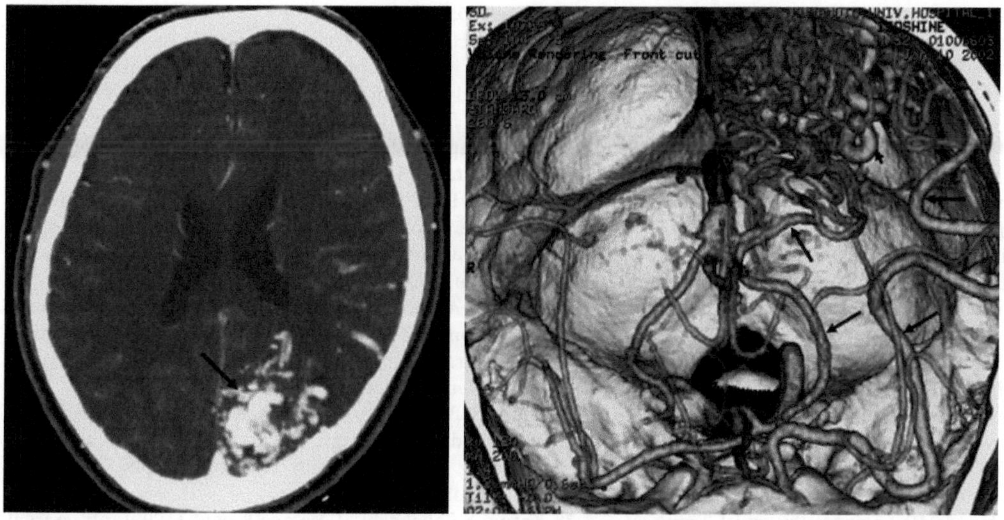

a b

Fig. 5.8a,b A 32-year-old man with left parietooccipital arteriovenous malformation. **a** Contrast-enhanced axial CT image shows abnormal enlarged vessels (*arrow*) in the parietooccipital region, which suggest cerebral arteriovenous malformation. **b** Volume-rendered CTA image from the front and above shows feeding arteries (*arrows*) from the middle and posterior cerebral arteries and draining veins (*arrowheads*).

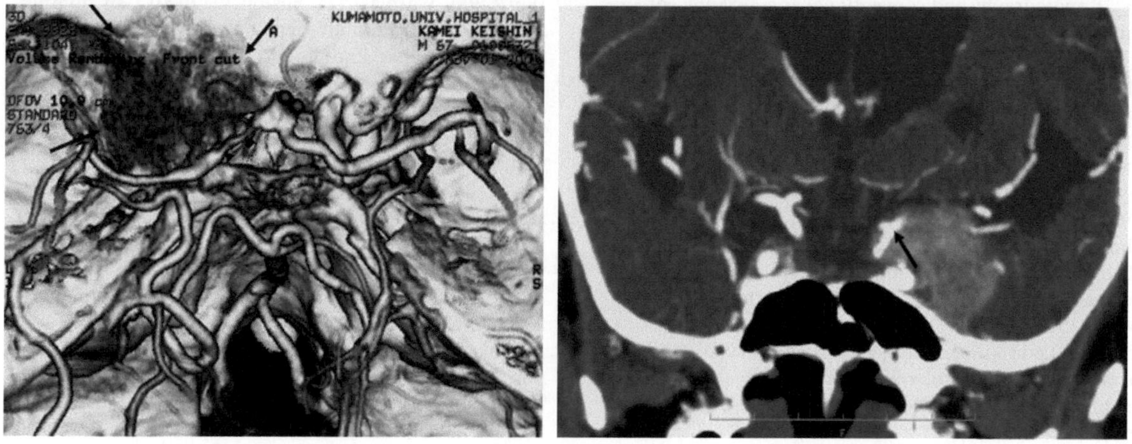

a b

Fig. 5.9a,b A 67-year-old man with left sphenoid ridge meningioma. **a** Volume-rendered CTA image from the above shows left sphenoid ridge mass (*arrows*) and wall irregularity of the left anterior cerebral artery (*arrowheads*) suggesting tumor encasement. **b** Multiplanar reconstruction image of CTA shows the encasement of the left carotid fork (*arrow*) in the tumor.

References

1. Reyberg J, Buckwalter KA, Caldemeyer KS et al. (2000) Multisection CT: scanning techniques and clinical applications. Radiographics 20:1787–1806
2. Bae KT, Heiken JP, Brink JA (1998) Aortic and hepatic peak enhancement at CT: effect of contrast medium injection rate-pharmacokinetic analysis and experimental porcine model. Radiology 206:455–464
3. Yamashita Y, Komohara Y, Takahashi M et al. (2000) Abdominal helical CT: evaluation of optimal doses of intravenous contrast material-a prospective randomized study. Radiology 216:718–723
4. Hope JKA, Wilson JL, Thomson FJ (1996) Three-dimensional CT angiography in the detection of intracranial berry aneurysms. AJNR Am J Neuroradiol 17:439–445
5. Ogawa T, Okudera T, Noguchi K et al. (1996) Cerebral aneurysms: evaluation with three-dimensional CT angiography. AJNR Am J Neuroradiol 17:447–454
6. Knauth M, Kummer R von, Jansen O et al. (1997) Potential of CT angiography in acute ischemic stroke. AJNR Am J Neuroradiol 18:1001–1010
7. Shrier DA, Tanaka H, Numaguchi Y et al. (1997) CT angiography in the evaluation of acute stroke. AJNR Am J Neuroradiol 18:1011–1020
8. Van Hoe L, Marchal G, Baert AL et al. (1995) Determination of scan delay-time in spiral CT-angiography: utility of a test bolus injection. J Comput Assist Tomogr 19:216–220
9. Hittmair K, Fleischmann D (2001) Accuracy of predicting and controlling time-dependent aortic enhancement from a test bolus injection. J Comput Assist Tomogr 25:287–294
10. Hirai T, Korogi Y, Ono K et al. (2001) Maximum stenosis of extracranial internal carotid artery: effect of luminal morphology on stenosis measurement by using CT angiography and conventional DSA. Radiology 221:802–809
11. Hirai T, Korogi Y, Ono K et al. (2002) Prospective evaluation of suspected stenoocclusive disease of the intracranial artery: combined MR angiography and CT angiography compared with digital subtraction angiography. AJNR Am J Neuroradiol 23:93–101
12. Hirai T, Korogi Y, Ono K et al. (2001) Preoperative evaluation of intracranial aneurysms: usefulness of intraarterial 3D CT angiography and conventional angiography with a combined unit-initial experience. Radiology 220:499–505
13. Ochi T, Shimizu K, Yasuharu Y et al. (1999) Curved planar reformatted CT angiography: usefulness for the evaluation of aneurysms at the carotid siphon. AJNR Am J Neuroradiol 20:1025–1030
14. Kuszyk BS, Heath DG, Ney DR et al. (1995) CT angiography with volume rendering: imaging findings. AJR Am J Roentgenol 165:1579–1580
15. Johnson PT, Heath DG, Kuszyk BS, Fishman EK (1996) CT angiography with volume-rendering: advantages and application in spanchnic vascular imaging. Radiology 200:564–568
16. Davis CP, Ladd ME, Romanowski BJ et al. (1996) Human aorta: preliminary results with virtual endoscopy based on three-dimensional MR imaging data sets. Radiology 199:37–40
17. Rubin GD, Beaulieu CF, Argiro V et al. (1996) Perspective volume rendering of CT and MR images: applications for endoscopic imaging. Radiology 199:321–330
18. Gorzer H, Heimberger K, Schindler E (1994) Spiral CT angiography with digital subtraction of extra and intra cranial vessels. J Comput Assist Tomogr 18:839–841
19. Venema HW, Hulsmans FJH, Heeten GJ den (2001) CT angiography of the circle of Willis and intracranial internal carotid arteries: maximum intensity projection with matched mask bone elimination-feasibility study. Radiology 218:893–898
20. Jayakrishnan VK, White PM, Aitken D et al. (2003) Subtraction helical CT angiography of intra- and extracranial vessels: technical considerations and preliminary experience. AJNR Am J Neuroradiol 24:451–455
21. Remonda L, Senn P, Barth A et al. (2002) Contrast-enhanced 3D MR angiography of the carotid artery: comparison with conventional digital subtraction angiography. AJNR Am J Neuroradiol 23:213–219
22. Heiserman JE, Drayer BP, Keller PJ, Fram EK (1992) Intracranial vascular stenosis and occlusion: evaluation with three-dimensional time-of-flight MR angiography. Radiology 185:667–673
23. Fürst G, Hofer M, Sitzer M et al. (1995) Factors influenceing flow induced signal loss in MR angiography: an in vitro study. J Comput Assist Tomogr 19:692–699
24. Setton A, Davis AJ, Bose A, Nelson PK, Berenstein A (1996) Angiography of cerebral aneurysms. Neuroimag Clin North Am 6:705–738
25. Alberico RA, Patel M, Casey S et al. (1995) Evaluation of the circle of Willis with three-dimensional CT angiography in patients with suspected intracranial aneurysms. AJNR Am J Neuroradiol 16:1571–1578
26. Zouaoui A, Sahel M, Marro B et al. (1997) Three-dimensional computed tomographic angiography in detection of cerebral aneurysms in acute subarachnoid hemorrhage. Neurosurgery 41:125–130
27. Velthuis BK, Rinkel GJE, Ramos LMP et al. (1998) Subarachnoid hemorrhage: aneurysm detection and preoperative evaluation with CT angiography. Radiology 208:423–430
28. Korogi Y, Takahashi M, Katada K et al. (1999) Intracranial aneurysms: detection with three-dimensional CT angiography with volume rendering-comparison with conventional angiographic and surgical findings. Radiology 211:497–506
29. White PM, Wardlaw JM, Easton V (2000) Can noninvasive imaging accurately depict intracranial aneurysms? Systematic review. Radiology 217:361–370
30. Velthuis BK, Leeuwen MS van, Witkamp TD et al. (1999) Computerized tomography angiography in patients with subarachnoid hemorrhage: from aneurysm detection to treatment without conventional angiography. J Neurosurg 91:761–767
31. Hochmuth A, Spetzger U, Schumacher M (2002) Comparison of three-dimensional rotational angiography with digital subtraction angiography in the assessment of ruptured cerebral aneurysms. AJNR Am J Neuroradiol 23:1199–1205
32. Sugahara T, Korogi Y, Nakashima K et al. (2002) Comparison of 2D and 3D digital subtraction angiography in evaluation of intracranial aneurysms. AJNR Am J Neuroradiol 23:1545–1552
33. Vieco PT, Morin III EE, Gross CE (1996) CT angiography in the examination of patients with aneurysm clips. AJNR Am J Neuroradiol 17:455–457

34. Van Loon JJ, Yousry TA, Fink U et al. (1997) Postoperative spiral computed tomography and magnetic resonance angiography after aneurysm clipping with titanium clips. Neurosurgery 41:851–856
35. Derdeyn CP, Graves VB, Turski PA, Masaryk AM, Strother CM (1997) MR angiography of saccular aneurysms after treatment with Guglielmi detachable coils: preliminary experience. AJNR Am J Neuroradiol 18:279–286
36. Kähärä VJ, Seppänen SK, Ryymin PS, et al. (1999) MR angiography with three-dimensional time-of-flight and targeted maximum-intensity-projection reconstructions in the follow-up of intracranial aneurysms embolized with Guglielmi detachable coils. AJNR Am J Neuroradiol 20:1470–1475
37. Weber W, Yousry TA, Felber SR et al. (2001) Noninvasive follow-up of GDC-treated saccular aneurysms by MR angiography. Eur Radiol 11:1792–1797
38. Sacco RL, Kargman DE, Gu Q, Zamanillo MC (1995) Race-ethnicity and determinants of intracranial atherosclerotic cerebral infarction. The Northern Manhattan Stroke Study. Stroke 26:14–20
39. Chimowitz MI, Kokkinos J, Strong J et al. (1995) The warfarin-aspirin symptomatic intracranial disease study. Neurology 45:1488–1493
40. Heiserman JE, Drayer BP, Keller PJ, Fram EK (1992) Intracranial vascular stenosis and occlusion: evaluation with three-dimensional time-of-flight MR angiography. Radiology 185:667–673
41. Korogi Y, Takahashi M, Mabuchi N et al. (1994) Intracranial vascular stenosis and occlusion: diagnostic accuracy of three-dimensional, Fourier transform, time-of-flight MR angiography. Radiology 193:187–193
42. Korogi Y, Takahashi M, Nakagawa T et al. (1997) Intracranial vascular stenosis and occlusion: MR angiographic findings. AJNR Am J Neuroradiol 18:135–143
43 Katz DA, Marks MP, Napel SA, Bracci PM, Roberts SL (1995) Circle of Willis: evaluation with spiral CT angiography, MR angiography, and conventional angiography. Radiology 195:445–449
44. Skutta B, Fürst G, Eilers J et al. (1999) Intracranial stenoocclusive disease: double-detector helical CT angiography versus digital subtraction angiography. AJNR Am J Neuroradiol 20:791–799
45. Del Zoppo G, Higashida R, Furlan A et al. (1998) PROACT: a phase II randomized trial of recombinant pro-urokinase by direct arterial delivery in acute middle cerebral artery stroke. PROACT Investigators. Prolyse in acute cerebral thromboembolism. Stroke 29:4–11
46. Furlan A, Higashida R, Wechsler L et al. (1999) Intra-arterial prourokinase for acute ischemic stroke. The PROACT II study: a randomized controlled trial. Prolyse in acute cerebral thromboembolism. JAMA 282:2003–2011
47. Libman R, Wirkowski E, Alvir J et al. (1995) Conditions that mimic stroke in the emergency department. Implications for acute stroke trials. Arch Neurol 52:1119–1122
48. Lev MH, Farkas J, Rodriguez VR et al. (2001) CT angiography in the rapid triage of patients with hyperacute stroke to intraarterial thrombolysis: accuracy in the detection of large vessel thrombus. J Comput Assist Tomogr 25:520–528
49. Suzuki J, Takaku A (1969) Cerebrovascular "moyamoya" disease: disease showing abnormal net-like vessels in base of brain. Arch Neurol 20:288-299
50. Taveras JM (1969) Multiple progressive intracranial arterial occlusions: a syndrome of children and young adults. AJR 106:235–268
51. Takahashi M (1980) Magnification angiography in moyamoya disease: new observations on collateral vessels. Radiology 136:379–386
52. Yamada I, Himeno Y, Suzuki S, Matsushima Y (1995) Posterior circulation in moyamoya disease: angiographic study. Radiology 197:239–246
53. Tsuchiya K, Makita K, Furui S (1994) Moyamoya disease: diagnosis with three-dimensional CT angiography. Neuroradiology 36:432–434
54. Hart RG, Easton JD (1983) Dissections of cervical and cerebral arteries. Neurol Clin 1:155–182
55. Caplan LR, Baquis GD, Pessin MS et al. (1988) Dissection of the intracranial vertebral artery. Neurology 38:868–877
56. Provenzale JM (1995) Dissection of the internal carotid and vertebral arteries: imaging features. AJR Am J Roentgenol 165:1099–1104
57. Shievink WI (2001) Spontaneous dissection of the carotid and vertebral arteries. N Engl J Med 344:898–906
58. Hosoya T, Watanabe N, Yamaguchi K, Kubota H, Onodera Y (1994) Intracranial vertebral artery dissection in Wallenberg syndrome. AJNR Am J Neuroradiol 15:1161–1165
59. Hirai T, Korogi Y, Murata Y et al. (2003) Intracranial artery dissections: serial evaluation with MR Imaging, MR angiography, and source images of MR angiography. Radiat Med 21:86–93
60. Lanzino G, Kaptain G, Kallmes DF, Dix JE, Kassell NF (1997) Intracranial dissecting aneurysm causing subarachnoid hemorrhage: the role of computerized tomographic angiography and magnetic resonance angiography. Surg Neurol 48:477–481
61. Leclerc X, Lucas C, Godefroy O, et al. (1998) Helical CT for the follow-up of cervical internal carotid artery dissections. AJNR Am J Neuroradiol 19:831–837
62. EC-IC Bypass Study Group (1985) Failure of extracranial-intracranial arterial bypass to reduce the risk of ischemic stroke. Results of an international randomized trial. N Engl J Med 313:1191–2000
63. Jack CR Jr, Sundt TM Jr, Fode NC et al. (1988) Superficial temporal-middle cerebral artery bypass: clinical pre- and postoperative angiographic correlation. J Neurosurg 69:46–51
64. Tsuchiya K, Aoki C, Katase S et al. (2003) Visualization of extracranial-intracranial bypass using multidetector-row helical computed tomography angiography. J Comput Assist Tomogr 27:231–234
65. Aoki S, Sasaki Y, Machida T et al. (1998) 3D-CT angiography of cerebral arteriovenous malformations. Radiat Med 16:263–271
66. Coskun O, Hamon M, Catroux G et al. (2000) Carotid-cavernous fistulas: diagnosis with spiral CT angiography. AJNR Am J Neuroradiol 21:712–716
67. Tsuchiya K, Hachiya J, Mizutani Y, Yoshino A (1996) Three-dimensional helical CT angiography of skull base meningiomas. AJNR Am J Neuroradiol 17:933–936

6 Carotid Arteries

Carlo Catalano, Federica Pediconi, Alessandro Napoli, Massimiliano Danti, Piergiorgio Nardis, and Linda Bertoletti

CONTENTS

6.1 Introduction

The two major reasons for the interest in the efficacious and noninvasive imaging of the extracranial carotid arteries are the relatively high incidence of atherosclerotic disease in Western countries [1] and the ease with which this disease can be treated [2–5]. Stroke is the third leading cause of severe disability and death in the Western world, creating an enormous economic burden on society. Ischemic cerebrovascular events are often due to atherosclerotic narrowing at the carotid bifurcation. Digital subtraction angiography (DSA) is the current standard of reference for the evaluation of carotid artery disease [6, 7]. However, because of the costs and risks of this procedure, noninvasive techniques such as computed tomography (CT) have been developed.

C. Catalano, MD, Associate Professor;
F. Pediconi, MD; A. Napoli, MD; M. Danti, MD;
P. Nardis, MD; L. Bertoletti, MD
Department of Radiological Sciences, University of Rome "La Sapienza," V. le Regina Elena 324, 00161 Rome, Italy

Investigators of several large clinical trials concluded that the risk of stroke can be reduced by performing carotid endarterectomy in symptomatic patients with a stenosis of more than 70% [8]. Furthermore, endarterectomy in patients with a symptomatic moderate carotid stenosis of 50–69% produced a moderate reduction in the risk of stroke. Investigators in the Asymptomatic Carotid Atherosclerosis Study (ACAS) [9] suggested that asymptomatic patients could benefit from carotid endarterectomy, even with a stenosis of 60%. However, high-grade stenoses may remain asymptomatic, and it is widely recognized that other factors are also important in determining whether a carotid lesion will remain clinically silent [10--15]. Plaque morphology and composition have been proposed as important risk factors for thromboembolic events, giving rise to the concept of unstable plaque. Plaques that are more prone to disruption, fracture, or fissuring may be associated with a higher risk of embolization, occlusion, and consequent ischemic neurological events [16, 17]. These studies have emphasized the importance of accurate delineation of the morphology of the carotid bifurcation, as well as the degree of stenosis.

The ability of catheter angiography to depict the vessel lumen is usually excellent. Multiple angiographic series in various projections, however, may be required to completely understand or resolve a complex area of luminal abnormality. Catheter angiography is reproducible from institution to institution, is able to accurately depict the morphology of the vessel lumen regardless of blood flow rates and can portray the arterial anatomy form the aortic arch to the very small intracranial vessels in a single examination. Important information regarding cerebral hemodynamics may also be obtained from the examination, including the presence of intracranial and extracranial collateral circulation; any noninvasive imaging modality for the evaluation of the carotid arteries should provide information similar to or better than catheter angiography [18, 19].

The need for a noninvasive imaging modality nevertheless is also related to the relatively high incidence of complications of diagnostic catheter angiography. In fact several studies have shown that related to catheter angiography there is a risk of transient ischemic attack or minor stroke up to 4%, a 1% risk of major stroke, and a small (<1%), but definite risk of death. Even patients without apparent neurological complications after DSA have been shown to develop minor asymptomatic infarctions due to microembolisms [20].

The importance of a reliable, noninvasive imaging modality is also related to the recent development of less invasive means than carotid endarterectomy to treat carotid artery occlusive disease with angioplasty and stenting. Relevant preoperative information can be achieved with CT.

Since the early 1990s, CT angiography has challenged DSA in the evaluation of many regions of the vascular system. In fact, CT angiography has proved a superior diagnostic accuracy over catheter arteriography in several applications [21–23]. Furthermore, CT angiography is significantly less invasive and expensive and allows three-dimensional (3D) visualization from any angle and view, which cannot be achieved with projection techniques such as DSA. Spiral CT angiography is a well-established technique for imaging atherosclerotic disease of the extracranial carotid artery and has also been proposed for evaluating plaque morphology and composition.

Since the introduction of spiral CT, several studies have demonstrated the efficacy of this technique in the assessment of the carotid arteries [24, 25]. In fact the carotid arteries lend themselves to be examined by CT angiography. They primarily run in the longitudinal plane of scanning, which limits the effect of decreased resolution along this plane, which is particularly present with single detector-row scanners. The cross section of the arterial lumen lies mainly in the axial plane. Motion of patients is easy to control and breath-hold studies are not necessary. Several studies have demonstrated that single-slice spiral CT is accurate as compared to DSA, although it has some drawbacks, represented by a limited volume of exploration, the use of large amount of iodinated contrast agent, and difficulties in assessing the degree of stenosis in the presence of heavily calcified plaques [26--28].

The recent introduction into the clinical practice of multidetector-row spiral CT (MDCT) with simultaneous acquisition of multiple channels has a substantial effect on CT angiography, providing acquisition of large volumes at high resolution, with excellent visualization also of small branches, reducing the amount of iodinated contrast agent [29–31]. Although there are several studies on the use of MDCT angiography in several vascular regions, there are limited data on its use in patients with suspected carotid artery stenosis, mainly concerning the feasibility but not the accuracy [32, 33].

Most, if not all, limitations of single-slice spiral CT have been overcome by MDCT, particularly regarding the length of the examined volume and the spatial resolution along all three axes of the acquisition.

6.2 Acquisition and Contrast-Agent Administration Techniques

The advent of multidetector-row spiral CT has enabled a significant increase in spatial and temporal resolution and reduced the limitations of single-slice spiral CT. In fact although excellent results were obtained even with single-slice spiral CT in the evaluation of the carotid arterial system, with demonstration of the presence of plaque and degree of stenosis, the examination was limited to the tract of the bifurcation with a volume coverage of 8–10 cm. With single-slice spiral CT studies, the collimation used ranged between 2 and 5 mm, with limited resolution along the *z*-axis [24, 25].

In the examination of the carotid arteries, a high-resolution protocol should be used to increase the spatial resolution along the *z*-axis. According to the type of equipment available (4-, 8-, or 16-detector-row scanners) a different protocol can be used (Table 6.1). In any case, 1.25 mm or less collimation should be used with an effective slice thickness of 1.25 mm and a reconstruction interval of 1–0.75 mm in order to have an overlap of 30–50%.

Patients are positioned supine with their head tilted back to avoid artifacts from dental hardware, which if possible should be removed. Upper arms are

Table 6.1 High-resolution computed tomography angiography study (volume coverage 30 cm)

	Detector configuration	Pitch	Scan time	Table speed (mm/s)
4-channel	4×1.25	1.5	32	9.375
	4×1	1.5	25	12
8-channel	8×1.25	1.5	11	27
16-channel	16×1.25	1.375	11	27.5
	16×0.75	1.5	7	43

positioned along the body of the patient, as for any other neck and head CT study.

Anteroposterior and lateral topograms are initially acquired in order to correctly position the volume of acquisition and include all vascular structures. The acquisition should include a volume from the aortic arch to the intracranial circulation. In the preparation of the acquisition of the CT angiogram, the delay time between contrast administration and start of the acquisition must be defined. Among all parameters the delay time appears to be the most important; in fact the carotid circulation time is extremely rapid, which means that the jugular veins generally are filled approximately 10 s after the carotid arteries. Therefore, in order to have an exclusive arterial enhancement, the delay time must be accurately determined either by using the test bolus technique or bolus triggering. We prefer the use of the test bolus, with sequential dynamic scans acquired at the level of the aortic arch after i.v. administration of a small contrast-agent volume of 16 ml at the flow rate that will be used during the acquisition (in our experience 4 ml/s); if a double-piston power injector is available or even two injectors are present in the CT suite, it can be helpful to flush the test bolus with saline solution. Otherwise the bolus-triggering technique can be used, although the delay time between visualization of the contrast agent and the start of the acquisition may determine venous contamination of the images. During the acquisition, patients are asked to hold their breath, although not strictly necessary, and especially to avoid swallowing.

The amount of contrast agent necessary for CT angiography of the carotid arteries is limited. We prefer to inject a volume of 60–70 ml of high-concentration contrast agent (370–400 mg I/ml) at a flow rate of 4 ml/s; exactly as in other vascular regions, the duration of the injection should correspond to that of the acquisition (i.e., injecting at 4 ml/s, for a scan duration of 20 s, the volume of contrast agent administered should correspond to 80 ml). In order to have a compact bolus of contrast agent traveling in the arteries and avoid hyperconcentration artifacts from the contrast agent in the superior vena cava, it is advisable to flush the contrast agent with saline solution, injected at the same flow rate as the contrast agent, with a volume of 20–30 ml.

Once the acquisition is completed, it may be useful to perform a reconstruction task at greater slice thickness (5 mm), with a dedicated kernel for the evaluation of the brain parenchyma, since most of the patients present with ischemic neurological disorders.

6.3 Image Evaluation

6.3.1 3D Reconstruction

In the evaluation of the carotid arteries, 3D reconstructions should be performed in order to display the entire supra-aortic vasculature. Different techniques are currently in use for carotid artery reconstructions: multiplanar reformation (MPR), maximum-intensity projections (MIP) and volume rendering (VR).

MPR and MIP are limited to external visualization of the vessels, while VR also performs the internal visualization and can be used for endoscopic-type applications.

MPR is a very convenient and available technique for displaying the data. One substantial limitation of traditional MPR is that visualized structures must lie in a plane. Because the carotid arteries for which 3D visualization is desired do not lie within a single plane, an MPR cannot be created that demonstrates the entirety of the vessel. As structures course in and out of the MPR, pseudostenoses can be created. The solution to this problem is to use curved planar reformations (CMPR) along the common and internal carotid artery that allow the entire visualization of the vessels (Fig. 6.1). MPR also is particularly useful in the carotid arteries when heavy parietal calcifications are present that impair visualization of the inner residual lumen of the vessel. A smooth window-level setting should also be used in these instances to distinguish calcifications from contrast agent.

MIP are created when a specific projection is selected (anteroposterior for example) and then rays are cast perpendicular to the view through the volume data, with the maximum value encountered by each ray encoded on a 2D output image. As a result the entire volume is collapsed, with only the brightest structures being visible. An advantage of MIP over MPR is that structures that do not lie in a single plane are visible in their entirety (Fig. 6.2). A limitation of MIP, however, is that bones or other structures which are more attenuative than contrast-enhanced blood vessels, for example, will obscure the blood vessels. The solution to this problem is to use MIP of a limited volume and especially to use different obliquities, similar to what is performed with catheter angiography. In most cases pre-defined projections cannot be used, although anteroposterior, lateral, and oblique (+45° and −45°) generally allow visualization of the carotid bifurcation and separation of the internal

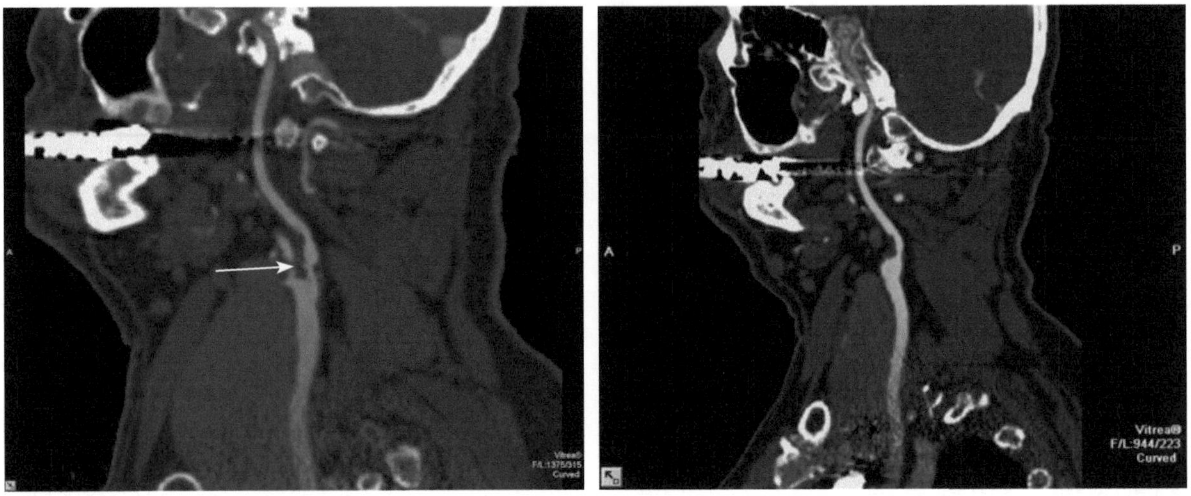

a b

Fig. 6.1a,b. Curved multiplanar reformations show, along their entire courses, both common and internal carotid arteries. Bilaterally there is evidence of the degree of stenosis. In **a** the plaque appears irregular *(arrow)*. In **b** also note the potential to follow the internal carotid artery either in the extra- or intracranial tract.

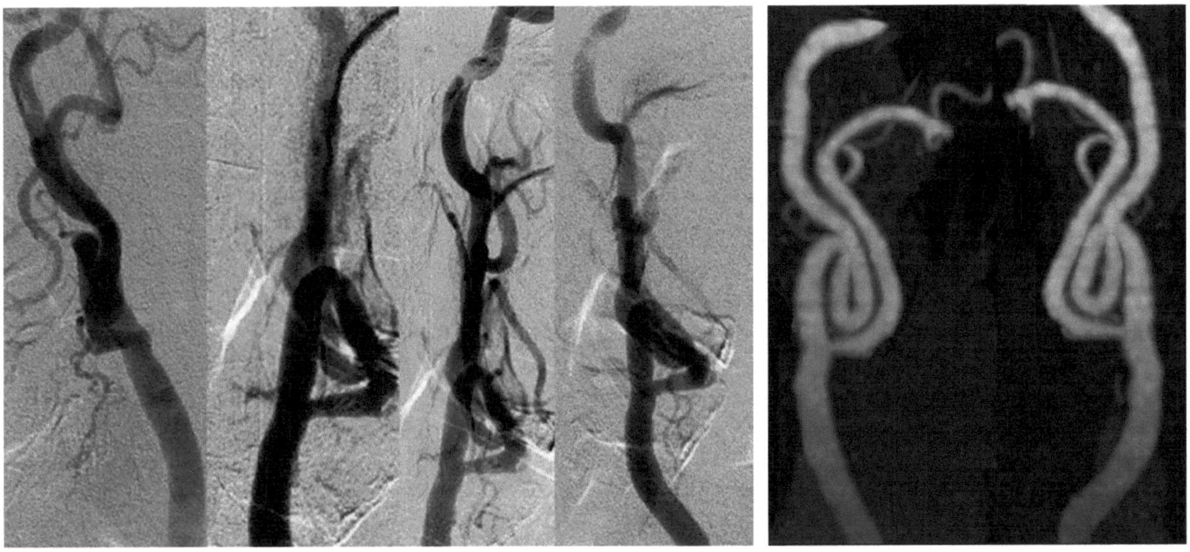

a b

Fig. 6.2a,b. Multiple-projection selective digital subtraction angiography (**a**) barely demonstrates the course of both internal carotid arteries, which is easily demonstrated, even in the presence of severe kinking, by multidetector-row computed tomography angiography with thin maximum-intensity projection reconstructions (**b**).

from the external carotid artery. Nevertheless in our experience the best approach is to interactively perform reconstructions at different rotations instead of just taking predefined images. Even in MIP the use of different rotations may allow distinction of inner residual lumen, which can be obscured when horseshoe heavy calcifications are present.

The final and most complex rendering technique is VR. There are many different versions and interfaces for VR, but the general approach is that all voxel values are assigned an opacity level that varies from total transparency to total opacity. Despite the theoretical interest of VR 3D display over the current postprocessing techniques, no definite advantage of this technique for the evaluation of carotid artery disease is found in most of the cases. VR appears particularly useful when carotid arteries are tortuous and present multiple kinkings and in all those cases in which the anatomical course of the vessels requires a perspective view for easier visualization (Fig. 6.3).

The analysis of transverse images is particularly useful in problem solving, such as when heavy parietal calcifications are present and when severe stenosis or pseudo-occlusions are present. By using the axial sections, the degree of narrowing can be correctly estimated if the scanning plane is roughly perpendicular to the vessel. Mural calcifications constitute a drawback for MIP reconstructions, but the combination of axial and MIP imaging enables an accurate estimation of the degree of stenosis severity in most cases (Fig. 6.4). The use of the VR technique may be useful when dense calcifications are located around or close to the residual lumen, because the arterial lumen may be viewed in its transparency through the surrounding structures. In clinical routine, all techniques should be used in association with the axial images. The most appropriate method of reconstruction has to be selected in each case also based on the different type of plaque.

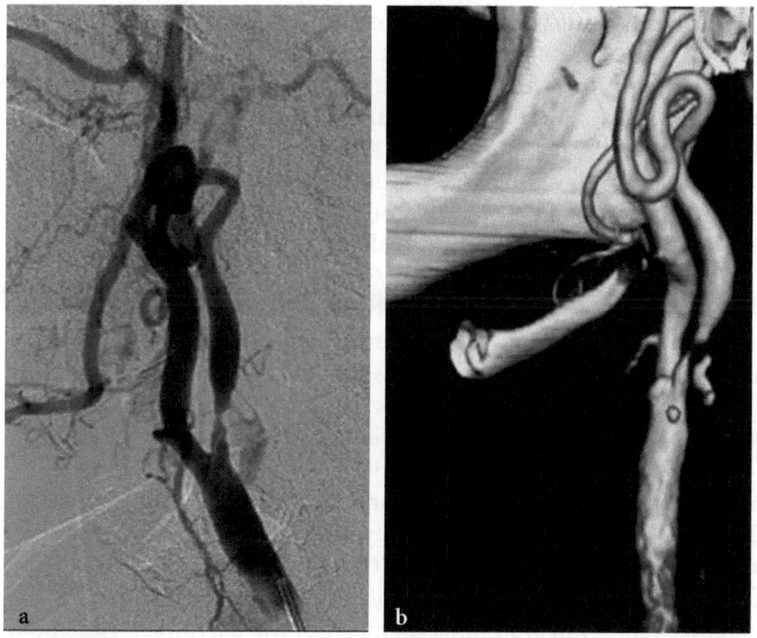

Fig. 6.3a,b Selective digital subtraction angiography (**a**) demonstrates the presence of a severe stenosis at the origin of the internal carotid arteries. Multidetector-row computed tomography angiography with volume-rendered reconstruction (**b**) confirms the presence of the severe stenosis, but also shows a severe kinking of the distal internal carotid artery.

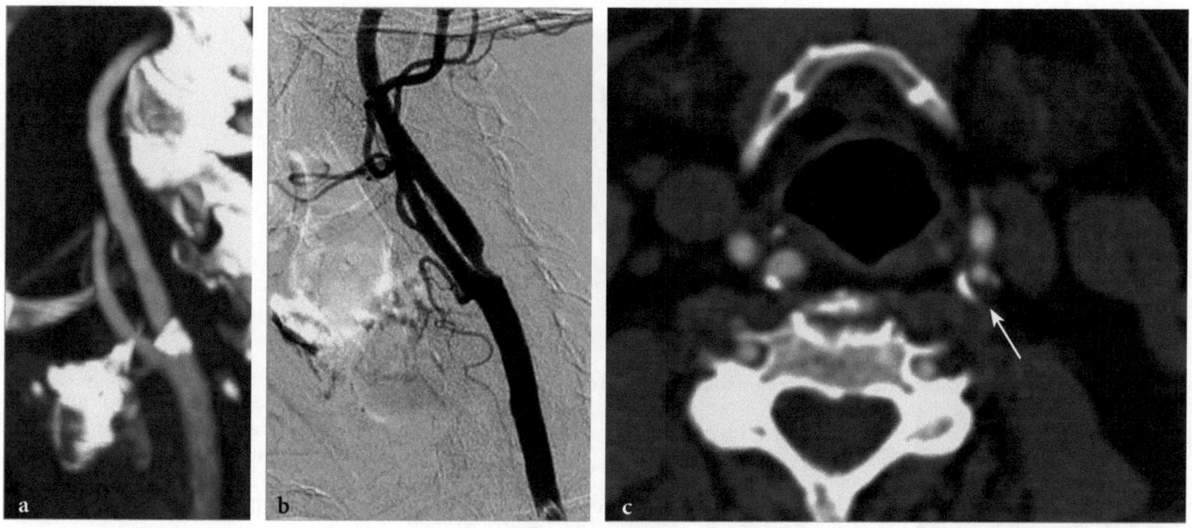

Fig. 6.4. a Multidetector-row computed tomography angiography with thin maximum-intensity projection reconstruction does not allow assessment of the entity of the stenosis in the presence of a heavy calcification. **b** Transverse image demonstrates the residual lumen and the presence of a fibro-lipidic plaque with parietal calcification *(arrow)*. **c** The entity of the stenosis is confirmed by selective digital subtraction angiography

More recently, automated 3D CT angiography analysis software has become available from various manufacturers. With the application of automated 3D CT angiography analysis software, it is possible to obtain both 3D visual evaluation and quantification of the vessels with automatic detection of minimal diameters at the level of maximal stenosis. The principle of automated 3D CT angiography analysis relies on region-growing techniques from a start point determined by the observer. The trajectory is built in an iterative way, step by step, going into the direction of the end point. The algorithm detects trajectories where the density along the trace remains high in amplitude. It also detects density changes perpendicular to the calculated trace, in order to create the vessel contours; thus, automated 3D CT angiography analysis is designed to make it easy to manipulate the vessels to be assessed by the observer. Most of the postprocessing work is thus done by the computer; however, the reproducibility and accuracy of this image-reconstruction technique in the evaluation of carotid artery stenosis still remains to be fully determined. There are some limitations to this method, mainly related to the presence of calcifications and severe irregularities of the vessels walls. Calcifications with high density lead to decreases in the density difference between intraluminal contrast media and calcification, making it difficult for the software to detect the exact boundary of enhanced carotids. It is sometimes difficult to determine the true contour of the carotid even by manual correction of the ROI indicator because of partial-volume effects.

6.3.2 Grading Methods for Carotid Artery Stenosis

Several different methods of measuring the degree of stenosis from carotid angiograms have evolved, each with different definitions of what constitutes a carotid stenosis. It is thus possible for the same angiogram to be reported as showing differing degrees of stenosis according to the particular method of measurement used.

The stenosis can be graded using the European Carotid Surgery Trial (ECST), North America Symptomatic Carotid Endarterectomy Trial (NASCET), and Common Carotid (CC) methods (Fig. 6.5).

ECST method calculates stenosis using the ratio of the linear luminal diameter of the narrowest segment of the diseased portion of the artery to the original internal carotid lumen, made at the point of maximal stenosis (not necessarily the bulb), and is an estimate: ECST = $(1-\text{md}/B)\times100\%$.

NASCET stenosis is calculated from the ratio of the linear luminal diameter of the narrowest segment of the diseased portion of the artery to the diameter of the artery beyond any poststenotic dilatation: NASCET = $(1-\text{md}/C)\times100\%$.

CC method calculates stenosis using the ratio of the linear luminal diameter of the narrowest segment of

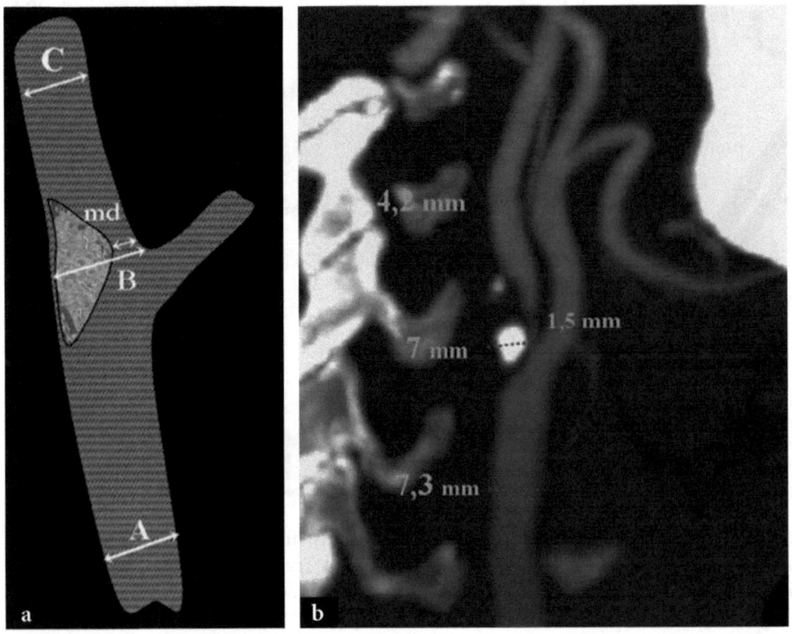

Fig. 6.5a,b. Scheme (**a**) and practical example on a thin maximum-intensity projection multidetector-row computed tomography angiography image (**b**) of the three different methods to calculate the degree of stenosis. *md* = minimal diameter; *A* = common carotid artery normal caliber; *B* = presumed carotid artery caliber at level of stenosis; *C* = normal internal carotid artery calibre

the diseased portion of the artery to the common carotid lumen, 3–5 cm proximal to the carotid bifurcation. CC method for angiographic assessment of carotid stenoses: CC = (1–md/A)×100%.

Some studies have used the NASCET criteria for grading of stenoses and others the ECST criteria [2, 34, 35]. Furthermore, additional methods for grading of stenoses have been proposed, and it has also been noted that there is interobserver variability in measuring the degree of stenosis. The most commonly used alternative is the CC method. This raises the question of which method is most reproducible. Even if all three methods demonstrated a high reproducibility, several studies showed the best reproducibility in the following order: CC, ECST, and NASCET [36, 37]. The ECST and CC methods grade stenoses similarly; the NASCET method tends to underestimate the degree of stenosis, classifies more stenoses in lower categories than the other methods, and has lower agreement with the ECST and CC methods. Significant discrepancies between the NASCET and the ECST angiographic methods are reported, such that a 50% stenosis by NASCET is equivalent to approximately 70% by ECST [38].

Both the NASCET and ECST methods have limitations. With the NASCET method, one problem is deciding the appropriate segment of distal internal carotid artery (ICA) on which to base a measurement. Inadequate contrast enhancement or the presence of overlying vessels may obscure the distal ICA. Furthermore, since the carotid bulb is larger than the distal ICA, minor degree of stenosis (<50% bulb diameter reduction) may result in a "negative stenosis." For ECST measurements, the problem lies in predicting the normal position of the carotid bulb; variations in anatomy or irregular stenoses can make this difficult even for the experienced observer. The principal difficulty, therefore, with both methods is establishing the diameter of the normal ICA.

The CC method demonstrated the best reproducibility in several studies and, when the methods are compared, almost identical results in different studies were obtained [19, 35, 39]. In one series a 70% NASCET stenosis corresponded to an 81% CC stenosis and a 78% ECST stenosis [39].

According to those results, the CC method appears to be the most preferable; it has the additional advantage that atheromatous changes are rare in the common carotid artery, and that the vessel is usually visualized on the images without overlap of the structures. Furthermore, in clinical routine it would be wise to base decisions on the other methods as well.

6.4 Clinical Applications

Two major categories of diseases of the carotid arteries are most often seen in clinical practice: atheromatous disease and the nonatheromatous diseases. In the West, atherosclerotic disease is the major cause of clinically silent vascular disease.

6.4.1 Atheromatous Disease

The most common area of atherosclerotic involvement of the supra-aortic vessels is at the carotid bifurcation. The basic histological feature of atherosclerosis is the deposition of fatty compounds in the intima. The atheromatous plaque (cells, fibrous connective tissue, and lipids) and the occasional complication associated with it (intraplaque hemorrhage and ulceration) are responsible for the development of significant stenoses of the vessel. In some cases, significant luminal irregularities without a hemodynamically significant stenosis lead to platelet aggregation and embolic phenomena to the brain. The composition of dangerous plaques in the carotid arteries is different from plaques elsewhere. High-risk carotid plaques are heterogeneous, very fibrous, and not necessarily lipid-rich. Less common, although they may also be present, are atherosclerotic changes of the carotid origin and intracranial vessels. A complete evaluation of the carotid arteries therefore requires visualization of the entire supra-aortic branches from the aortic arch to the intracranial circulation, assessment of vascular stenoses, and evaluation of plaque morphology.

Few studies have evaluated the accuracy of multidetector-row spiral CT angiography in the evaluation of carotid artery stenosis. On the contrary, in the mid-1990s, several studies compared single-slice spiral CT angiography with catheter angiography. Leclerc et al. found a very good correlation between catheter and CT angiography, with correct classification of the degree of stenosis in 95% of the cases [25]. Cumming et al also found a high degree of correlation with catheter angiography (r=0.928, p<0.001), with good morphological definition of carotid stenosis and demonstration of all occlusions and ulcerated plaques [24].

Randoux et al. performed a more complete study, evaluating several parameters, among which were the degree and length of stenosis, and the presence of plaque irregularities and ulcerations [40]. The sensitivity and specificity of CT angiography for the demonstration of stenosis greater than 70% were, respectively, 100% and 100%, with a very good correlation for what regards the length of the stenosis. CT angiography showed more plaque irregularities and ulcerations than catheter angiography, in consideration of the limited number of views obtained with catheter angiography.

An important aspect of all CT angiography studies of the carotid arteries is the very high accuracy in the detection of pseudo-occlusions, with no problems in the visualization of slow residual flow (Fig. 6.6). Chen et al. recently demonstrated a 100% accuracy in diagnosing near versus total occlusions, classifying stump or retrograde flow of total occlusions and recognizing stenoses of near occlusions [41]. In addition CT angiography provided, in this study performed on 57 carotid arteries, information on the underlying pathology, such as dissection or thrombosis.

In our extensive experience with multidetector-row CT angiography of the carotid arteries, we have found a very high correlation with DSA. The interobserver (four observers with different experience in vascular imaging) agreement, in the evaluation of 109 carotid arteries, was almost perfect in the evaluation of the degree and length of stenosis and the morphology of the plaque. At consensus reading the sensitivity, specificity, and accuracy of MDCT angiography, as compared to DSA, for grades of stenosis greater than 70% were, respectively, 100%, 96%, and 94%, with a κ-value of 0.812 (almost perfect agreement). On DSA, 82 diseased segments (75.2%) were identified: 16 with mild disease, 12 with moderate (<50%) stenosis, 11 with moderate (>50%) stenosis, 30 with severe stenosis, and 9 occluded internal carotid arteries. In 3 cases (3 moderate stenosis at DSA diagnosed as with severe stenosis at MDCT), the degree of stenosis was overestimated by MDCT angiography by 1 grade. In 1 patient the degree of stenosis (moderate stenosis at DSA diagnosed as with mild stenosis at MDCT angiography) was underestimated by 1 grade. Regarding the length of stenosis, there was a perfect correlation between MDCT angiography and DSA. The length of stenosis was underestimated of 1 grade in two cases at MDCT angiography, in which the stenosis appeared to extend for less than 10 mm while turned out to be between 10 and 15 mm long at DSA. In 1 case the length of stenosis was overestimated by 1 grade at MDCT angiography, in which the stenosis seemed to extend between 10 and 15 mm.

Tandem lesions can be easily demonstrated with MDCT angiography if a large volume is acquired; in fact they can be located in all supra-aortic vessels, from the aortic arch to the intracranial circulation, and may contribute to the symptoms. Their identification is also important, since it can modify treatment choice. In our experience with 55 patients, all four tandem lesions were correctly demonstrated by MDCT angiography. In 2 cases a severe stenosis affected the proximal right subclavian artery and in 1 the left common carotid artery; in another case a moderate stenosis was found in the basilar artery (Fig. 6.7).

6.4.1.1 Plaque Imaging

Plaque morphology and composition have been proposed as important risk factors for thromboembolic events, giving rise to the concept of unstable plaque [12, 13, 42]. It is suggested that embolic phenomena are associated with thinning and subsequent ulceration of the fibrous cap on the surface of the atherosclerotic plaque, resulting in release into the parent vessel of necrotic lipoid debris from the plaque substance. Several studies have established a correlation between plaque ulceration and irregularity with clinical presentation, outcome, and prognosis [12, 15, 16, 43]. Recent analysis of the European Carotid Surgery Trial collaborative group data has shown that surface irregularity and ulceration seen on catheter angiography are associated with more frequent symptoms [4]. Controversy exists regarding the importance of other pathological features; for instance there is no evidence to correlate intraplaque hemorrhage with symptoms [15]. Other authors have proposed a high plaque lipid content to correlate with clinical presentation, especially if located just beneath a thin fibrous cap [43].

In imaging the carotid arteries, it is therefore becoming increasingly important to identify factors other than the simple degree of stenosis. The widespread use of spiral CT has led to its proposal as a method for plaque evaluation, and a small number of preliminary studies have been performed to define its role in this area [44]. Studies from Estes et al. [45] and Oliver et al. [46], although performed in a relatively small number of patients, have suggested a role for CT in differentiation of fibrous stroma from lipid-rich areas within plaques. Cinat et al. [21] have also proposed a role for CT in the identification of plaque ulceration. Walker et al. [47] showed a correlation between lower attenuation values and the amount of intraplaque lipid, supporting the suggestion that low-density plaques are more likely to be lipid-rich. Nevertheless the same authors observed a

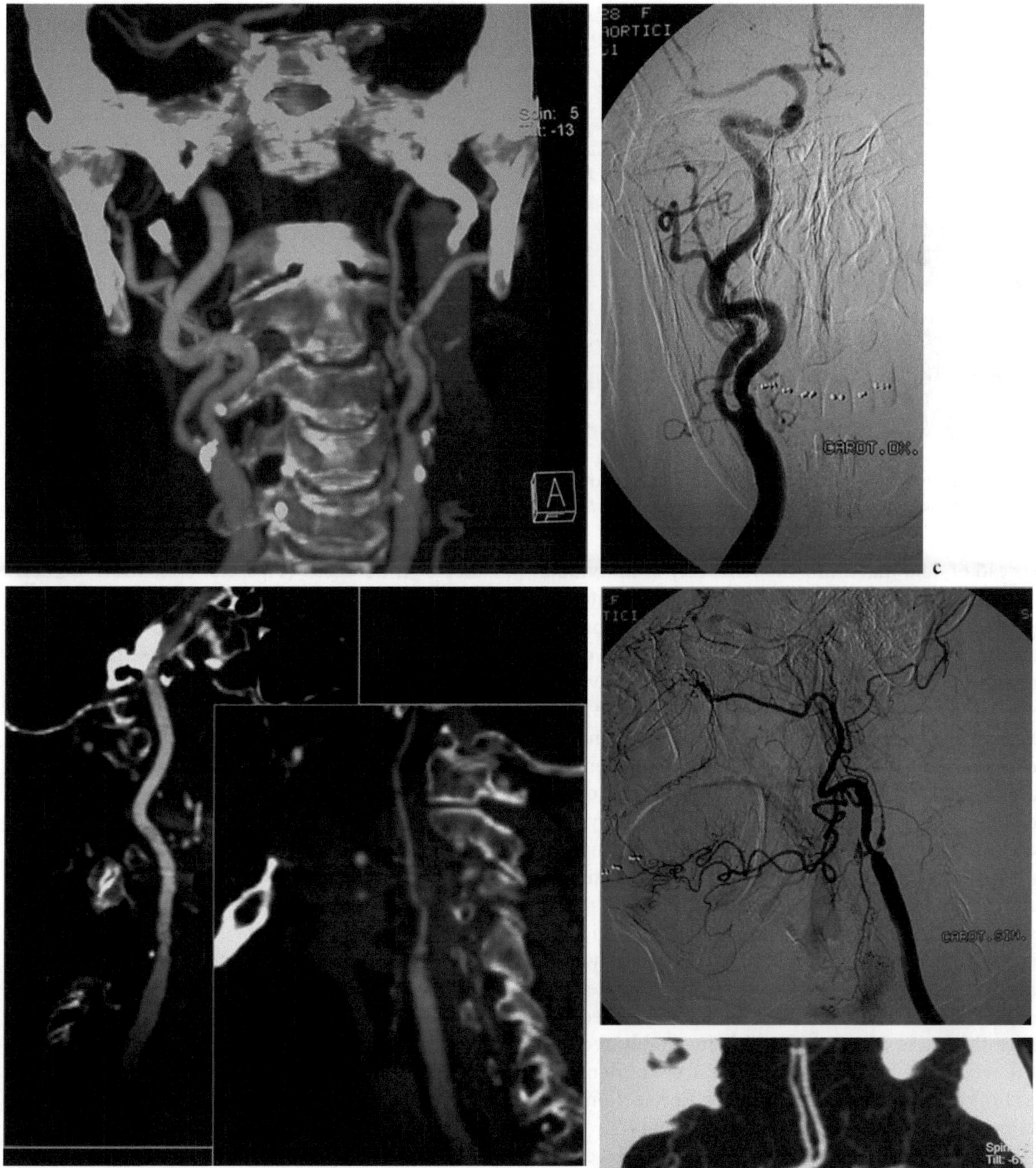

a

b

c

d

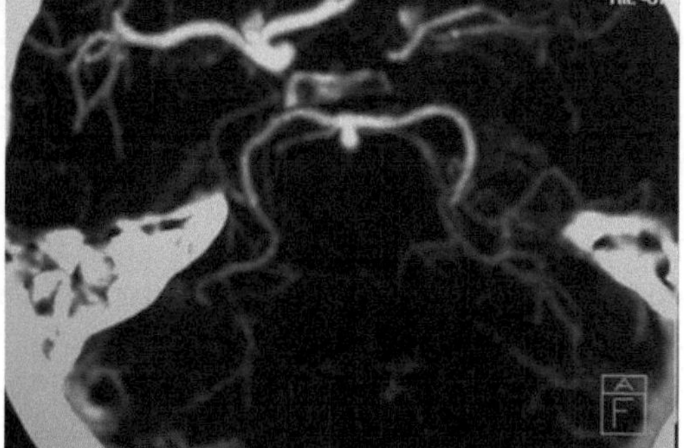

e

Fig. 6.6a–e. Coronal thin maximum-intensity projection (MIP) multidetector-row computed tomography angiography (**a**) demonstrates normal common carotid arteries and right carotid bifurcation, with severe stenosis and pseudo-occlusion of the left internal carotid artery, as better demonstrated by curved multiplanar reformations (**b,c**). The findings are confirmed by selective digital subtraction angiography of the right (**d**) and left (**e**) carotid arteries. e Thin MIP reconstruction of the circle of Willis demonstrates patency of the intracranial circulation.

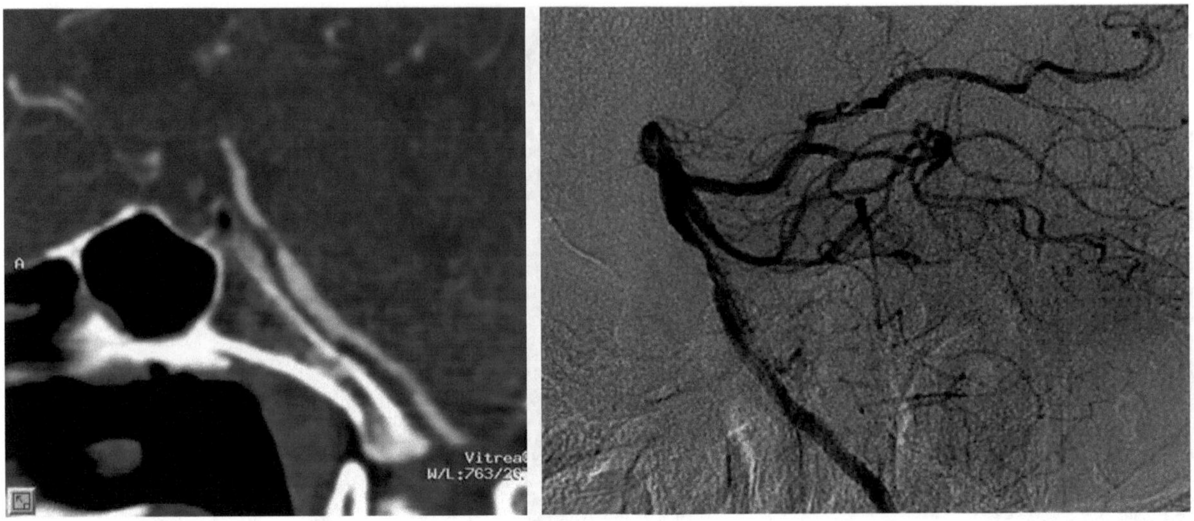

Fig. 6.7a,b. Multidetector-row computed tomography angiography with thin MIP reconstruction (**a**) demonstrates a moderate stenosis of the basilar artery (arrow), as confirmed by selective digital subtraction angiography (**b**)

spread of data that limits the reliability of individual Hounsfield unit (HU) readings as an indicator of plaque lipid or fibrous tissue. The relatively poor reliability of HU measurements for the prediction of the amount of lipid or fibrous tissue within an individual plaque may be explained at least partly by the great heterogeneity observed on histological examination of individual plaques. The relatively homogeneous appearance of plaque on CT imaging does not adequately represent the plaque heterogeneity evident on microscopic analysis. Regarding the visualization of plaque ulceration, only studies with single-slice spiral CT have been performed; the most recent study performed on plaque morphology provided a sensitivity of 60%, with a specificity of 74%, with a moderate positive predictive value for the detection of ulcerations, with a technical limitation related to a slice thickness of 1.5 mm, which inevitably reduces the sensitivity for small fissures or areas of denuded or broken fibrous cap visible on the fine sections obtained with histopathological processing [47].

In our experience with 100 carotid arteries, evaluated in comparison with MDCT angiography and catheter angiography, plaque morphology was correctly assessed in 90 of the 100 cases. MDCT angiography identified wall irregularities in 9 cases in which DSA demonstrated regular vascular walls and lumen. In 1 case normal at MDCT angiography, DSA demonstrated the presence of wall irregularities. The sensitivity and specificity for plaque morphology were, respectively, 98 and 83%, with a positive predictive value of 84% and a negative predictive value of 98%. MDCT angiography correctly identified the presence of ulcers in 26 cases (Figs. 6.8, 6.9), while demonstrating smooth plaques in 68 patients (Fig. 6.10). In 5 cases which turned out to be normal at DSA, MDCT angiography incorrectly demonstrated the presence of a ulcer, while, in 1 case apparently normal at MDCT angiography, DSA showed a small ulcer. The sensitivity and specificity for presence of ulcers were, respectively, 96 and 93%, with a positive predictive value of 84% and a negative predictive value of 98%.

6.4.2 Nonatheromatous Disease

Nonatheromatous disease of the carotid circulation is less frequent than atherosclerotic disease, but remains an important cause of cerebrovascular disease. Nonatheromatous processes are always suspected in patients with the appropriate clinical history or in younger subjects with acute ischemic symptoms.

Carotid dissection is a particularly important cause of stroke in young patients [48–50]. Dissections result from hemorrhage into the wall of a vessel. Most commonly the vessel responds to the hemorrhage in two ways: the lumen is compromised, but the vessel wall diameter is enlarged. Dissection may be either traumatic or spontaneous, although in most of the cases even spontaneous dissection derives from unrecognized, minor traumas. Carotid dissection can occur as a result of blunt or penetrating trauma, and pseudoaneurysms can complicate dissections. Dissection can cause transient ischemic attacks or strokes and/or unilateral headache and Horner syndrome.

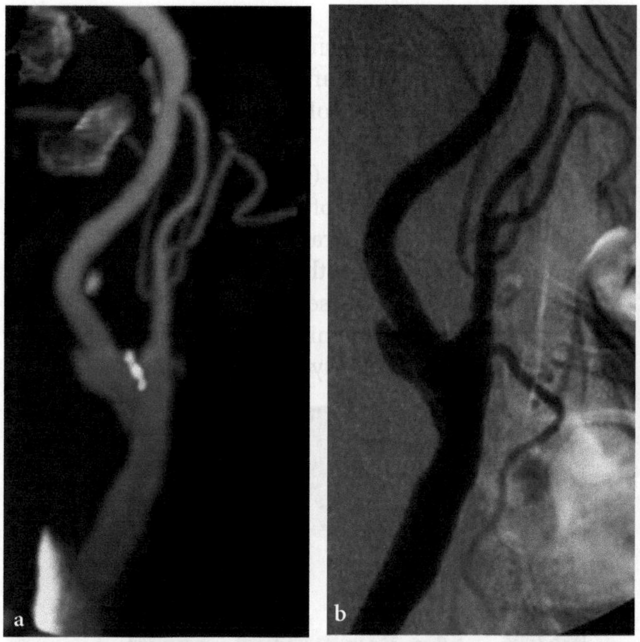

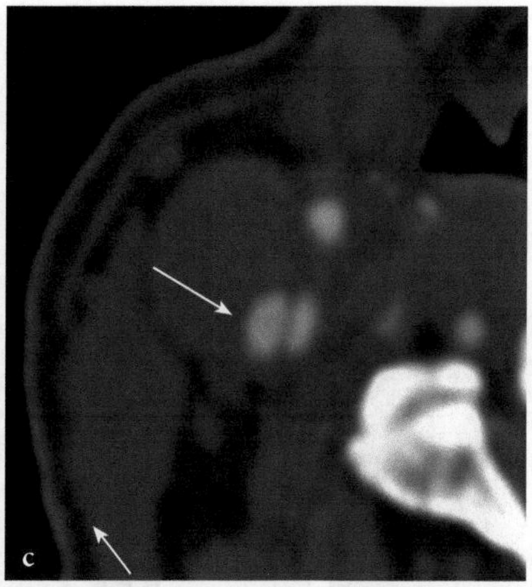

Fig. 6.8. **a** Multidetector-row computed tomography angiography with thin MIP reconstruction demonstrates the presence of a large ulcer of the proximal internal carotid artery. **b** The same finding (*arrow*) can be depicted on a transverse image (**b**). **c** Selective digital subtraction angiography confirms the presence of the large ulcer.

a

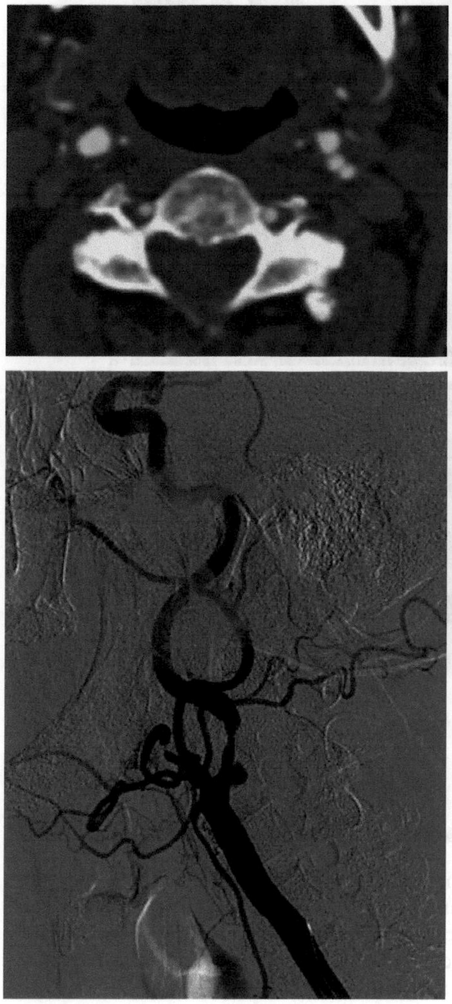

b

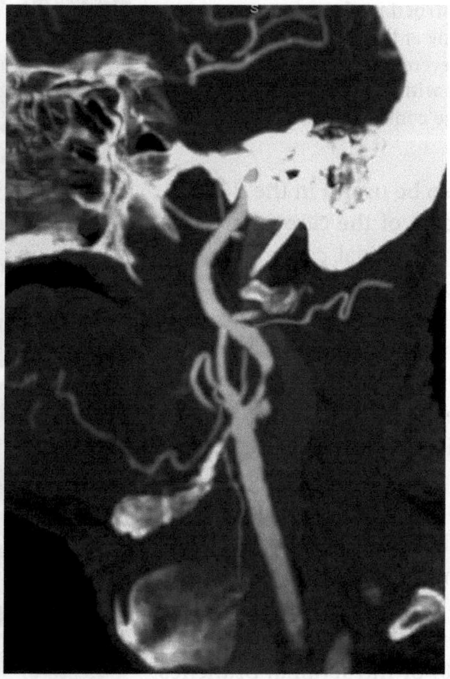

c

Fig. 6.9. **a** Multidetector-row computed tomography angiography with thin MIP reconstruction shows a severe stenosis of the proximal internal carotid artery, due to a complex plaque also presenting an ulcer (*arrow*). **b** The ulcer is confirmed by transverse image (*arrow*). **c** All findings are confirmed by selective DSA.

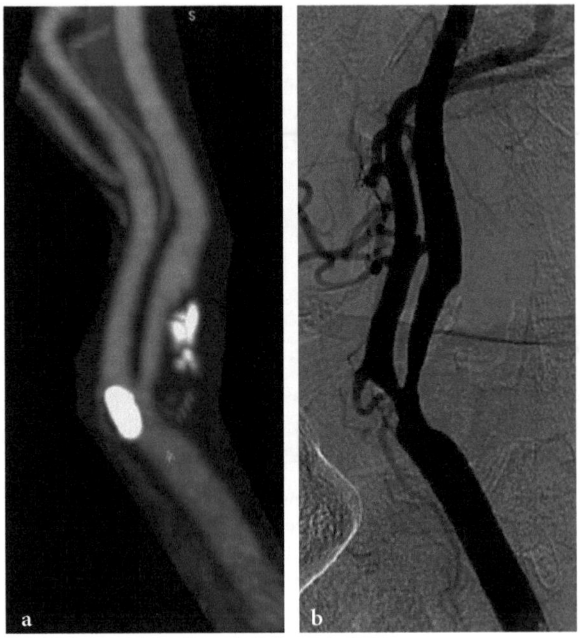

Fig. 6.10. **a** Multidetector-row computed tomography angiography with thin MIP reconstruction demonstrates an eccentric, partially calcified plaque at the origin of the internal carotid artery determining a severe stenosis. **b** Selective DSA confirms the degree of stenosis without any potential to demonstrate the calcifications or the content of the plaque.

CT angiography may also be useful in the diagnosis of inflammatory disorders of the carotid arteries (Fig. 6.11). Abnormalities in arterial caliber, arterial occlusion, and irregularities of vessel margins are seen with these disorders. Typically vasculitis results in tapering of vessels over long segments; however, vasculitis can also cause focal stenoses and dilatations that result in a beaded appearance.

Fibromuscular dysplasia is another cause of vascular disease in younger patients, resulting from a vasculopathy of unknown cause that typically affects medium-sized arteries. Fibromuscular dysplasia is more common in women, and involvement of the carotid arteries is second only to the renal arteries [51]. In a minority of patients, there is involvement of the vertebral arteries (15%) or intracranial branches (10%). The appearance has been likened, as in the renal arteries, to a string of beads. Fistulas, including carotid-cavernous fistulas, may develop as a complication of the disease.

Uncommon congenital anomalies, postoperative anastomotic strictures, and poststenting stenoses can be easily demonstrated with CT angiography [52]. Other nonspecific and uncommon vasculopathies may also be diagnosed. Radiation-induced arteritis may be seen in patients with history of radiation therapy for neck primary cancers, in most of the cases 10 years or more after treatment, and results in long-segment stenoses of the distal common carotid arteries [53, 54].

Carotid body tumors (also known as chemodectomas or paragangliomas of the carotid body) are rare lesions that arise from paraganglionic cells that migrate from the neural crest in the adventitia of the common carotid bifurcation. These cells are scattered throughout the body, thus explaining their ubiquitous distribution. Lesions grow slowly, gradually encroaching and

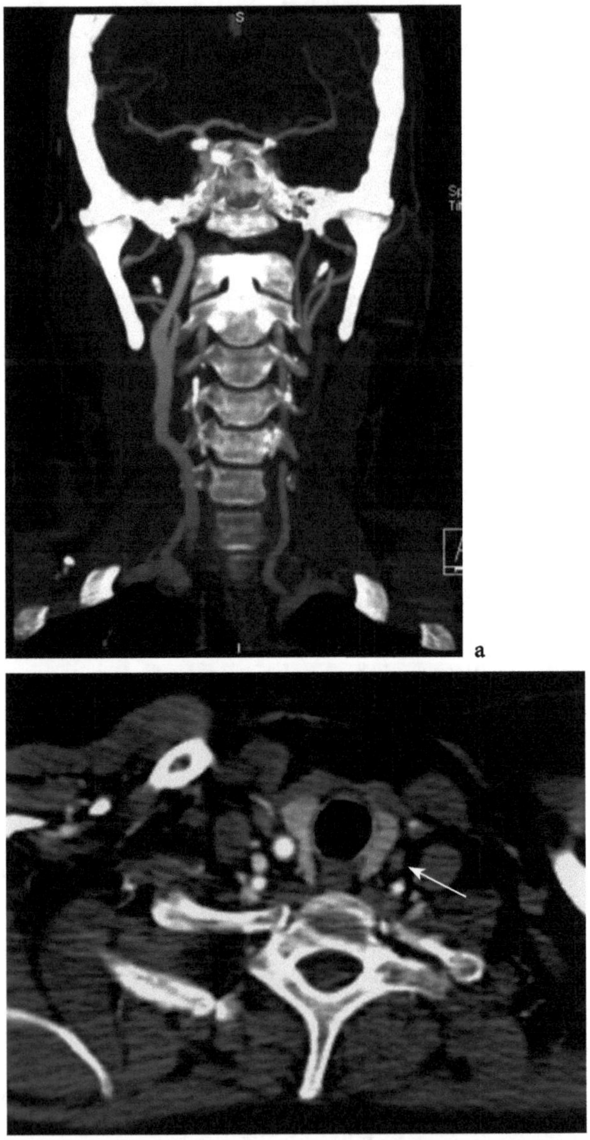

Fig. 6.11. **a** Coronal thin MIP multidetector-row computed tomography angiography shows occlusion of the proximal left common carotid artery with reconstitution immediately below its bifurcation. **b** Transverse image *(arrow)* confirms occlusion and significant lumen reduction.

encasing the carotid bifurcation, with a characteristic splaying of the internal and external carotid arteries. By histological criteria most cases can be classified as malignant, contradicting the benign clinical course of these neoplasms (less than 10% metastasize). A familial incidence, with an autosomal dominant role of transmission, has been reported (approximately 20% of the cases), and, in these patients, bilateral tumors are often present (26–33%). Both sexes, particularly in the fourth and fifth decades of life, can be affected.

An asymptomatic, slow-growing, lateral cervical pulsing mass, is the most common clinical presentation. Sometimes, patients complain about physical symptoms such as pain, dyspnea, dysphagia, nerve palsy, dizziness, and hearing loss. On physical examination the lesion has a laterolateral, but not vertical, mobility (the so-called Fontain's sign). A bruit or a superficial thrill may be present, because of the rich vascular supply.

For many years, digital subtraction angiography has been the only method for the diagnosis of carotid body tumors. At present, other less invasive imaging modalities, including ultrasonography, CT, magnetic resonance, and scintigraphy, have been developed and can be used for the evaluation of carotid body tumors. Surgery is the most effective treatment, with complications rate related to the size and to the vascular encirclement by the tumor.

CT angiography has several advantages compared with conventional angiography, including minimal invasiveness, cost, better patient compliance, and reduced ionizing radiation exposure for both patients and staff. At present, multidetector-row CT angiography combined with VR algorithm provides complete assessment of the carotid arteries in both a two-dimensional and a three-dimensional fashion. Thus, this technique is extremely useful in the preoperative evaluation of carotid body tumors. With the use of thin-slice collimation protocols, even very small (≤5 mm) lesions can be accurately depicted. CT effectively confirms the diagnosis, allowing excellent evaluation of tumor size, relationship with carotid arteries, and adjacent structures. Although conventional angiography was considered the standard of reference in the diagnosis of carotid body tumors, its current use should be limited to those patients with indeterminate findings on other less invasive imaging modalities and aimed at providing access for preoperative embolization. Imaging studies are essential to differentiate carotid body tumors from other masses of the neck (lymphadenopathies, tumors, cysts, etc.) and, once the diagnosis is established, to precisely plan the surgical excision.

6.4.3 CT Angiography in Treatment Planning

In the last decade there has been an increasing interest in less invasive means (angioplasty and stenting) to treat carotid artery occlusive disease than endarterectomy. As a general rule, PTA (Percutaneous Transluminal Angiplasty) with endovascular stents can be suggested for patients with smooth, relatively short (less than 15 mm) internal carotid artery stenosis, small ulcerations, and slight irregularity of plaques. Surgery is suggested for patients with heavily calcified plaques with a horseshoe appearance, with irregular ulcerated plaques, longer stenoses, and with multiple stenotic lesions.

All the information needed for treatment planning can be easily achieved with CT angiography, as our experience and that of other authors have demonstrated; in particular the length of the stenosis together with the morphology of the plaque and of heavy circumferential calcifications appear to be particularly useful. In treatment planning, it is also crucial to distinguish occlusions from pseudo-occlusions, which can be performed accurately with MDCT angiography and with less positive results with other noninvasive imaging modalities.

In treatment planning, MDCT angiography seems to provide superior information as compared to other imaging modalities; in fact CT seems to be unique in determining with good accuracy the anatomy and course of the vessels, the degree of the stenosis, and the morphology of the plaque, especially in terms of presence and entity of calcifications, irregularities, and ulcerations.

6.4.4 Follow-Up after Therapy

In the past few years, the clinical trials performed to demonstrate the efficacy of carotid endarterectomy have stressed the indications for treating carotid artery stenosis (Fig. 6.12). Along with surgical and anesthesiological improvements that have minimized the risks of carotid endarterectomy, the development of endovascular therapies and material for interventional radiology, particularly metallic stents, has significantly increased the potentials of minimally invasive treatment even for the carotid arteries [55]. Carotid artery stenting has now become a routine procedure in many institutions, with excellent results (Fig. 6.13) and minor complications. Problems related with stenting, although materials have sig-

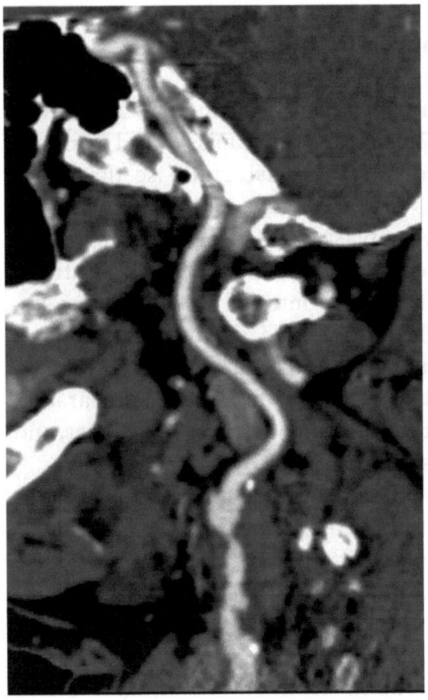
a

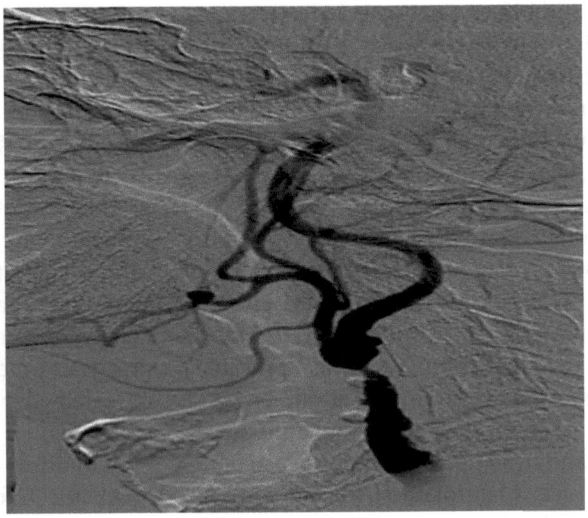
b

Fig. 6.12a,b. Postendarterectomy restenosis with involvement of the distal common carotid artery and bifurcation, as shown by curved multiplanar reformation multidetector-row computed tomography angiography (a) and selective digital subtraction angiography (b).

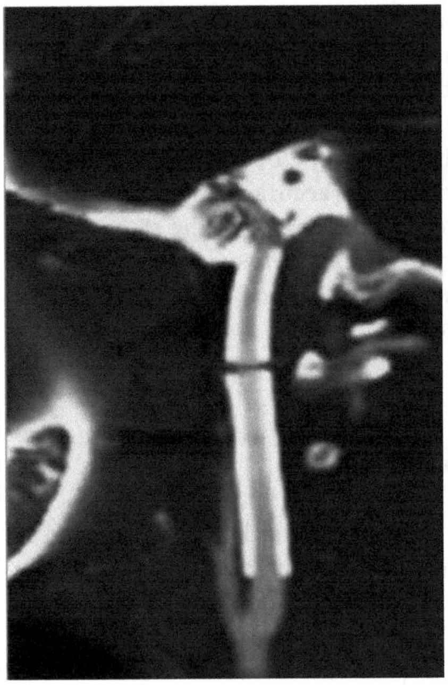
a

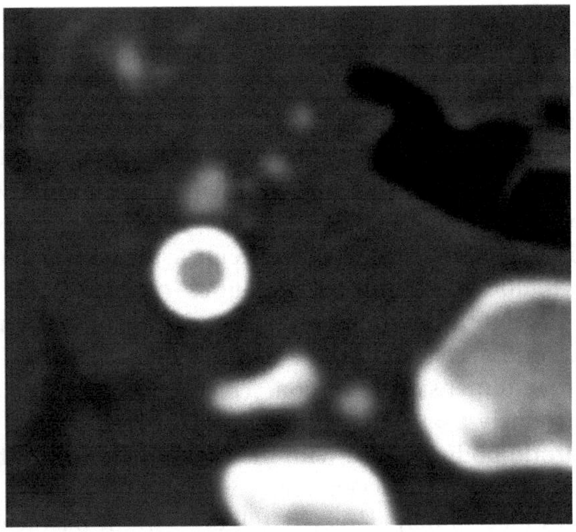
b

Fig. 6.13a,b. Patient with acute dissection treated with double stenting; stents patency assessed by a curved multiplanar reformation (MPR) reconstruction (a) and transverse MPR (b).

nificantly improved, are mainly related to restenosis for neointimal hyperplasia (Fig. 6.14). Metallic stents may cause artifacts and therefore examinations must be evaluated adequately, choosing the correct algorithm of postprocessing. A recent study performed by Leclerc et al. demonstrated that VR, based on a selection of voxels of the image with adjustment of opacity for each selected material and change in the transparency allows assessment of residual arterial lumen through arterial wall calcifications. Based on this observation, VR algorithm was also applied to follow up patients treated with carotid angioplasty and stenting, because the arterial lumen can be analyzed theoretically despite the high-attenuation values of

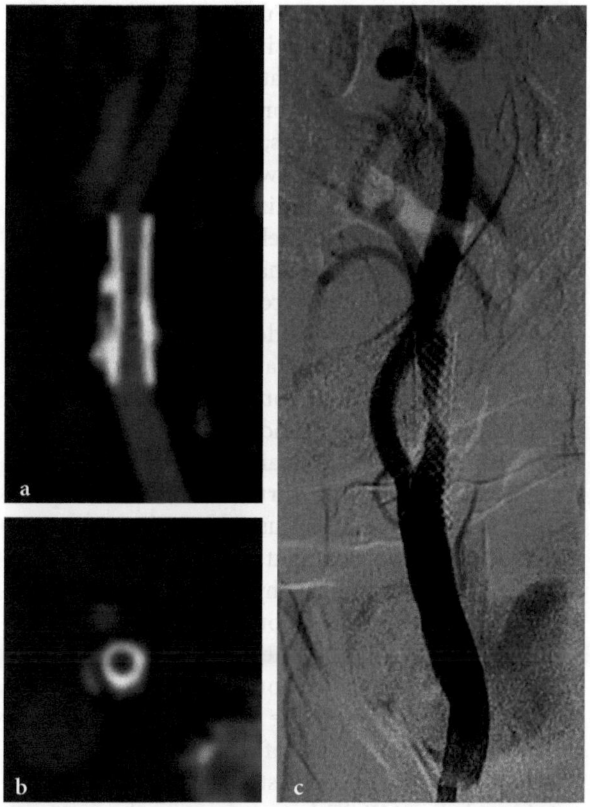

Fig. 6.14a–c. Patient with atherosclerotic stenosis treated with stenting. a Curved MPR multidetector-row computed tomography angiography demonstrates a low density within the stent, indicating restenosis due to neointimal hyperplasia. b In-stent, low-density tissue can also be assessed by transverse MPR. c Restenosis is then confirmed by selective digital subtraction angiography.

the stent. The use of a high spatial-frequency convolution algorithm and appropriate windows allowed the authors to differentiate the wall of the stent from the enhanced arterial lumen within the prosthesis in all patients. However, axial source images showed an apparent increase in the thickness of the stent wall and maximum intensity-projection reconstructions did not allow the visualization of the arterial lumen owing to the higher attenuation values of the stent compared with those of the enhanced arterial lumen. On the contrary, volume-rendered images showed accurate delineation of the enhanced arterial lumen through the stent, despite the thickness of the stent wall, which appeared uniformly increased. By applying a VR algorithm, the authors classified voxels according to the probability that they contained a tissue type. The two selected materials (contrast material and stent) were retained by using trapezoid functions with specific adjustments of parameters. However, this method determines an overestimation of the thickness of the stent wall in all cases despite having separate trapezoids for the arterial lumen and the stent wall. This overestimation is probably related to a partial volume effect of voxels at the border of the stent, including portions of both the arterial lumen and the stent wall. This misclassification of voxels depends on the position of the trapezoids and can be minimized by using thin slices, overlapping reconstruction, and a high-resolution matrix. Despite this limitation, the high-attenuation values related to the stent can be assessed in their transparency by applying a low-opacity value; this technique allowed accurate delineation of the arterial lumen through the stent. Volume-rendered images, according to the experience of Leclerc et al, provide 3D angiographic appearance with good analysis of the relationship between arterial lumen and stent and therefore might be useful to evaluate the carotid artery after angioplasty with stenting and especially to detect restenosis in the long-term follow-up after treatment.

6.5 Advantages and Limitations Versus Other Imaging Modalities

6.5.1 Advantages

In the examination of the supra-aortic vessels, good image quality is essential. CT angiography enables excellent image quality in most of the cases, provided that the patient does not move or swallow during the few seconds of acquisition. A breath-hold acquisition is not necessary, although, especially if a 16-row-detector scanner is used, the acquisition time is so short that any patient can hold their breath at least during acquisition up to the base of the skull [32, 56].

Another advantage of CT angiography is to allow observations of bony structures. Catheter angiography can hint at a hypoplastic ICA, while CT angiography can confirm the diagnosis by finding a hypoplastic carotid canal.

The transverse mode of acquisition represents an advantage; in fact the possibility to follow the flow direction allows to discriminate even very slow residual flow from thrombosed vessels, which is crucial in determination of treatment planning. As compared to other imaging modalities commonly utilized in the assessment of the carotid arteries, MDCT angiography provides excellent results even in pseudo-occlusions, which are difficult to differentiate from occlusions either with color-Doppler ultrasound (US) or flow-based and contrast-enhanced MR angiography [41].

The analysis of transverse images provides information that is harder to achieve with other imaging modalities and even with catheter angiography. In fact the visualization of the vessel wall and composition of the plaque, although, as previously demonstrated, not highly specific in comparison with pathological examination, provide an added value, especially useful when planning treatment and evaluating the possibility of performing an endovascular stenting. The presence of heavy calcifications may constitute a limitation in the assessment of the true degree of stenosis with color-Doppler US, and is not detected with MR angiography. Color-Doppler US may also present difficulties in the evaluation of the carotid bifurcation when it is located higher, as compared to bony structures, than normal. Furthermore, with color-Doppler US, it is in most of the cases impossible to exclude the presence of tandem lesions, involving either the origin of the supra-aortic vessels or the intracranial circulation. Finally, as stressed by several authors, the technique is limited by a significant operator-dependency [57].

MR angiography provides excellent results in vascular pathologies and has proved accurate in the evaluation of the supra-aortic vessels. Contrast-enhanced sequences overcome most of the limitations of flow-based sequences in terms of overestimation of the degree of stenosis and length of vascular involvement, although even with these sequences there might be dephasing artifacts with a slight overestimation of the stenosis [57]. In MR angiography, unless dedicated studies with high-resolution coils and sequences are performed, the visualization of the plaque and its morphology and composition is generally difficult, although the presence of ulcerations and irregularities can generally be well documented.

6.5.2 Limitations

Two are the major limitations of MDCT angiography in the evaluation of patients with suspected carotid artery stenosis: the use of ionizing radiations and iodinated contrast agents. Regarding the radiation issue, it has been noted recently [58] that it is not that important in older individuals, who are the typical patients with cerebrovascular insufficiency, and that the radiation dose, as compared to that of DSA is significantly lower [31]. Furthermore it might be possible, as has been shown in other areas, to reduce the radiation dose to the patient by optimizing the acquisition protocol [59]. For what concerns the use of iodinated contrast agents, it must be considered that several patients present with poor renal function and cannot tolerate an administration of a possibly nephrotoxic agent; nevertheless the nephrotoxicity of nonionic contrast agents has been significantly reduced as compared to ionic contrast agents, and their administration can be considered safe and well tolerated, even in high-risk populations [60]. Furthermore the amount of iodinated contrast agent needed for CT angiography of the carotid arteries is significantly lower with multidetector scanners than with single-slice spiral CT, and the further increase in speed of new MDCTs will allow use of smaller amounts. Another disadvantage is that, in contrast to US, and catheter and MR angiography, CT angiography cannot provide information about flow velocity.

It is difficult to determine which will be the role of MDCT angiography as compared to contrast-enhanced MRA. Although the latter presents several advantages, such as the use of nonionizing radiations and nonnephrotoxic contrast agent [61], it must be considered that MDCT has, at least at the moment (but rapid improvements are expected also in this area), superior spatial resolution as compared to MRA, and the diffusion of MDCT scanners is increasing faster than that of high field-strength MR equipment with powerful gradients, and all software and hardware capabilities to perform optimal MRA of the entire supra-aortic vessels. Furthermore the ease with which the morphology and composition of the plaque are evaluated appears particularly useful now that more and more endovascular treatment is performed in these patients. MDCT angiography of the carotid arteries is very accurate and reproducible and has the potential to substitute in most cases for catheter-based DSA.

References

1. Robins M, Baum H (1981) National survey of stroke: incidence. Stroke 12:45–57
2. Barnett HJ, Taylor DW, Eliasziw M et al. (1998) Benefit of carotid endoarterectomy in patients with symptomatic moderate or severe stenosis. North American Symptomatic Carotid Endoarterectomy Trial Collaborators (comments). N Engl J Med 339:1415–1425
3. European Carotid Surgery Trialists' Collaborative Group (1991)

4. European Carotid Surgery Trialists' Collaborative Group (1998)5. Taylor et al. (1991)
5. Taylor DC (1991). Duplex Ultrasound in the assessment of vascular disease in clinical Hypertension. Am J Hypertens, 4: 550-6
6. Estol C, Claasen D Hirsch W, Wechsler L, Mossy J (1991). Correlative angiographic and pathologic findings in the diagnosis of ulcerated plaque in the carotid artery. Arch Neurol. 48: 692-4
7. Ricotta JJ, Schenk ED, Ekholm SE, De Weese JA (1986). Angiographic and pathologic correlates in carotid artery disease. Surgery 99: 284-92.
8. North American Symptomatic Carotid Endoarterectomy Trial Collaborators (1991) Beneficial effect of carotid endarterectomy in symptomatic patients with high grade stenosis. N Engl J Med 325:445–453
9. Executive Committee for the Asymptomatic Carotid Atherosclerosis Study (1995)
10. Streifler JY, Eliaszwiw M, Fox AJ, Benavente OR, Hachinsky VC, Ferguson GG, Barnett HJ (1994). Angiographic detection of carotid plaque ulceration. Comparison with surgical observation in a multicenter study. North American Symptomatic carotid endoarterectomy Trial. Stroke, 25: 1130-1132.
11. Rothwell PM, Pendlebury ST, Wardlaw J, Warlow CP (2000). Critical appraisal of the design and reporting of studies of imaging and measurement of carotid stenosis. Stroke 31: 1144-50.
12. Carr S, Farb A, Pearce W, Virmani R, Yao J (1996) Atherosclerotic plaque rupture in symptomatic carotid artery stenosis. J Vasc Surg 23:755–766
13. Seeger J, Barratt E, Lawson G, Klingman N (1995) The relationship between carotid plaque composition, plaque morphology, and neurological symptoms. J Surg Res 58:330–336
14. Longstreth WT Jr, Shemansky L, Lefkowitz D, O'Learly DH, Polak SF, Wolfson SK Jr (1998). Asymptomatic internal carotid artery stenosis defined by ultrasound and the risk of subsequent stroke in the elderly. The cardiovascular health study. Stroke 29: 2371-6.
15. Golledge J, Greenhalgh R, Davies A (2000) The symptomatic carotid plaque. Stroke 31:774–781
16. Eliasziw M, Streifler JY, Fox AJ Hachiniski VC, Ferguson GG, Barnett HJM (1994) Significance of plaque ulceration in symptomatic patients with high-grade carotid stenosis. Stroke 25:304–308
17. Hatsukamy TS, Ferguson MS, Beach KW, Gordon D, Detmer P, Burns D, Alpers C, Strandness DE Jr (1997). Carotid plaque morphology and clinical event. Stroke 28: 95-100.
18. Bladin CF, Alexandrov AV, Murphy S, Maggisano R, Norris JW (1995). A new method of measuring internal carotid artery stenosis. Stroke 26: 230-4.
19. Rothwell PM, Gibson RJ, Slattery J, Sellar RJ, Warlow CP, for the European Carotid Surgery Trialists' Collaborative Group (1994) Equivalence of measurements of carotid stenosis: a comparison of three methods on 1001 angiograms. Stroke 25:2435–2439
20. Davies KN, Humphrey PR (1993). Complications of cerebral angiography in patients with symptomatic carotid territory ischaemia screened by carotid ultrasound. J Neurol Neurosurg Psychiatry 56: 967-72
21. Cinat M, Lane CT, Pham H, Lee A, Wilson SE, Gordon I (1998) Helical CT angiography in the preoperative evaluation of carotid artery stenosis. J Vasc Surg 28:290–297
22. Kaatee R, Beek FJ, de Lange EE et al. (1997) Renal artery stenosis: detection and quantification with spiral CT angiography versus optimized digital subtraction angiography. Radiology 205:121–127
23. Van Hoe L, Baert AL, Gryspeerdt S et al. (1996) Supra- and juxtarenal aneurysms of the abdominal aorta: preoperative assessment with thin section spiral CT. Radiology 198:443–448
24. Cumming MJ, Morrow IM (1994). Carotid artery stenosis: a prospective comparison of CT angiography and conventional angiography. AJR Am J Roentgenol 163: 517-23.
25. Leclerc X, Godefroy O, Pruvo JP, Leys D (1995) Computed tomography angiography for the evaluation of carotid artery stenosis. Stroke 26:1577–1581
26. Schwartz RB, Jones KM, Chernoff DM, Mukherji SK, Khorasani R, Tice HM, Kikinis R, Hooton SM, Stieg PE (1992). Common carotid artery bifurcation: evaluation with spiral CT. Work in progress. Radiology 185: 435-9.
27. Castillo M (1993). Diagnosis of disease of the common carotid artery bifurcation: CT angiography vs catheter angiography. AJR Am J Roengenol 161: 395-8.
28. Dillon EH, Van Leeuwen MS, Fernandez MA, Eikelboom BC Mali WP (1993). CT angiography: application to the evaluation of carotid artery stenosis. Radiology 189: 211-9.
29. Hu H (1999) Multi-slice helical CT: scan and reconstruction. Med Phys 6:5–18
30. Klingenbeck-Regn K, Schaller S, Flohr T, et al. (1999) Subsecond multislice computed tomography: basics and applications. Eur J Radiol 31:110–124
31. Rubin GD, Shiau MC, Leung AN, Kee ST, Logan LJ, Sofilos MC (2000) Aorta and iliac arteries: single versus multiple detector-row helical CT angiography. Radiology 215:670–676
32. Ertl-Wagner B, Hoffmann RT, Bruning R, Dichgans M, Reiser MF (2002) Diagnostic evaluation of the craniocervical vascular system with a 16-slice multi-detector row spiral CT. Protocols and first experiences. Radiologe 42:728–732
33. Lell M, Wildberger JE, Heuschmid M, Flohr T, Stierstorfer K, Fellner FA, Lang W, Bautz WA, Baum U (2002) CT-angiography of the carotid artery: first results with a novel 16-slice-spiral-CT scanner. Rofo Fortschr Geb Rontgenstr Neuen Bildgeb Verfahr 174:1165–1169
34. Chang YJ, Golby AJ, Albers GW (1995) Detection of carotid stenosis. From NASCET results to clinical practice. Stroke 26:1325–1328
35. Chang YJ, Golby AJ, Albers GW (1995). Detection of carotid artery stenosis. From NASCET results to clinical practice. Stroke 26: 1325-8.
36. Rothwell PM, Gibson RJ, Slattery J, Warlow CP, for the European Carotid Surgery Trialists' Collaborative Group (1994) Prognostic value and reproducibility of measurements of carotid stenosis: a comparison of three methods on 1001 angiograms. Stroke 25:2440–2444
37. Williams MA, Nicoliades AN (1987) Predicting the normal dimension of the internal and external carotid arteries form the diameter of the common carotid. Eur J Vasc Surg 1:91–96
38. Alexandrov AV, Bladin CF, Maggisano R, Norris JW (1993)

Measuring carotid stenosis. Time for reappraisal. Stroke 24:1292–1296

39. Staikov IN, Arnold M, Mattle HP, et al. (2000) Comparison of the ECST, CC and NASCET grading methods and ultrasound for assessing carotid stenosis. J Neurol 247:681–686
40. Randoux B, Marro B, Koskas F, Duyme M, Sahel M, Zouaoui A, Marsalt C (2001). Carotid artery stenosis : prospective comparison of CT, Three-dimensional gadolinium enhanced MR and conventional angiography. Radiology 220: 179-85.
41. Chen CJ, Lee TH, Hsu HL, et al. (2004) Multi-slice CT angiography in diagnosing total versus near occlusions of the internal carotid artery: comparison with catheter angiography. Stroke 35:83–85
42. CASANOVA Study Group (1991) Carotid surgery versus medical therapy in asymptomatic carotid stenosis. Stroke 22:1229–1235
43. Gronholdt M (1999) Ultrasound and lipoproteins as predictors of lipid-rich, rupture prone plaques in the carotid artery. Arterioscler Thromb Vasc Biol 19:2–13
44. Anderson GB, Ashfort R, Steinke DE, Ferdinandy R, Findlay JM (2000) CT angiography for the detection and characterization of carotid artery bifurcation disease. Stroke 31:2168–2174
45. Estes JM, Quist WC, Lo Gerfo FW, Costello P (1998) Noninvasive characterization of plaque morhology using helical computed tomography. J Cardiovasc Surg 39:527–534
46. Oliver TB, Lammie GA, Wright AR, et al. (1999) Atherosclerotic plaque at the carotid bifurcation: CT angiographic apperance with histopathologic correlation. Am J Neuroradiol 20:897–901
47. Walker LJ, Ismail A, Mc Meekin W, Lambert D, Mendelow DA, Birchall D (2002). Computed Tomography Angiography for the evaluation of carotid atherosclerotic plaque: correlation with hystopatology of endoarterectomy specimens. Stroke 33: 977-98.
48. Bogousslavsky J, Pierre P (1992). Ischemic stroke in patient under age 45. Neurol Clin 10: 113-24.
49. Houser OW, Mokri B, Sundt TM, Baker HL Jr, Reese DF (1984). Spontaneous cervical cephalic arterial dissection and its residuum: angiographic spectrum. AJNR Am J Neuroradiol 5: 27-34.
50. Bousson V, Levy C, Brunereau L, Djoury H, Tubiana JM (1999). Dissection of the internal carotid artery: Three dimensional Time-of-flight MR angiography and MR imaging features. AJR Am J Roentgenol 173: 139-43.
51. Heiserman JE, Drayer BP, Fram EK, Keller PJ (1992). MR angiography of cervical fibromuscolar displasia. AJNR Am J Neuroradiol 13: 1457-61
52. Wagner AL (2001). Isolated stenosis of a persistent hypoglossal artery visualized at 3D CT Angiography. AJNR Am J Neuroradiol 22: 1613-4.
53. Silverberg GD, Britt RH, Goffinet DR (1978). Radiation-induced carotid artery disease. Cancer jan 41: 130-7
54. Elerding SC, Fernandez RN, Grotta JC, Lindberg RD, Causay LC, Mc Murtrey A (1981). Carotid artery disease following external cervical irradiation. Ann Surg 194: 609-15.
55. Roubin GS, New G, Iyer SS, et al. (2001) Immediate and late clinical outcomes of carotid artery stenting in patients with symptomatic and asymptomatic carotid artery stenosis. A 5-year prospective analysis. Circulation 103:532–537
56. Hollingworth W, Nathens AB, Kanne JP, et al. (2003) The diagnostic accuracy of computed tomography angiography for traumatic or atherosclerotic lesions of the carotid and vertebral arteries: a systematic review. Eur J Radiol 48:88–102
57. Sameshima T, Futami S, Morita Y, Yokogami K, Miyahara S, Sameshima Y, Goya T, Wakisaka S (1999). Clinical usefulness of and problems with three dimensional CT angiography for the evaluation of arteriosclerotic stenosis of the carotid artery: comparison with conventional angiography, MRA and ultrasound sonography. Surg Neurol 51: 301-9.
58. Katz DS, Hon M (2001) CT angiography of the lower extremities and aortoiliac system with a multi-detector row helical CT scanner: promise of new opportunities fulfilled. Radiology 221:7–10
59. Macari MJ, Bini E, Milano A, et al. (2001) Low-dose CT colonography in colorectal polyp detection. Radiology 221:403
60. Lorusso V, Taroni P, Alvino S, Spinazzi A (2001) Pharmacokinetics and safety of Iomeprol in healthy volunteers and in patients with renal impairment or end-stage renal disease requiring hemodialysis. Invest Radiol 36:309–316
61. Rofsky NM, Adelman MA (2000) MR angiography in the evaluation of atherosclerotic peripheral vascular disease. Radiology 214:325–338
62. Barnett HJM, Warlow CP (1995) Carotid endoarterectomy and the measurement of stenosis. Stroke 24:1281–1284
63. Rubin GD, Schmidt AJ, Logan LJ, Sofilos MC (2001) Multidetector row CT angiography of lower extremity arterial inflow and runoff: initial experience. Radiology 221:146–158

7 Thoracic Aorta

Michael D. Dake, Jeffrey C. Hellinger, and Jonathan M. Levin

CONTENTS

7.1 Introduction

The introduction of 16-channel multidetector-row computed tomography (MDCT) has made a tremendous impact upon the diagnosis and treatment of diseases of the thoracic aorta. At the current spatial and temporal resolution offered by MDCT, there are very few indications for conventional diagnostic angiography. CT angiography (CTA) provides an accurate analysis of the vessel lumen, as well as a unique window into the morphological analysis and pathophysiology of vascular disease. This type of information is critical to the surgeon or interventionalist in planning treatment strategies. CT also provides information beyond vessel-wall morphology and pathology, by demonstrating the normal anatomical relationship of mediastinal structures, as well as the extent of disease processes (such as hematoma or tumor invasion) in relationship to the thoracic aorta.

M. D. Dake, MD; J. C. Hellinger, MD; J. M. Levin, MD
Department of Radiology, Stanford University Medical Center, 300 Pasteur Drive, SHS H3647, Stanford, CA 94305-5642, USA

Volumetric CT data acquisition with single-detector-row spiral CT has been in practice for a number of years, but only recently has the implementation of MDCT had a revolutionary impact on the technique of CTA. The advantages of MDCT over single-channel CT include significantly faster image acquisition, allowing for greater axial coverage at a substantially improved *z*-axis resolution. These technological advances have led to near-complete suppression of respiratory and cardiac motion artifacts. With current state-of-the-art, 16-channel MDCT units, we are routinely able to generate all images at submillimeter collimation. Essentially, isotropic imaging becomes the standard rather than the goal. Isotropic volumetric data sets refer to equal spatial resolution as viewed in the *x*-, *y*-, and *z*-dimensions. This subsequently allows for improved quality in multiplanar reformations as well as three- (3D) and four-dimensional (4D) imaging.

7.2 Technique

Performing effective CTA of the thoracic aorta requires a solid understanding of the pathophysiology of vascular disease and a basic understanding of the different approaches to treatment. It is critical to form a general assessment of the patient in relationship to their disease process. There is a fine art to the balance of user-dependent variables (collimation, pitch, table feed, radiation dose) and user-independent variables (heart rate, breath-hold capability, cardiac function, body habitus).

When evaluating user-dependent variables, one must consider the disease process at hand and volume of coverage required to document such pathology. Being that vascular structures tend to be long and "systemic in nature," it is advisable to obtain large volumes of coverage. It is best to begin the scan at the thoracic inlet, allowing for adequate coverage of the supra-aortic vessels. As many diseases of the thoracic aorta extend into the abdomen, it is useful to image caudally through the iliac vessels and groin. This provides additional information for the interventionalist contemplating an endovascular procedure [1, 2]. There are certain exceptions where limiting scan coverage to only the thoracic aorta is recommended; these include follow-up scans where the anatomy of the abdomen and pelvis has already been documented. In addition, it is always advisable to limit the radiation dose whenever possible, particularly in children and young adults.

Determining adequate collimation is very important in performing effective CTA. For imaging of most thoracic aortic pathology, 1- to 2-mm collimation with 50% overlap of the reconstructed images offers optimal spatial resolution and the ability to generate fine-detailed multiplanar reformations. Thicker collimation may be useful for faster scanning requirements, such as would occur in acute trauma or in an obese patient where the signal-to-noise ratio (SNR) is the limiting factor in image quality. Maintaining adequate SNR at a reasonable radiation exposure to the patient is the main limiting factor for thin-collimation acquisitions with MDCT. As collimation decreases, there is a substantial increase in patient dose that is required to maintain effective SNR [3]. Another practical limitation of acquiring thin-section data sets involves the postprocessing of such large volumes of data and an effective medium to view these studies.

Pitch is defined as the ratio of the table feed per tube rotation divided by total slice collimation. A larger pitch allows for a faster acquisition and a shorter scan time. In CTA, the pitch selection will range between 1.2 and 1.8, depending on the volume of coverage desired within a specified scan time. Scanning at lower pitch values will produce an overlapping scan pattern with higher image quality, but at the expense of increased radiation exposure to the patient. Overlapping acquisitions are necessary for retrospective ECG-gated acquisitions, which will be addressed subsequently. Scanning at pitches greater than 2 leads to undersampling of the data and is not recommended.

The reconstruction interval is selected independently of the slice collimation. Overlapping reconstruction intervals will increase the number of images that must be interpreted, processed, and stored. However, it is quickly realized that with increasing reconstruction overlap there is more than a theoretical benefit in the quality of multiplanar and 3D reconstructions. For practical purposes, a reconstruction interval of 50% of the section width will provide a more than adequate data set for the interpretation and postprocessing of CTA studies of the thoracic aorta. Larger reconstruction intervals (nonoverlapping reconstruction) waste an important advantage of spiral CT, and small lesions may be missed due to partial volume effects [3]. Obviously, hard-copy interpretation of CTA studies with thin collimation and fine overlapping reconstruction intervals is not practical due to the tremendous number of images generated that are routinely between 600 and 1000 images per study.

Optimizing techniques on the administration of contrast medium in CTA requires a separate chapter. Attention to contrast injection parameters becomes more critical when high-velocity, 16-channel MDCT scanners are used with lower volumes of contrast at faster table feeds. High flow rates are required (typically between 4 and 5 ml/s) via at least a 20-gauge catheter, most conveniently placed in the right antecubital position. In patients with poor venous access, however, we have been able to obtain reasonable results with flow rates of 3 ml/s. It is preferable to achieve access through the right antecubital approach, as it reduces the characteristic streaking artifacts from the left brachiocephalic vein that potentially limits visualization of disease processes affecting the ascending and transverse aorta. With the very short scanning delays used in CTA, we routinely use extravasation detector kits, which substantially reduce the risk of subcutaneous infiltration.

There are many variables involved in determining the ideal scan delay. Most of these are easily manipulated by the user. They include injection rate, contrast volume delivered, and the target region of interest. There are some patient-dependent factors that are not as easy to manipulate, such as heart rate, cardiac output, and body habitus. These factors have traditionally been more difficult to control and have, in the past, required elaborate test bolus injection techniques. With the introduction of bolus-tracking techniques (standard on all commercially available scanners), we are no longer hampered by the variability of these patient-related factors. Bolus-tracking techniques use a monitoring scan (with a substantially reduced dose) at a predefined region of interest to initiate the diagnostic scan when the detection of the contrast bolus has occurred [3]. The user has control over such variables such as monitoring delay (the time at which the monitoring phase begins, typically 8–10 s) and the interscan delay (the time between scans during the monitoring phase, typically 2–5 s). The actual scan will then be triggered by either the user on the basis of enhancement curves or automatically by the scanner on the basis of a predetermined attenuation threshold within the vessel of interest. There is an additional contrast detection to scan delay that occurs between the time contrast has been detected in the vessel at the predefined region of interest (for example at the level of the aortic arch) and the time it takes for the scanner to reset into proper position to begin the actual scan (at the level of the thoracic inlet). This contrast detection to scan time delay varies, and can range anywhere from 3–9 s. If for example there is a greater than 5-s delay, you must take this into account during the monitoring phase and set the enhancement curves or attenuation thresholds lower to account for such delays. An alternative approach is to define the location of the monitoring phase and scan initiation at the same level, therefore eliminating the inherent contrast detection to scan delay. This can potentially decrease the scan time by 5 s and result in a decrease in amount of contrast administered.

There is an important relationship between collimation, pitch, and the patient's capacity for a reasonable breath-hold (reasonable being 45 s). Traditionally, with the use of single- and even 4-channel MDCT, we have been forced to increase the collimation or increase the pitch in order to image the thoracic aorta within a reasonable breath-hold period. For example, with a 4-channel unit, we are limited to scanning the thoracic aorta with 2.5-mm collimation in order to complete the scan within a single breath-hold. However, with current 8- and 16-channel MDCT units, most CTA studies of the thorax with 1-mm collimation can be performed in less than 10 s. CTA of the thorax with ECG gating can be performed in approximately 30 s. In fact, in our practice, we frequently perform an ECG-gated chest CTA immediately followed by a CTA of the abdomen and pelvis, all within a reasonable breath-hold of approximately 45 s (Fig. 7.1).

Currently, at Stanford University, all CTA routine studies of the thoracic aorta are being effectively performed on an 8- or 16-channel MDCT unit. If we plan to perform ECG gating as part of our protocol, then we will routinely use the faster 16-channel MDCT units. Our typical protocol of CTA of the thorax (which varies slightly depending on the vendor-specific scanner being used) includes 1.25-mm collimation, gantry rotation time of 0.4–0.5 s (depending on scan time), table feed of 52–68 mm/s, pitch factor of 1.3–1.7, typical milliampere-seconds of 350, and typical kVp of 120. Reconstruction intervals are typically 50% of the slice collimation. The field of view is variable depending on scan volume, with an image matrix of 512×512 pixels. Contrast dose administration can vary anywhere from 80 to 160 ml of 350 mg/ml of iodinated contrast, depending on the scan time.

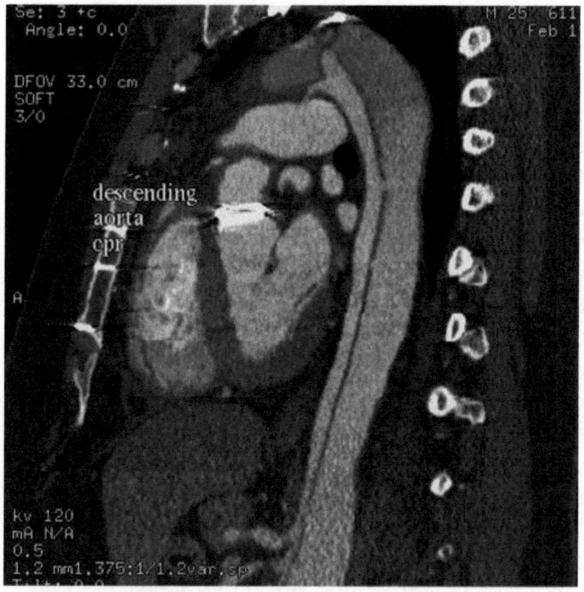

Fig. 7.1 Type B aortic dissection. Gated chest computed tomography angiography performed on a General Electric 16-channel detector and 3D reconstruction on ADV Windows 4.1. Curved planar reformation demonstrates a type B dissection that extends through a patent ductus arteriosus. Patient is also status post-AVR.

For example, a routine CTA limited to the thoracic aorta with an estimated scan time of 10 s on our current 16-slice MDCT will require an estimated contrast dose of approximately 80 ml of 350 mg/ml of iodinated contrast, the goal being to administer an intravenous bolus of contrast medium throughout the duration of the scan. This amount of contrast is calculated based upon the scan time added to contrast detection to scan delay multiplied by the injection rate (usually 4 ml/s).

When performing an ECG-gated study of the thoracic aorta, there are a few variations to our standard protocol. The gated portion of the study will increase the length of the scan by approximately a factor of 3. Obviously, this will necessitate a longer breath-hold, as well as an increase in the contrast dose to cover the longer scan time. Considering a standard 8-channel MDCT that takes 20 s to cover the thorax, adding ECG gating would increase the total scan time to 60 s. A 60-s breath-hold is not realistic for most patient populations. However, with a 16-channel MDCT unit, a nongated CTA of the entire thorax can be performed within a 10-s breath-hold. With ECG-gating, this will increase the scan time to approximately 25–30 s, well within a reasonable breath-hold capacity for most patient populations. Therefore, all ECG-gated studies of the thoracic aorta are effectively performed on a 16-channel MDCT unit.

We are increasingly being asked to perform an ECG-gated study of the thoracic aorta followed by a CTA study of the abdomen and pelvis, as many diseases of the thoracic aorta extend into the aortoiliac vessels. Obviously, it is a challenge to perform a study with such a long scan time within a single breath-hold. The previous generation of MDCT units (4 and 8 channels) simply do not allow for large enough z-axis coverage within a reasonable scan time with our current MDCT scan parameters. Allowing the patient to breath between the two studies would lead to unacceptable respiratory artifacts as well as necessitate the administration of an additional contrast bolus. When optimizing a protocol for such studies, there are many issues to consider. The most important being how one will acquire the entire data set within a single breath-hold. This includes not only the individual scan lengths of the gated chest and abdomen/pelvis components of the study, but also the amount of time it takes for the scanner to reset into proper position during the two scans. Our standard ECG-gated thoracic aorta study on the 16-channel MDCT unit takes approximately 25–30 s. A CTA study of the abdomen and pelvis on the 16-channel MDCT unit takes approximately 10 s. The amount of time it takes for the scanner to reset between the individual scans varies between 5 and 10 s. Therefore, the total scan time of a gated chest followed by abdomen and pelvis CTA can take between 40 and 50 s. Depending upon the volume of coverage, certain parameters may need to be modified to reduce the scan length. A typical gantry rotation time for CTA studies is 0.6 s, but the newer generation of scanners will permit a rotation of 0.4–0.5 s, resulting in a faster scan. Keep in mind that faster gantry rotation times are not always advisable, as there is an increased radiation dose required to maintain image noise at acceptable levels. Additionally, the pitch factor can be increased, which will result in a decreased scan time, but this results in a decrease in overlapping scan pattern, with subsequent loss in image quality. Finally, one may simply choose to reduce the total scan volume.

7.3 ECG Triggering Techniques

There are multiple challenges to obtaining accurate CTA studies of the thoracic aorta. The two most formidable are respiratory artifacts and cardiac pulsation. Respiratory artifacts have been addressed previously. When imaging the thoracic aorta, cardiac pulsation usually only becomes a problem during short segments of systole. ECG-gated techniques have made tremendous strides in improving the motion artifacts caused by cardiac pulsation (Fig. 7.2). The ability to effectively suppress cardiac motion allows for improved visualization of not only the thoracic aorta, but also major branch vessels, including the coronary arteries and supra-aortic vessels. Some of the immediate implications include accurate analysis of the wall of the thoracic aorta and its subsequent disease processes. Additionally, ECG-gated techniques improve evaluation of the proximal coronary arteries and the supra-aortic vessels, as well as their disease processes (Fig. 7.3).

ECG gating to appropriate segments of the diastolic phase, coupled with fine collimation and rotation gantry times less than 0.5 s can provide a temporal resolution approaching 125 ms, and thus effectively eliminate the effects of cardiac pulsation upon the thoracic aorta [4]. There are two fundamentally different methods of cardiac gating, and the intricacies of each technique are far beyond the scope of this chapter.

The first method is prospective cardiac gating. This method allows the user to preselect a gate during the R-R interval that characteristically has the least motion artifacts, such as end-diastole. This usually coincides with anywhere between 40% and 80% of the R-R interval. Acquisition of data will only occur throughout the predefined window of the R-R interval.

Alternatively, the user may retrospectively select a gate during the R-R interval which optimally displays the data with the least pulsation artifacts. In this technique, continuous acquisition of data throughout all phases of the cardiac cycle is obtained, permitting phase selective reconstructions. This requires the use of very low pitch factors and overlapping scan data, with the understanding that radiation dose concerns are sacrificed for image quality. The user subsequently has the option to view all ten phases or only those phases that coincide with end-diastole. There are many advantages to retrospectively gating a CTA of the chest. The most obvious advantage is that the user has acquired all of the data throughout the R-R interval and has the flexibility to view the phase of the cardiac cycle with the least cardiac pulsation artifacts [4]. Additional advantages are realized at the workstation, where the user can reconstruct data from all consecutive phases of the cardiac cycle to

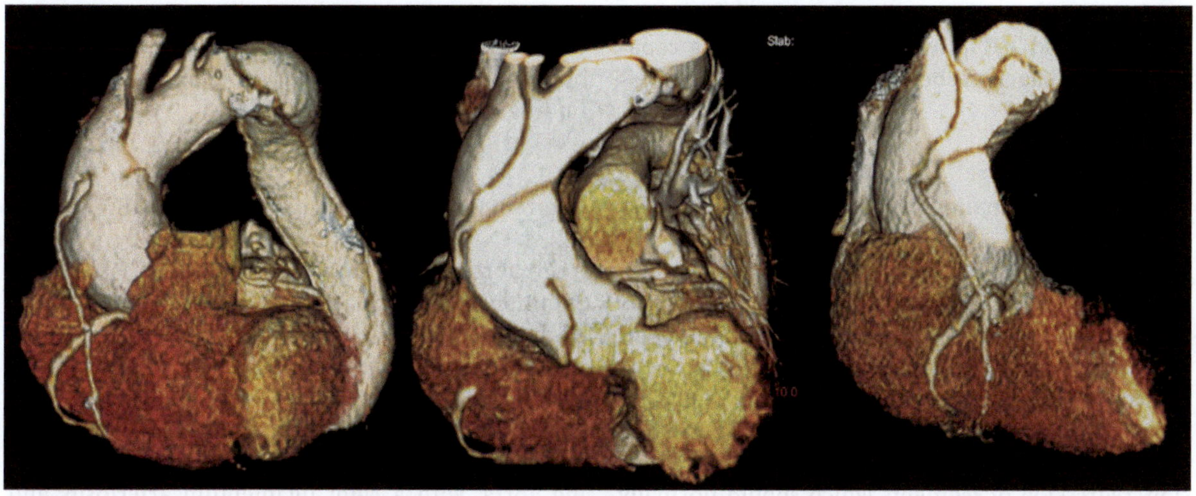

Fig. 7.2 Type A aortic dissection. Gated chest computed tomography angiography performed on a GE 16-channel detector, images reconstructed at 10% intervals throughout cardiac cycle. 3D reconstructions performed on a TeraRecon workstation. Patient is status post-right coronary artery saphenous venous bypass graft. At subsequent coronary angiography, there was a resultant type A dissection which extends into the right coronary artery bypass graft as well as caudally toward the aortic annulus. Operative findings correlate with the radiographic report.

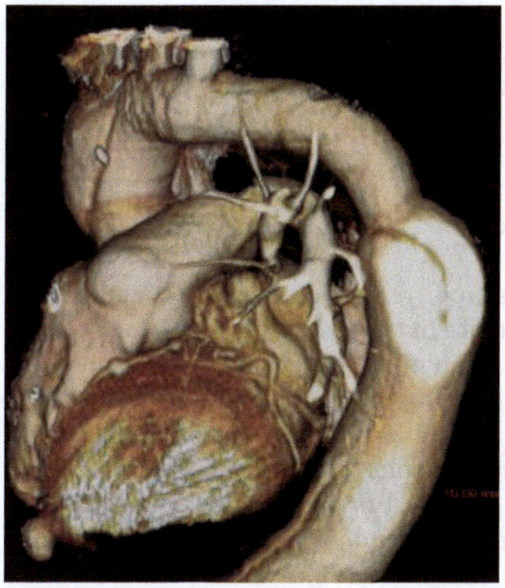

Fig. 7.3 Patient with Marfan's syndrome who underwent elephant trunk procedure. Multidetector-row CT demonstrates residual type A dissection extending into brachiocephalic artery. Also, incidental note is made of tandem aneurysms of the left anterior descending coronary artery as well as focal outpouching of the left ventricular apex consistent with pseudoaneurysm formation s/p iatrogenic left ventricular cannulation at time of aortic repair.

demonstrate real-time imaging [5]. This allows for accurate evaluation of the mechanics of aortic wall and cardiac valvular motion [6]. The major disadvantage to retrospective gating is the necessary increase in radiation dose.

7.4 Four-Dimensional Cine Imaging

ECG-gated 4D real-time imaging affords us our first opportunity at evaluating the mechanics of aortic wall and aortic valvular motion [7]. The four dimensions refer to the three spatial axes resolved by the time axis. In essence, we have now moved from routine volumetric imaging to *dynamic time-resolved* volumetric imaging of the thoracic aorta and the aortic valve. 4D imaging consists of reconstructing a 3D, retrospectively ECG-gated volumetric data set into a predetermined number of cardiac phases based upon a set trigger point in the R-R interval. Each data set corresponds to a specific phase of the cardiac cycle, and all phases are reconstructed at the same speed, corresponding to the original heart rate. 4D imaging capabilities, currently only available on selected workstations, allow the user to interpret 3D volumetric sets based upon multiphase data. Applying this technology to imaging of the thoracic aorta has many important utilities. We currently use 4D imaging to evaluate for aortic valve motion as well as for competency of prosthetic aortic valves. With 4D imaging we have been able to visualize a real-time assessment of the motion of aortic dissection flaps and their relationship to the coronary and supra-aortic vessels. We have also been able to evaluate the hyperkinetic wall motion of the thoracic aorta commonly seen in Marfan's patients at the level of the sinotubular junction.

The following sections illustrate clinical applications where MDCT provides unique imaging capabilities and diagnostic benefits.

7.4.1 Congenital Anomalies

Aortic arch and branch vessels, as well as the pulmonary arteries, develop during the first 4–8 weeks of gestation through a series of transformations involving the embryological paired aortic arches, dorsal aortae, and 7th intersegmental arteries. This involves differential regression and then growth of persisting tissue. Anomalies result from failure of normal regression, regression of segments which should normally persist, or combinations thereof [8]. Traditionally, anomalies have been investigated with digital subtraction angiography. CTA, however, is an alternative noninvasive means to obtain the same structural information. With superior spatial resolution, faster scanning to allow acquisitions of the chest in a single breath-hold, and the ability for cardiac synchronization with ECG-gating, MDCT has become an excellent modality to detect and depict congenital thoracic aortic anomalies. Isotropic data sets provide robust 3D displays, allowing integration from any projection of potentially complex structural morphology. Axial transverse source images in turn provide high definition of the aortic wall. Acquiring MDCT source images with decreased motion artifacts not only benefits assessment of vascular structures, but also aids in the assessment of nonvascular structures, which are crucial interpretive elements for complete evaluation of congenital heart disorders and thoracic anomalies.

As thin-section high-resolution technique becomes the standard for routine thoracic aortic CTA, knowledge of the congenital aortic arch anomalies is important for the cardiovascular imager. In adults, findings may be incidental, but identification and correct interpretation is essential. In both children and adults, one will now be asked to exclude an anomaly as a cause for clinical symptoms (i.e., respiratory difficulty, hypertension). Once an anomaly is identified, search should be made for any associated congenital heart disease (CHD). The purpose of this section, therefore, is to offer an overview of common thoracic aortic anomalies, including left aortic arch with an aberrant right subclavian artery (RSCA); right aortic arch with either mirror-image branching or an aberrant left subclavian artery (LSCA); double arch; coarctation; and pseudocoarctation. The rare cervical aortic arch will also be discussed. Finally, although not considered an arch anomaly, patent ductus arteriosus (PDA) will be discussed here, given its embryological arch origin and also the occasional PDA finding on routine thoracic CTA.

7.4.1.1 Aberrant Right Subclavian Artery

A left aortic arch with an aberrant RSCA is the most common aortic arch anomaly, occurring in 0.4–2.3% of the population [9]. The RSCA arises distal to the LSCA as the last branch off the arch. The aberrant vessel courses retroesophageal, obliquely and superiorly, left to right (Fig. 7.4). Three variations exist: with a left ligamentum arteriosus and left-sided descending aorta, with a right ligamentum arteriosus and left-sided descending aorta, and with a right ligamentum arteriosus and right-sided descending aorta. All may be associated with origin dilatation, known as a diverticulum of Kommerall [10].

An aberrant RSCA usually is asymptomatic. Rarely, extrinsic tracheal and esophageal compression may occur from either (1) ectatic and aneurysmal caliber or (2) vascular ring formation with a right ligamentum arteriosum. In these instances, symptoms include stridor, dyspnea, and dysphagia.

7.4.1.2 Right Aortic Arch

This results from regression of the left aortic arch with persistence of the right arch, occurring in up to 0.2% of the population [10, 11]. Regression, however, is not uniform, providing two types of right aortic arches: (1) without a retroesophageal segment, and (2) with a retroesophageal segment. The former has mirror-image vessel branching, typically with a right ligamentum arteriosum, and is a counterpart to a normal left aortic arch (Fig. 7.5). It is more common in the pediatric population, given the high association with CHD (up to 98%). Most commonly, associated CHD includes truncus arteriosus, tetralogy of Fallot, ventricular septal defect with pulmonary atresia, double-outlet right ventricle, and transposition of the great arteries (TGA) [10, 11].

Right aortic arch with a retroesophageal segment has an aberrant LSCA and is the counterpart to the left aortic arch with aberrant RSCA. It is most commonly seen in adults, with only 12% having associated CHD (tetralogy of Fallot, septal defects, and coarctation) [11]. Those without CHD are usually asymptomatic. However, a vascular ring may form if there is a left ligamentum arteriosum [10].

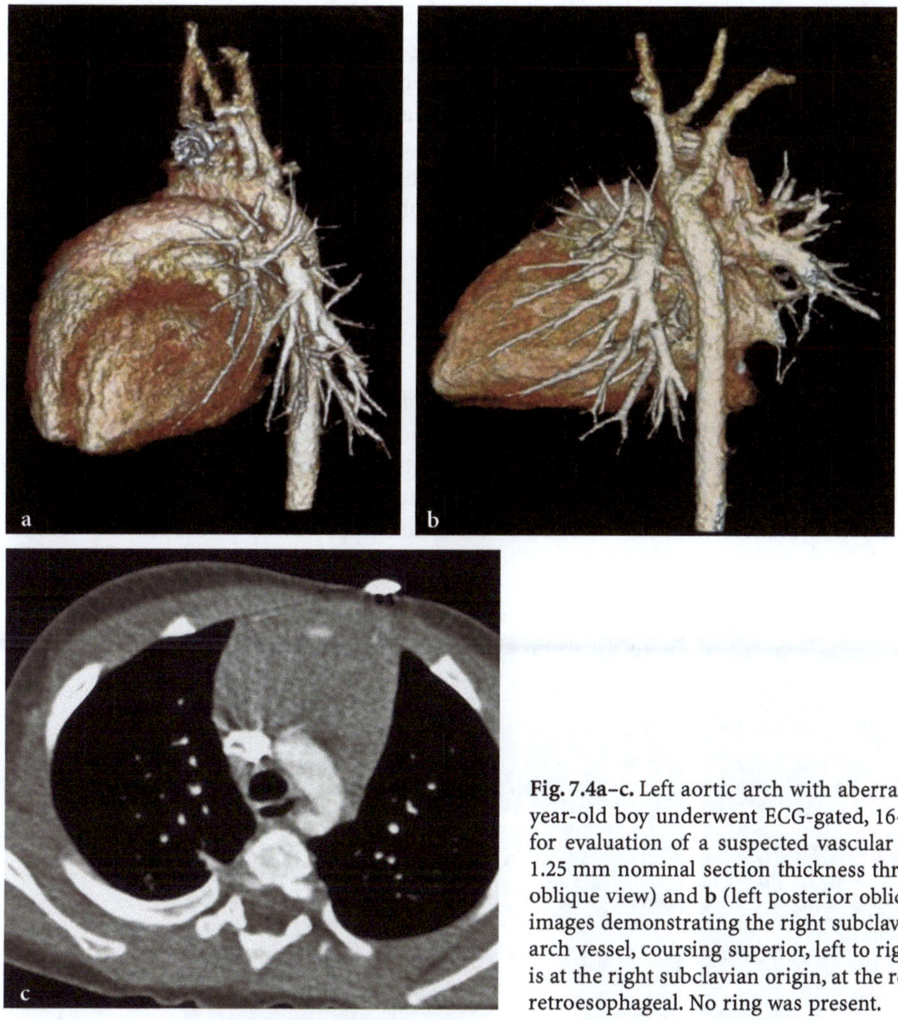

Fig. 7.4a–c. Left aortic arch with aberrant right subclavian artery. A 2-year-old boy underwent ECG-gated, 16-channel multidetector-row CT for evaluation of a suspected vascular ring. Images were acquired at 1.25 mm nominal section thickness through the chest. **a** (left anterior oblique view) and **b** (left posterior oblique view) are volume-rendered images demonstrating the right subclavian arising as the fourth aortic arch vessel, coursing superior, left to right. The axial source image in **c** is at the right subclavian origin, at the region where it begins to course retroesophageal. No ring was present.

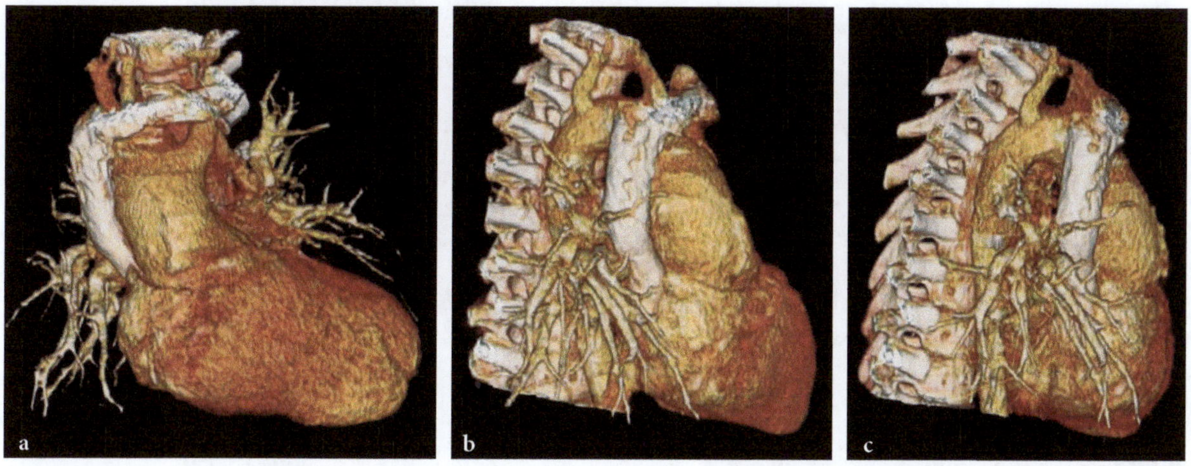

Fig. 7.5a–c. Right aortic arch with mirror-image branching. To evaluate postsurgical repair morphology in a 3-year-old boy with tetralogy of Fallot, 0.625-mm retrospectively gated images were acquired through the chest using 16-row multidetector-row CT . High-resolution volume-rendered images confirm a right aortic arch with mirror-image branching. The left brachiocephalic artery arises first, followed by the right common carotid and subclavian arteries. Note the uplifted cardiac apex, characteristic of tetralogy of Fallot.

7.4.1.3 Double Arch

A double aortic arch results from failure of right or left aortic arch involution, occurring in up to 0.3% of the population [12]. The arches arise from the aortic root and then join to form a single descending thoracic aorta, which most commonly is left sided (Fig. 7.6). The ligamentum arteriosum may connect to either arch.

In a double arch, the right arch is usually larger in size and superior in location than the left arch. The right arch passes posterior to the esophagus, while the left arch courses anterior to the trachea. In some instances, the anterior arch may have an atretic segment. Common carotid and subclavian arteries arise symmetrically from the respective arches, with the carotid arteries anterior and the subclavian arteries posterior in origin [10].

The double arch is the most common cause of a complete vascular ring, with both arches encircling the trachea and esophagus. Depending on the severity of constriction, stridor, dyspnea, recurrent pneumonia, and dysphagia may ensue. Associated CHD is rare [10, 12].

7.4.1.4 Coarctation

Coarctation is defined by narrowing of the aorta in the region of the ductus or ligamentum arteriosum. It is subdivided into two types: preductal and postductal.

In the preductal type, also known as infantile form, constriction is proximal to the ductus and is

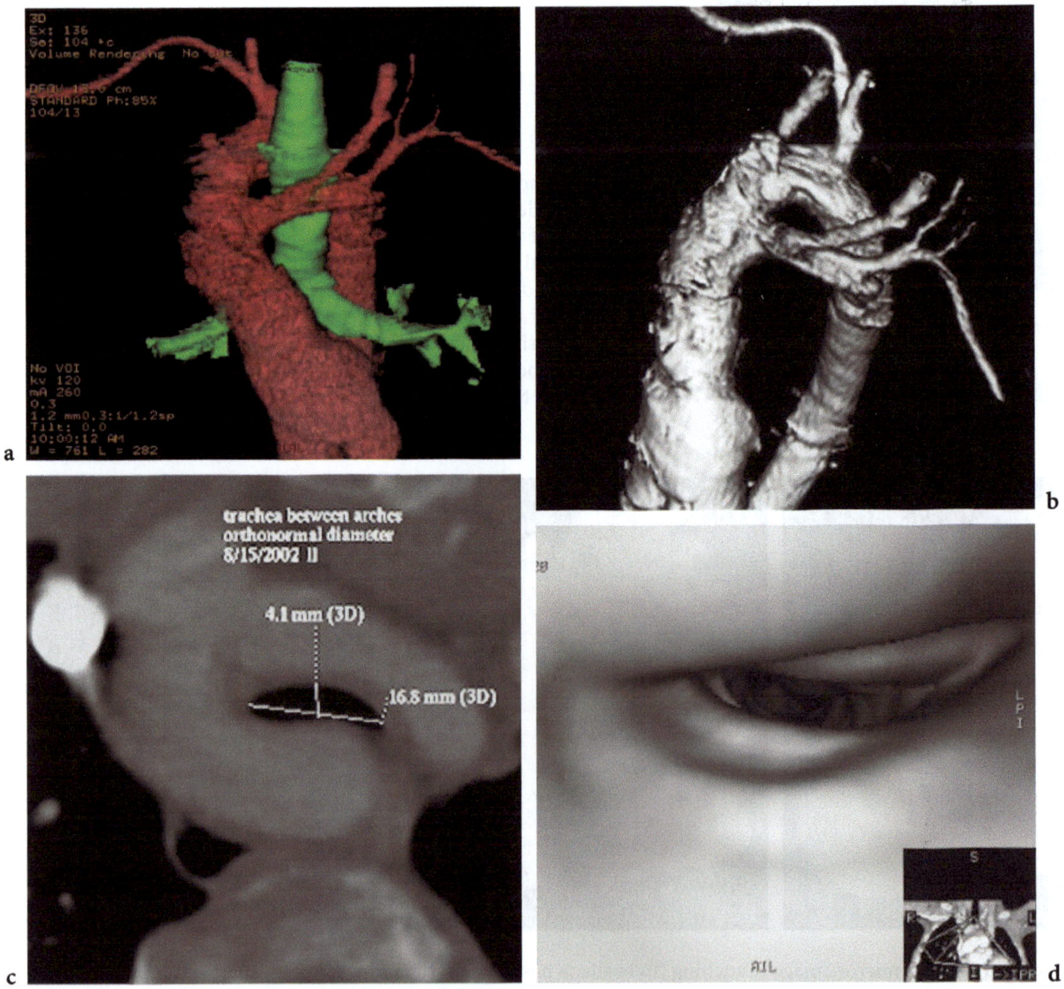

Fig. 7.6a–d. Double arch. Experiencing respiratory difficulties, a 6-year-old boy underwent retrospectively ECG-gated 16-channel multidetector-row CT with 1.25-mm nominal section thickness. **a** and **b** confirm a double arch with a complete ring. This results in tracheal narrowing, as demonstrated by the source images and also the virtual endobronchoscopy (**c** and **d**).

associated with tubular hypoplasia of the aortic arch distal to the brachiocephalic artery. The ductus arteriosum often remains patent (PDA) and there is high CHD association. Bicuspid aortic valve, ventricular septal defect (VSD), hypoplastic left heart, and TGA are most common. The diffuse arch involvement commonly results in significant left ventricular (LV) afterload. This leads to neonatal LV dysfunction, LV dilatation, congestive heart failure, and dependence for LV decompression and systemic perfusion on both the VSD and PDA [10].

In the postductal type, localized constriction is present just distal to the ductus arteriosum. The ductus arteriosum often closes and CHD is less common. Presentation usually is in adults, but may be in neonates and older children. Clinical findings include claudication, hypertension, and differential extremity blood pressure. An aberrant RSCA artery will result in decreased right upper-extremity systolic blood pressure, relative to the left.

CTA findings reflect not only the aortic constriction, but also the physiological response to the coarctation. A search should be made for a collateral network involving internal mammary, thyrocervical, scapular, intraspinal, and intercostal arteries that directs blood from the high-pressure aorta above the constriction to the low-pressure aorta below the constriction. Attention should also be made toward identifying CHD, LV hypertrophy (response to afterload resistance), and inferior rib scalloping with sclerosis (response to enlarged, pulsatile intercostal arteries).

7.4.1.5 Pseudocoarctation

Pseudocoarctation is defined as an asymptomatic localized buckling at the level of the ligamentum arteriosum, resulting from thoracic aorta elongation and redundancy (Fig. 7.7) [13]. Unlike coarctation, in pseudocoarctation, there are no hemodynamic

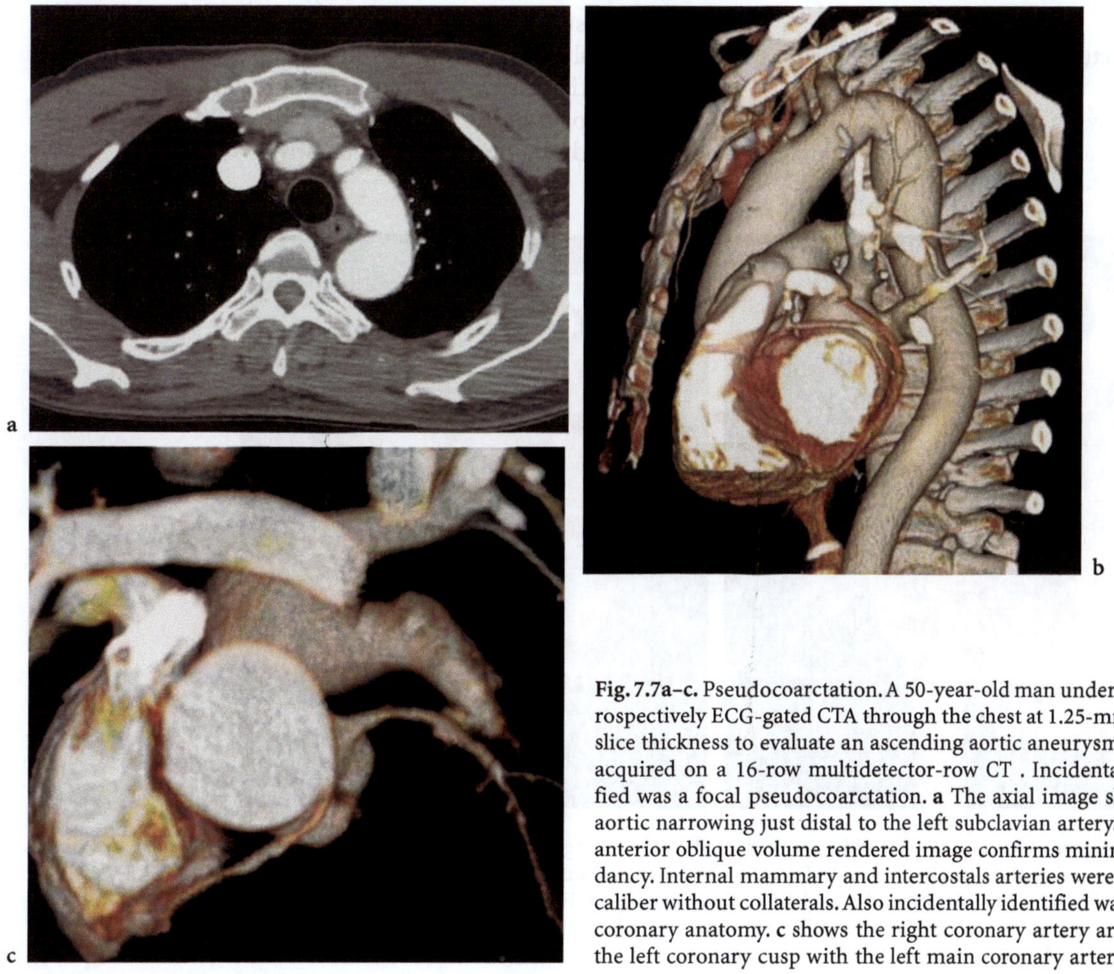

Fig. 7.7a–c. Pseudocoarctation. A 50-year-old man underwent a retrospectively ECG-gated CTA through the chest at 1.25-mm nominal slice thickness to evaluate an ascending aortic aneurysm. Data was acquired on a 16-row multidetector-row CT . Incidentally identified was a focal pseudocoarctation. **a** The axial image shows focal aortic narrowing just distal to the left subclavian artery. **b** The left anterior oblique volume rendered image confirms minimal redundancy. Internal mammary and intercostals arteries were normal in caliber without collaterals. Also incidentally identified was aberrant coronary anatomy. **c** shows the right coronary artery arising from the left coronary cusp with the left main coronary artery.

changes. Upper- and lower-extremity blood pressures are symmetrically normal, there is no collateral network, and inferior ribs show no scalloping or sclerosis. Similar to coarctation, there is a slightly increased prevalence of CHD, including PDA, VSD, and bicuspid aortic valve [14].

7.4.1.6 Cervical Arch

Cervical arch is a rare congenital anomaly, with the transverse aorta extending into the neck (Fig. 7.8). Haughton classified cervical aortic arches into five types (types A–E), based on aortic configuration, brachiocephalic branching, and embryogenesis [15]. Association with aneurysm formation is not uncommon, particularly in a type D. Proposed etiologies for this include embryological development, abnormal connective tissue, altered hemodynamics and aortic wall stress, and trauma [16]. Depending on the type and presence of an aneurysm, patients may present with a pain, dysphagia, and/or a pulsatile mass.

7.4.1.7 Patent Ductus Arteriosum

A PDA may be easily overlooked. With situs solitus and a left aortic arch, the PDA communicates between the left pulmonary artery and inferior aspect of the distal transverse and proximal descending thoracic aorta, opposite the LSCA origin. If identified, a search should be made for other congenital heart and aorta anomalies.

7.4.2 Intervention

Indications for thoracic aorta surgical or endovascular repair include aneurysms, dissection, penetrating atherosclerotic ulcers, intramural hematoma, traumatic aortic injury, and coarctation. With the ability to assess vessel wall morphology, vascular calcifications, perivascular disease, and vessel relationships with adjacent bone and soft tissue, similar to its role in planning surgical and endovascular interventions, MDCT angiography is paramount in assessment of the thoracic aorta postintervention. With regard to image display, while MDCT 3D postprocessing (MPR, CPR, MIP, VR) provides invaluable understanding of the reconstructed anatomy, the greatest advance in postintervention CTA has been ECG gating with 4D real-time imaging. Cardiac motion artifact is reduced; native and reimplanted coronary arteries as well as bypass grafts can be evaluated; and valve structure and function can be qualitatively examined.

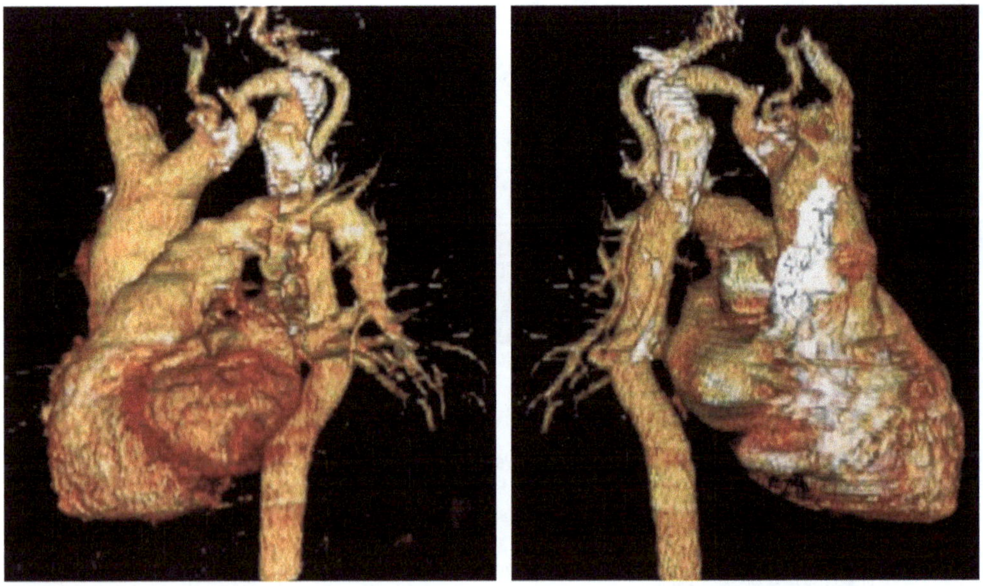

a b

Fig. 7.8a,b. Cervical arch. A 67-year-old man presented to the emergency department with chest pain. To evaluate for acute aortic syndrome, routine 16-channel multidetector-row CT angiography was performed at 1.25-mm nominal thickness with a gantry speed of 0.6 s per rotation and a pitch of 1.375. Although no dissection, penetrating atherosclerotic ulcer, or intramural hematoma was present, images identified atherosclerosis with a left cervical arch. Note the hypoplastic appearance of the cervical transverse arch with normal ordered arrangement of the supra-arch vessels.

The primary interpretive goals of MDCT angiography postintervention, whether by surgical or endovascular means, include: identifying complications; confirming luminal patency (native aorta, graft, endograft); confirming aneurysm exclusion (inclusion grafts or stent grafts); and providing disease surveillance. Since patients with repaired dissection or aneurysm may have underlying connective tissue disorders, the immediate postintervention study serves as a baseline for subsequent studies – these patients are at risk for future aneurysmal dilatation, dissection progression, and/or new dissection. Recognition of the normal postsurgical and postendovascular thoracic aorta facilitates the postintervention diagnoses.

7.4.2.1 Surgical

Surgical options for the thoracic aorta include interposition and inclusion grafts. The interposition technique, as applied to the ascending aorta and aortic arch, involves excision of the diseased segment and then graft replacement with an end-to-end anastomosis (Fig. 7.9). The inclusion technique involves aortotomy, graft insertion, and wrapping the diseased aorta around the graft, resulting in a potential space, which affords graft protection.

When an ascending aorta aneurysm or dissection extends into the aortic root, additional steps

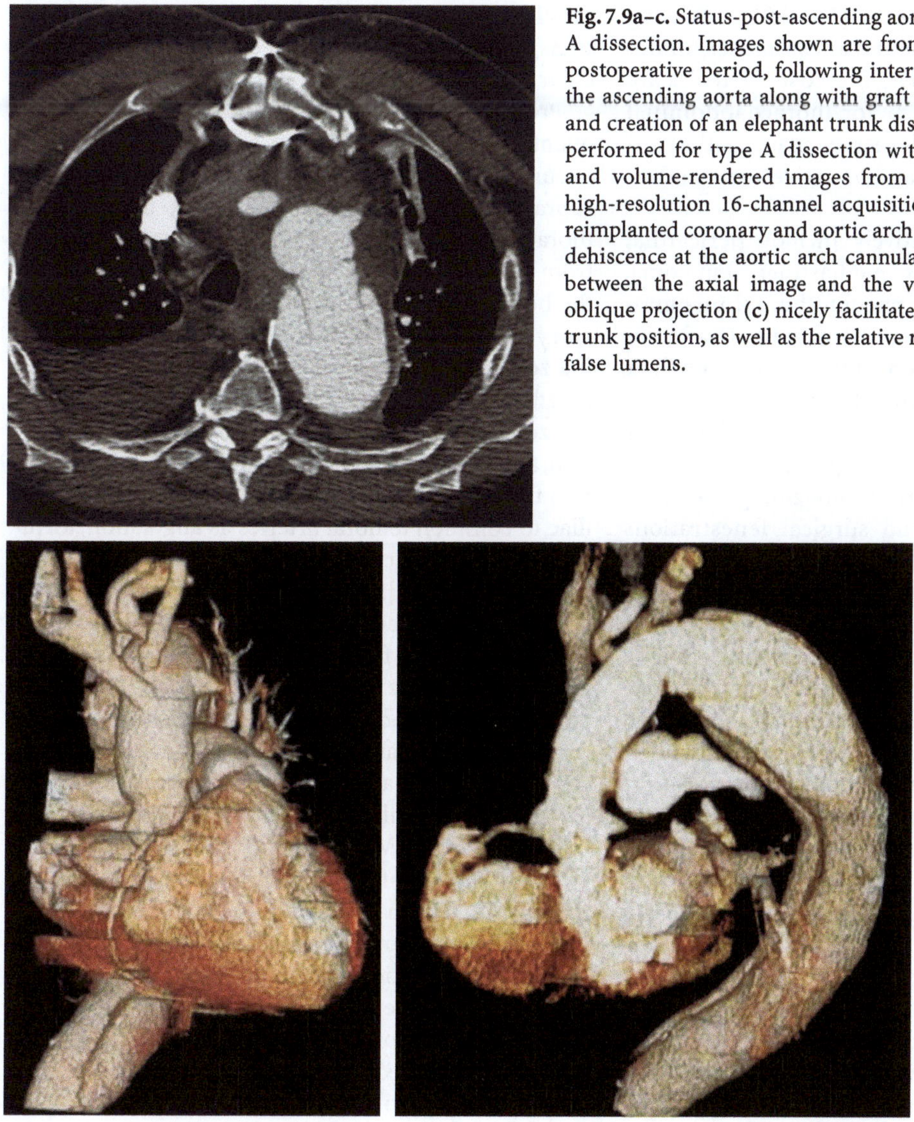

a b c

Fig. 7.9a–c. Status-post-ascending aorta interposition graft for type A dissection. Images shown are from a patient in the immediate postoperative period, following interposition graft replacement of the ascending aorta along with graft repair of the transverse aorta and creation of an elephant trunk distally. Operative treatment was performed for type A dissection with aneurysm formation. Axial and volume-rendered images from a retrospectively ECG-gated, high-resolution 16-channel acquisition identify patent grafts and reimplanted coronary and aortic arch vessels, with a focal contained dehiscence at the aortic arch cannulation site (*arrow*). Correlation between the axial image and the volume-rendered left anterior oblique projection (c) nicely facilitates appreciation of the elephant trunk position, as well as the relative relations between the true and false lumens.

to graft replacement include either resuspension of the aortic valve or prosthetic valve replacement (Bentall composite graft procedure), both with coronary artery reimplantation. If the coronary arteries cannot be reimplanted, vein bypass grafts are the option of choice. The grafts may be placed separately or as a single conduit (Cabrol graft). When valve leaflets show normal morphology, valve-spearing replacement is an option (Tirone David procedure). Ascending aortic graft anastomosis to the aortic arch can be made with an end-to-end or hemiarch approach. For aortic arch replacement, an island of native arch tissue, containing ostia for the supra-arch vessels, is anastomosed to the graft. Arch graft repair can be performed as a single-stage (end-to-end anastomosis) or a two-stage procedure (elephant trunk), depending on the underlying pathology and extent of disease (Fig. 7.9). Following proximal and distal end-to-end anastomoses for descending aorta replacement, intercostal arteries are often reimplanted. Similarly for thoracoabdominal grafts, visceral and renal vessels may need reimplantation, either as an island of native aorta and/or individually [17].

CT findings postoperatively include pericardial effusion, pleural effusions, mediastinal hematoma, atelectasis, consolidation, pneumothorax, pneumomediastinum, and chest wall hematoma. Grafts are readily identified on the noncontrast images by their regular circular contour with slightly higher density ring. Noncontrast images should also be reviewed for the presence and location of surgical clips.

On the contrast-enhanced images, graft transitions to native aorta and surgical fenestrations should be recognized. Graft lumens, native vessels, and reimplanted arteries should be patent, without kinking, thrombus, or occlusion. In addition to graft and vessel luminal compromise, other complications to identify include anastomotic dehiscence with contrast extravasation and pseudoaneurysm formation, either from the graft or coronary artery suture lines. With inclusion grafts, there should be no perigraft flow. If there is anastomotic dehiscence or temporary transgraft leakage, the perigraft space will contain contrast in addition to thrombus. Access sites for cardiopulmonary bypass (i.e., aorta, pulmonary veins, atrial appendages, left ventricle, femoral artery/vein) are assessed for any dehiscence or thrombus (Fig. 7.10). 4D real-time imaging is most commonly applied in our practice to assess aortic valves following aortic valve sparing surgery (Tirone David procedure). Valve leaflets are assessed for thickening and closure.

7.4.2.2
Endovascular

Current approved devices for thoracic aortic stent-grafting are Talent (Medtronic AVE, Sunrise, Fla.), Aneurx (Medtronic AVE, Sunrise, Fla.), and Excluder (Gore, Flagstaff, Ariz.) stent-graft systems. Imagers should be familiar with the individual appearances. For instance, the Talent device has uncovered superior struts, which afford fixation above the left subclavian ostium.

Success of thoracic aorta endovascular repair relies on device and patient selection. Noninvasive imaging, in turn, plays a major role in deciding whether patients meet inclusion criteria. Although both MRA and CTA are the principal modalities for this objective, and CTA employs iodinated contrast, CTA offers superior resolution for depicting wall morphology, provides reliable assessment of vascular calcifications, and allows for simultaneous 3-D display of vascular and nonvascular structures.

Preendovascular CTA focuses on qualitative and quantitative assessment. The aortic pathology (i.e., aneurysm, dissection) is defined with reference to the supra-arch vessels. More importantly, the maximal thoracic aorta dimension, the proximal neck – distance from a reference vessel (i.e., left subclavian artery) to the beginning of the aortic pathology (i.e., aneurysm, entry tear for dissection) – and the planned distal landing zone are all measured for maximal diameter and length. In addition, the proximal neck and distal landing zone are evaluated for thrombus burden, angulation, and aneurysm formation, all of which are factored into the selection process. Imaging should include the iliac to common femoral arteries as angulation, tortuosity, heavy calcification, and stenosis all impact success negatively [11]. In these instances, a surgical retroperitoneal iliac or aorta conduit may be required.

Complications from stent-graft repair may occur early or late. As the technology and procedure are still young, patients require life-long surveillance. In our practice, unless patients have renal insufficiency, for routine thoracic aorta anatomical assessment, following endovascular repair, it is our choice to also employ CTA over MRA. Primary goals of imaging are to assess stent-graft position and patency while confirming aneurysm sac size stability or a decrease in size; excluding rupture and endoleaks; and excluding stent-graft migration, thrombus, kinking, and occlusion (Fig. 7.11). Identification of an endoleak requires comparison with precontrast images. Delayed images are useful for detecting slow perigraft flow. Attempts should be made to characterize the endoleak: type I, incomplete proximal or distal seal with aortic wall;

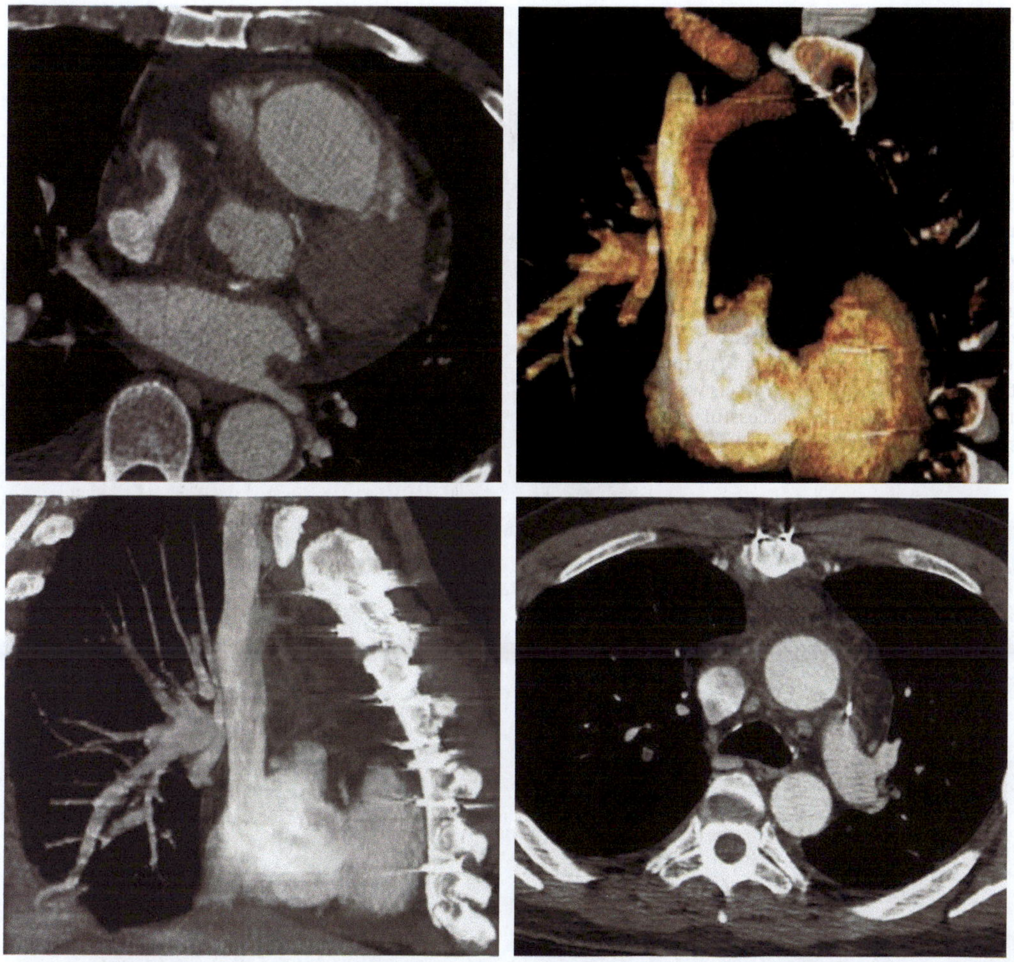

Fig. 7.10a–d. Right atrial appendage thrombus with pulmonary embolism. After a patient underwent interposition graft replacement for an ascending aortic aneurysm, postoperative imaging was performed with a retrospective ECG-gated 16-row acquisition. While the graft was patent (not shown), incidentally identified on axial (**a,d**), volume-rendered (**b**), and maximum-intensity projection images (**c**) was a right-sided atrial appendage thrombus, related to bypass cannulation (*arrows*) associated with right upper lobe pulmonary embolism (*arrowheads*).

type II, retrograde flow via patent aortic branches; type III, stent graft modular/structural failure; type IV, graft porosity. Dimensions of the aorta, neck, and landing zone should be correlated with any demonstrated stent-graft migration, kinking, or endoleak. Noncovered supra-arch, abdominal aorta and accessed iliofemoral vessels should be well opacified, without emboli or dissection. Another complication to exclude is a retroperitoneal hematoma [18].

7.5 Conclusion

These applications of MDCT demonstrate the unique imaging capabilities currently available with this modality. With such powerful technology at our disposal, not only are we able to challenge, but in most cases, surpass the diagnostic acumen of conventional angiography.

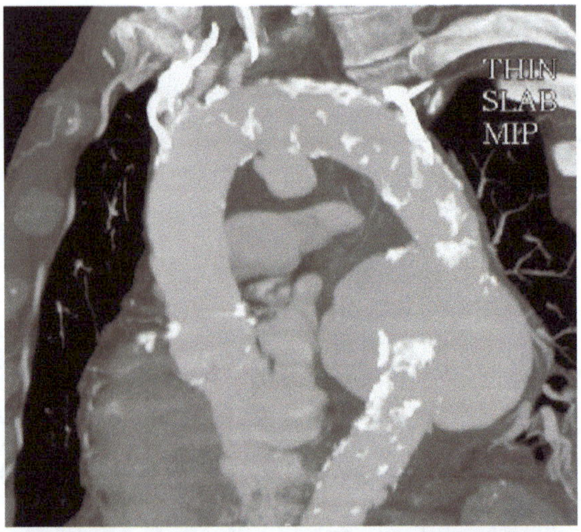

a

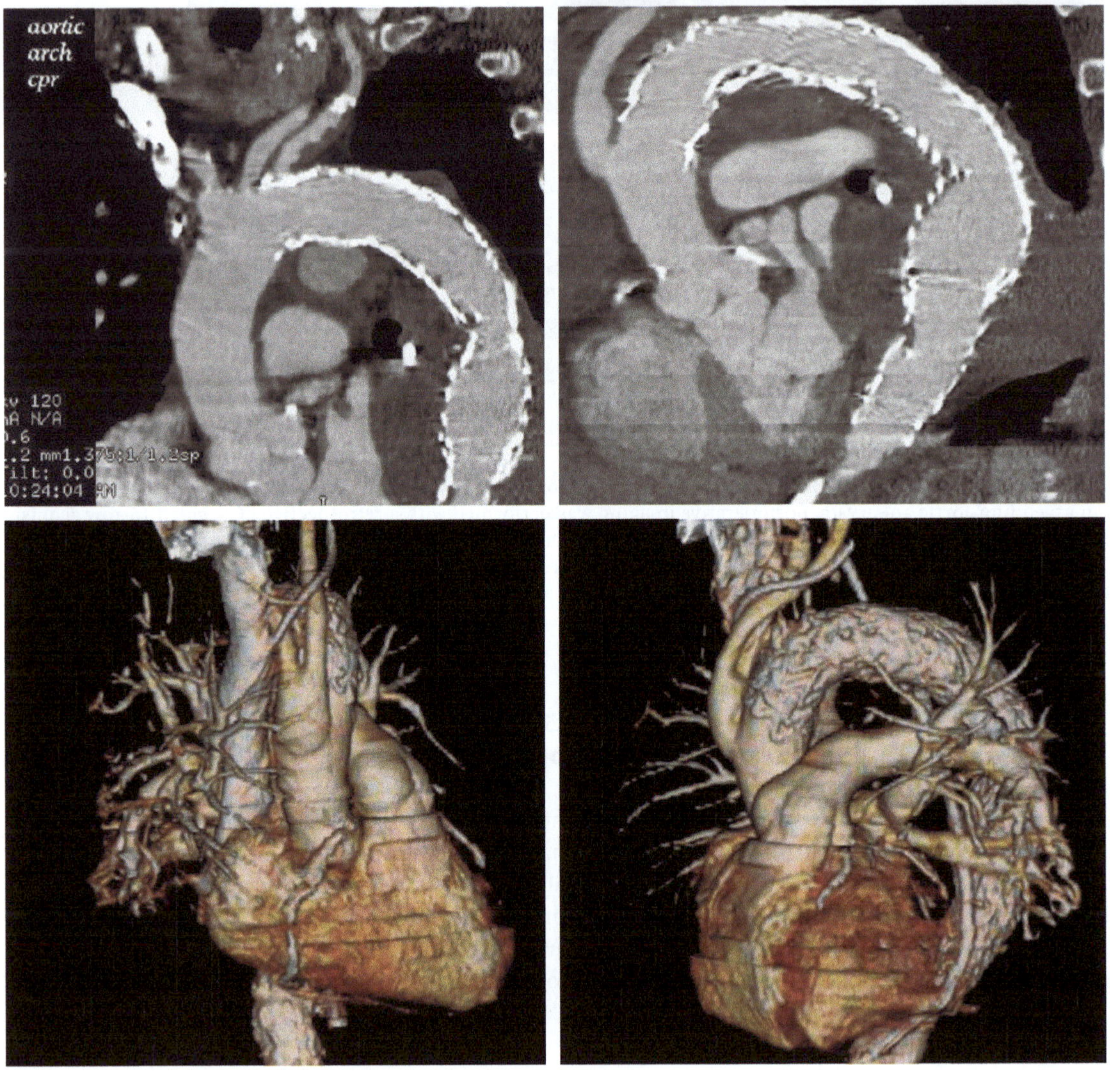

b c d e

Fig. 7.11a–e. Thoracic aortic aneurysm pre and postendovascular repair. **a** A patient with transverse and descending mycotic aortic aneurysms, who was not a surgical candidate, underwent endovascular repair. **b** Immediate poststent-graft CTA showed successful exclusion of the descending aortic aneurysm, but a type I leak at the transverse aorta. In an attempt to minimize the physiological stress of complete thoracic aortic graft repair, it was elected to extend the stent graft into the ascending aorta, covering the left subclavian artery and anastomosing a Y-bypass graft from the ascending aorta to the brachiocephalic and left common carotid arteries. **c-e** Retrospectively ECG-gated 1.25-mm sections provided high-resolution postprocessed images, confirming patency of the stent graft and the surgical Y-graft, as well as the coronary arteries, along with now-successful exclusion of the transverse aorta aneurysm.

References

1. Rubin GD (2001) Techniques in performing MDCT. Techn Vasc Interv Radiol 4:2–14
2. Rubin GD (2003) Paper presented at: Fourth International Symposium on Multidetector-Row CT, San Francisco, CA
3. Prokop M, Galanski M (2003) Spiral and multislice CT of the body. Thieme, New York
4. Willmann JK et al. (2002) Electrocardiographically gated multi-detector row CT for assessment of valvular morphology and calcification in aortic stenosis. Radiology 225:120–128
5. Roos JE et al. (2002) Thoracic aorta: motion artifact reduction with retrospective and prospective electrocardiography-assisted multi-detector row CT. Radiology 222:271–277
6. Morgan-Hughes G, Roobottom C, Marshall AJ (2002) Aortic valve imaging with computed tomography: a review. J Heart Valve Dis 11:604–611
7. Saito K, Saito M, Komatu S, Ohtoma K (2003) Real-time four dimensional imaging of the heart with multi-detector row CT. Radiographics. 23:8–18
8. Moore KL, Persaud TVN (2003) The circulatory system. In: Moore KL, Persaud TVN (eds) The developing human: clinically oriented embryology, 7th edn. Saunders, Philadelphia
9. Proto AV, Cuthbert NW, Raider L (1987) Aberrant right subclavian artery: further observations. AJR Am J Roentgenol 148:253–257
10. Spindola-Franco H, Fish BG (1991) Abnormalities of the great arteries. In: Elliot LP (ed) Cardiac imaging in infants, children, and adults. Lippincott, Philadelphia
11. Knight L, Edwards JE (1974) Right aortic arch: types and associated cardiac anomalies. Circulation 50:1047–1051
12. Predy TS, Mcdonald V, Demos TC et al. (1989) CT of congenital anomalies of the aortic arch. Semin Roentgenol 14:96–111
13. Amplatz K, Moller JH, Castaneda-Zuniga W (1986) Coarctation of the aorta. In: Amplatz K, Moller JH , Casteneda-Zuniga WR (eds) Radiology of congenital heart disease. Thieme, New York
14. VanDyke CW, White RD (1994) Congenital abnormalities of the thoracic aorta presenting in the adult. J Thoracic Imaging 9:230–245
15. Haughton VM, Fellows KE, Rosenbaum AE (1975) The cervical arches. Radiology 114:675–681
16. Pearson GD, Kan JS, Neill CA, et al. (1997) Cervical aortic arch with aneurysm formation. Am J Cardiol 79:112–114
17. Kaiser LR, Kron IL, Spray TL (1998) Thoracic aorta disease. In: Kaiser LR, Kron IL, Spray TL (eds) Mastery of cardiothoracic surgery. Lippincott-Raven, Philadelphia
18. Whitaker SC (2001) Imaging of abdominal aortic aneurysm before and after endoluminal stent-graft repair. Eur J Radiol 39:3–15

8 Multidetector-Row CT Angiography of the Pulmonary Circulation

U. Joseph Schoepf

CONTENTS

Introduction

The introduction of multidetector-row CT (MDCT) into clinical radiology has decisively reemphasized and reinvigorated the cardinal role of CT as the premier imaging modality for imaging the pulmonary circulation. The specific requirements of diagnostic imaging in the high-resolution environment of the chest, with fast-moving organs and the need for image acquisition during apnea, are ideally met by MDCT technology. The scan speed of current-generation MDCT scanners translates into the ability to scan the entire chest within a few seconds. Despite submillimeter resolution, this results in motion-free images even in the sickest of patients. Use of thin slices was shown to significantly improve the detection of minute vascular pathology such as small, peripheral pulmonary emboli [21, 78]. For a comprehensive diagnosis of focal and diffuse lung disease, both contiguous images and high-resolution CT (HRCT) can be reconstructed from the same single acquisition, without scanning the patient twice [75]. ECG synchronization with MDCT is a valuable tool to improve image quality and diagnostic accuracy by reducing motion artifacts as potential sources of diagnostic error [72]. However, while MDCT provides innumerable opportunities, its unique characteristics also pose hitherto unknown challenges to its users. The large-volume data sets generated by current and future generations of HRCT scanners are a logistical problem that threatens to overburden the radiologist with diagnostic information. Also, although MDCT can be used in ways that result in a reduction of patient radiation dose, with many applications the patient dose is likely to increase if no adequate precautions are taken. Solutions, however, are on the horizon and are comprehensively discussed throughout this book. The discipline of radiology is quickly adapting to novel concepts of data visualization, embracing 2D and 3D display techniques. Effective means for reducing radiation dose are being implemented. Tools for facilitating the analysis of large-volume MDCT data sets for accurate detection of pathology are continuously being refined. In the following we will discuss specific improvements, novel challenges, and sophisticated solutions, which the advent of ever-faster MDCT acquisition techniques has brought about for imaging of the pulmonary circulation.

U. J. Schoepf, MD
Department of Radiology, Medical University of South Carolina, 169 Ashley Avenue, Charleston, SC 29425, USA

8.1 Multidetector-Row CT Angiography of Pulmonary Embolism

8.1.1 Imaging Pulmonary Embolism: The Paradigm is Shifting

Although increasingly sophisticated clinical algorithms for "bedside" exclusion of pulmonary embolism (PE) are being developed, mainly based on a negative D-dimer test [6, 11, 42, 92], there is a high and seemingly increasing demand for imaging tests for suspected PE.

Invasive pulmonary angiography is still regarded by some as the "gold standard" technique, but in reality is rarely ever used as such [8, 40, 60, 71]. The main reason for the latter appears to be the invasiveness of this procedure, although the incidence of complications with contemporary techniques is low [79, 98]. More importantly there is mounting evidence for the limitations of this technique for the unequivocal diagnosis of isolated peripheral pulmonary emboli: At two recent analyses, the interobserver agreement rates for detection of subsegmental emboli by selective pulmonary angiography ranged between only 45% and 66% [10, 82]. Given such limitations, use of this test as an objective and readily reproducible tool for the verification of findings at competing imaging modalities as to the presence or absence of PE seems questionable, and the status of pulmonary angiography as the standard of reference for diagnosis of PE is tarnished.

Use of nuclear medicine imaging, once the first study in the diagnostic algorithm of PE, appears to be declining [44, 70] due to the high percentage of indeterminate studies (73% of all performed [59]) and poor interobserver correlation [4]. Revised criteria for the interpretation of ventilation-perfusion scans [80, 81] and novel technologies in nuclear medicine such as single photon-emission tomography (SPECT) [3, 56] can decrease the ratio of indeterminate scintigraphic studies, but cannot offset the limitations inherent to a mere functional imaging test [18].

Contrast-enhanced magnetic resonance (MR) angiography has been evaluated for the diagnosis of acute PE [30, 48, 55, 69]. However, the acquisition protocols that are currently available for MR pulmonary angiography lack sufficient spatial resolution for reliable evaluation of peripheral pulmonary arteries [30, 55]. More importantly, this modality has not seen widespread use in the acutely ill patient with suspected PE due to lack of general availability, relatively long examination times, and difficulties in patient monitoring.

This leaves us with CT, which, for most practical purposes, has become the first-line imaging test after lower-extremity ultrasound for the assessment of patients with suspected PE in daily clinical routine. The most important advantage of CT over other imaging modalities is that both mediastinal and parenchymal structures are evaluated, and thrombus is directly visualized [31, 95] (Fig. 8.1). Studies have shown that up to two-thirds of patients initially suspected to have PE receive another diagnosis [35], some with potentially life-threatening diseases such as aortic dissection, pneumonia, lung cancer (Fig. 8.2), and pneumothorax [89]. Most of these differential diagnoses are amenable to CT visualization, so that in many cases a specific etiology for the patients' symptoms or important additional diagnoses can be established [18]. The interobserver agreement for CT is better than for scintigraphy [90]. In a recent study, interobserver agreement for the diagnosis of PE was excellent for spiral CT angiography (κ=0.72) and only moderate for ventilation–perfusion lung scanning (κ=0.22) [4]. CT also appears to be the most cost-effective modality in the diagnostic algorithm of PE compared with algorithms that do not include CT but are based on other imaging modalities (ultrasound, scintigraphy, pulmonary angiography) [88]. Also, there is some indication that CT may not only be used for evaluating thoracic anatomy in suspected PE, but also could to some degree allow deriving physiological parameters on lung perfusion at single-slice, electron-beam, and MDCT [28, 73, 93]. The main impediment for the unanimous embrace of computed tomography as the modality of choice for the diagnosis of acute PE has been limitations of this modality for the accurate detection of small peripheral emboli. Early studies comparing single-slice CT with selective pulmonary angiography demonstrated CT's high accuracy for the detection of PE to the segmental arterial level [23, 63, 65, 85] but suggested that subsegmental pulmonary emboli may be overlooked by CT scanning. The degree of accuracy that can be achieved for the visualization of subsegmental pulmonary arteries and for the detection of emboli in these vessels with single-slice, dual-slice, and electron-beam CT scanners was found to range between 61% and 79% [23, 61, 66, 74].

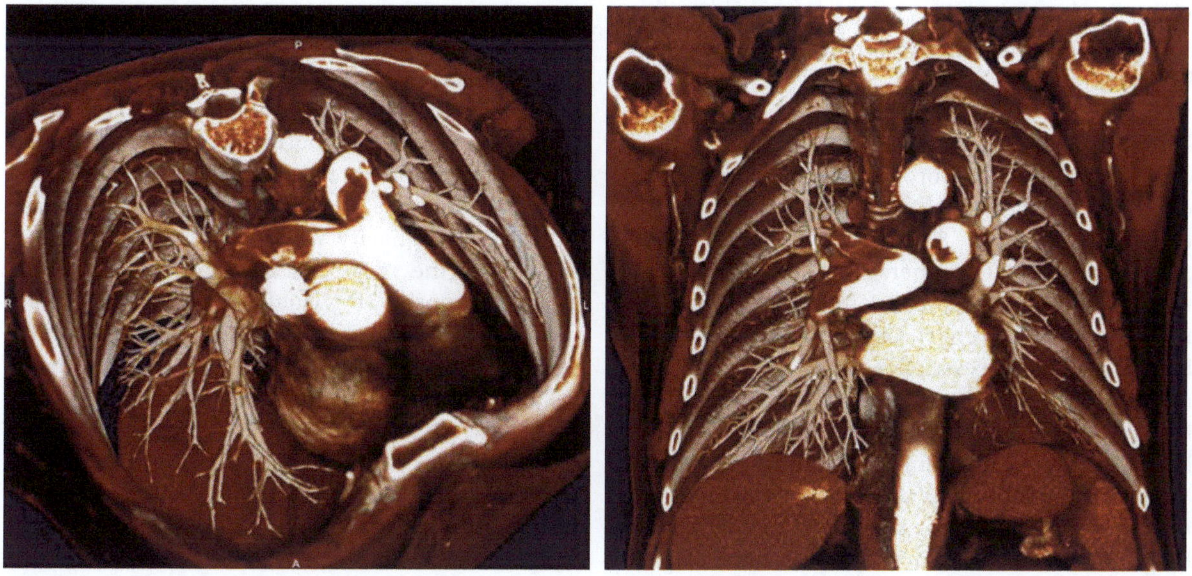

a b

Fig. 8.1a,b Seventy-two-year-old man with extensive, acute central pulmonary embolism with "saddle embolus" extending into both central pulmonary arteries. Contrast-enhanced 16-slice CT images. Colored volume-rendering technique seen from a frontal cranial (**a**) and coronal (**b**) perspective allows intuitive visualization of location and extent of embolism and facilitates communication with referring physicians

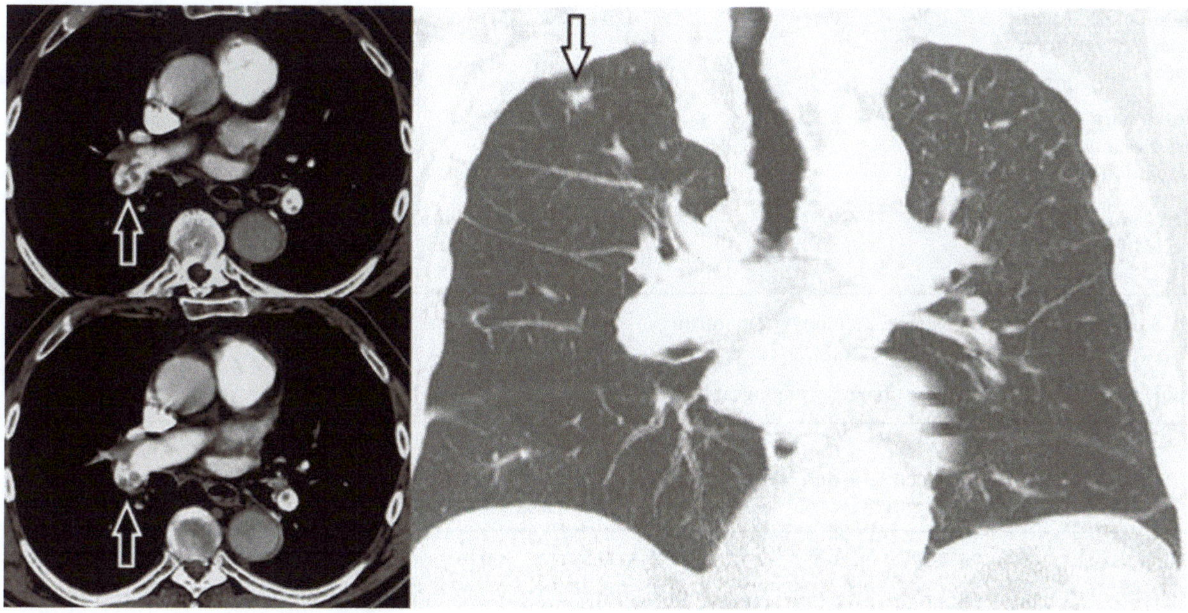

Fig. 8.2 Incidentally found T1 peripheral adenocarcinoma (*arrow, right panel*) in the right upper lobe of a patient with central pulmonary embolism (*arrows, left panels*). Contrast-enhanced 4-slice MDCT study. Axial sections (*left panels*) and coronal multiplanar reformat (*right panel*). Direct visualization of emboli and relevant alternative or additional disease is the key advantage of CT over competing modalities for the diagnosis of PE

8.1.2 Advantages of Multidetector-Row CT for PE Imaging

In the last few years, CT has seen decisive dynamic developments, mainly brought about by the advent of MDCT technology [34, 47]. The current generation of 4-slice (Table 8.1), 8-slice, 10-slice, and 16-slice (Table 8.2) CT scanners now allows for acquisition of the entire chest with 1-mm or submillimeter resolution within a short, single breath-hold of now less than 10 s in the case of 16-slice CT (Fig. 8.3). The ability to cover substantial anatomical volumes with high in-plane and through-plane spatial resolution has brought with it a number of decisive advantages. Short breath-hold times were shown to benefit imaging of patients with suspected PE and underlying lung disease and should reduce the percentage of nondiagnostic CT pulmonary angiography investigations [63]. The near-isotropic nature of high-resolution MDCT data lends itself to 2D and 3D visualization; this may in some instances improve PE diagnosis [64]. Potential pitfalls for PE diagnosis that have been cited relate to the incorrect interpretation of hilar lymphatic tissue as intraluminal filling defects. However, even for less experienced observers, diagnostic errors such as this are easy to avoid if familiarity with this potential pitfall is ensured. In the very few cases with a residual insecure diagnosis, 3D visualization of MDCT data may be helpful in clarifying the relationship of hilar lymphatic tissue to the central pulmonary arteries, aid diagnosis in such instances, and help avoid diagnostic pitfalls [67] (Fig. 8.4). 3D visualization is generally of greater importance for conveying information on localization and extent of embolic disease to referring clinicians in an intuitive and acceptable manner (Fig. 8.1).

Probably the most important advantage of high-resolution MDCT pulmonary angiography is the

Table 8.1 Four-slice MDCT pulmonary angiography protocols

	Colli mation (mm)	Table feed (mm/s)	Gantry Rotation (s)	Pitch	kV	mAs	Contrast volume (ml)	Flow (ml/s)	Delay (s)	Recon/ Increm. (mm)
Pulmonary arteries: high speed	4×2.5	30	0.5	6	120	120	80	4	18 or Bolus trigger	3/2 6/6 (lung)
Pulmonary arteries: high resolution	4×1	12	0.5	6	120	120	120	4	18 or Bolus trigger	1.25/1 6/6 (lung)
Veins in suspected PE and DVT	4×5 mm	70	0.5	7	120	120	No additional contrast	-	150-s total delay	6/6

DVT deep venous thrombosis, PE pulmonary embolism

Table 8.2 Sixteen-slice MDCT pulmonary angiography protocols

	Collimation (mm)	Table feed (mm/s)	Gantry rotation (s)	Pitch	kV	mAs	Contrast volume (ml)	Flow (ml/s)	Delay (s)	Recon/ Increm. (mm)
Pulmonary arteries	16×0.75	30	0.5	20 (1.25)	120	100	100	4	Bolus trigger	1.0/0.7 5/5 (lung)
Pulmonary arteries: ECG gating	12×0.75	6.7	0.42	3.7 (0.31)	120	500	120	4	Bolus trigger	0.75/0.4 1.0/0.5
Veins in suspected PE and DVT	16×1.5	72	0.5	24 (1.5)	120	100	No additional contrast	-	150-s total delay	5/5

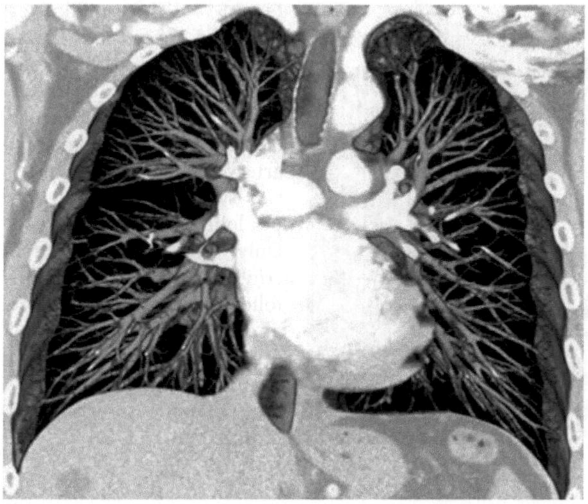

Fig. 8.3 Normal pulmonary vessels in a 56-year-old man presenting with mild chest pain after a long-distance flight. Contrast-enhanced 16-slice CT examination covers the entire chest within a scan time of 10 s, allowing analysis of even the most peripheral pulmonary vessels in exquisite detail

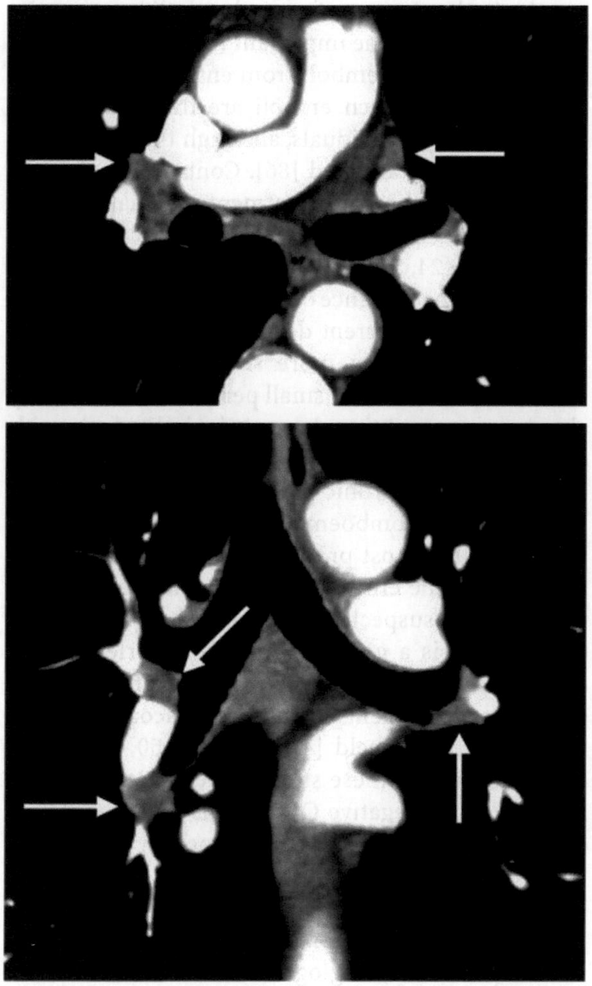

improved diagnosis of small peripheral emboli. Still with single-slice CT, it could be shown that superior visualization of segmental and subsegmental pulmonary arteries can be achieved with thinner slice widths (e.g., 2 mm versus 3 mm) [66]. However, with single-slice CT, the range, which can be covered with thin slice widths within one breath-hold, is rather limited [66, 73]. The high spatial resolution of 1-mm or submillimeter collimation data sets now allows evaluation of pulmonary vessels down to 6th-order branches [21] and significantly increases the detection rate of segmental and subsegmental pulmonary emboli [77] (Fig. 8.5). This increase in the rate of detection is probably due to reduced volume averaging and the accurate analysis of progressively thinner vessels by use of thinner sections. Improved visualization with high-resolution MDCT is most striking in peripheral arteries with an anatomical course parallel to the scan plane. Such vessels tend to be most affected by volume averaging if thicker slices are used [77] . The high spatial resolution along the scan axis of a thin-collimation, MDCT data set, however, allows an accurate evaluation of the full course of such vessels. The interobserver correlation for confident detection of subsegmental emboli with high-resolution MDCT by far exceeds the reproducibility of other imaging modalities, i.e., invasive pulmonary angiography [77].

Fig. 8.4a,b. Contrast-enhanced CT pulmonary angiography in a patient with suspected acute pulmonary embolism. Lymphatic tissue in the mediastinum and in the pulmonary hilum (*arrows*) may be misinterpreted as embolic filling defects in central pulmonary vessels by less experienced observers if only axial sections (**a**) are used for diagnosis. Coronal multiplanar reformats of a high-resolution 4-slice multidetector-row CT acquisition (**b**) allow better differentiation of lymphatic tissue, and vessels and may reduce sources of diagnostic error

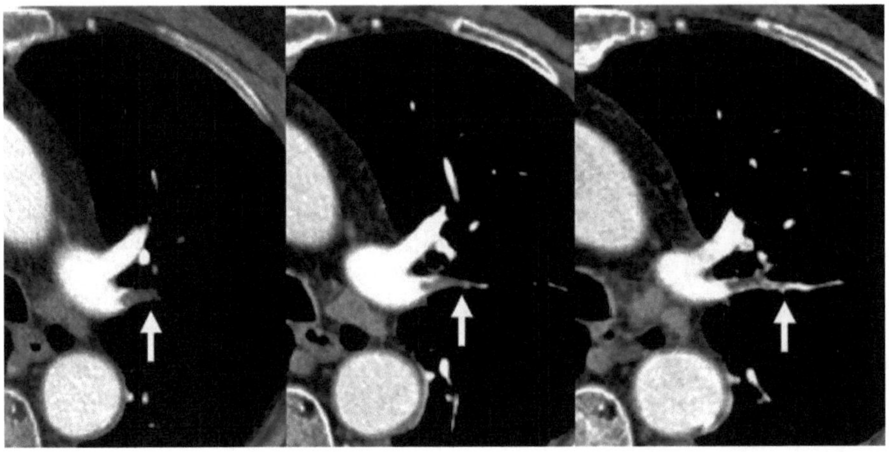

Fig. 8.5 Three-millimeter (*left*) and 2-mm (*middle*) axial reconstructions of a contrast-enhanced multislice CT data set suggest the presence of thrombus in a segmental artery supplying the posterior segment of the left upper lobe of the lung (*arrow*). Only 1-mm reconstruction (*right*) of the data set allows following the entire course of the segmental artery and unanimous visualization of the filling defect within the posterior subsegmental branch

8.1.3 The Quandary of the Isolated Subsegmental Embolus

While traditional technical limitations of CT for the diagnosis of pulmonary emboli appear successfully overcome with the advent of MDCT, we are now facing new challenges that are a direct product of our increased technical prowess. Small peripheral clots that might have gone unnoticed in the past are now frequently detected (Fig. 8.6).

While, based on a good quality MDCT scan, there may be no doubt in the mind of the interpreting radiologists as to the presence of a small isolated clot, such findings will be increasingly difficult to prove in a correlative manner. Animal experiments that use artificial emboli as an independent gold standard indicate that high-resolution, 4-slice MDCT is at least as accurate as invasive pulmonary angiography for the detection of small peripheral emboli [2]. However, it appears highly unlikely that pulmonary angiography will be performed on a patient merely to prove the presence of an isolated embolus. Also, given the limited interobserver correlation of pulmonary angiography, which was pointed out earlier [10, 82], it appears doubtful that this latter test, even if performed, would provide useful and adequate correlative proof for findings at high-resolution MDCT. Broad-based studies such as PIOPED II, which set out to establish the efficacy of MDCT in suspected PE, account for this latter fact by using a composite reference test based on ventilation/perfusion scanning, ultrasound of the lower extremities, pulmonary angiography, and contrast venography to establish the PE status of the patient [26].

Perhaps more importantly there is a growing sense of insecurity within the clinical community about how to manage patients in whom a diagnosis of isolated peripheral embolism has been established. It has been shown that 6% [59] to 30% [53] of patients with documented PE present with clots only in subsegmental and smaller arteries, but the clinical significance of small peripheral emboli in subsegmental pulmonary arteries in the absence of central emboli is uncertain. It is assumed that one important function of the lung is to prevent small emboli from entering the arterial circulation [31]. Such emboli are thought to form even in healthy individuals, although this notion has never been substantiated [86]. Controversy also exists about whether the treatment of small emboli, once detected, may result in a better clinical outcome for patients [24, 52, 65]. There is little disagreement though that the presence of peripheral emboli may be an indicator for current deep vein thrombosis, thus potentially heralding more severe embolic events [35, 53, 58]. A burden of small peripheral emboli may also have prognostic relevance in individuals with cardiopulmonary restrictions [24, 31, 53] and for the development of chronic pulmonary hypertension in patients with thromboembolic disease [53].

Perhaps the most practical and realistic scenario for studying the efficacy of CT for the evaluation of patients with suspected PE is assessing patient outcome. There is a growing body of experience concerning the negative predictive value of a negative CT study and patient outcome if anticoagulation is subsequently withheld [4, 19, 24, 25, 50, 54, 63, 84, 87]. According to these studies, the negative predictive value of a negative CT study is high, regardless of whether multidetector-row technology is used [63] or whether underlying lung disease is present [87]. The frequency of a subsequent clinical diagnosis of PE or deep venous thrombosis (DVT) after a negative CT pulmonary angiogram is low and lower than

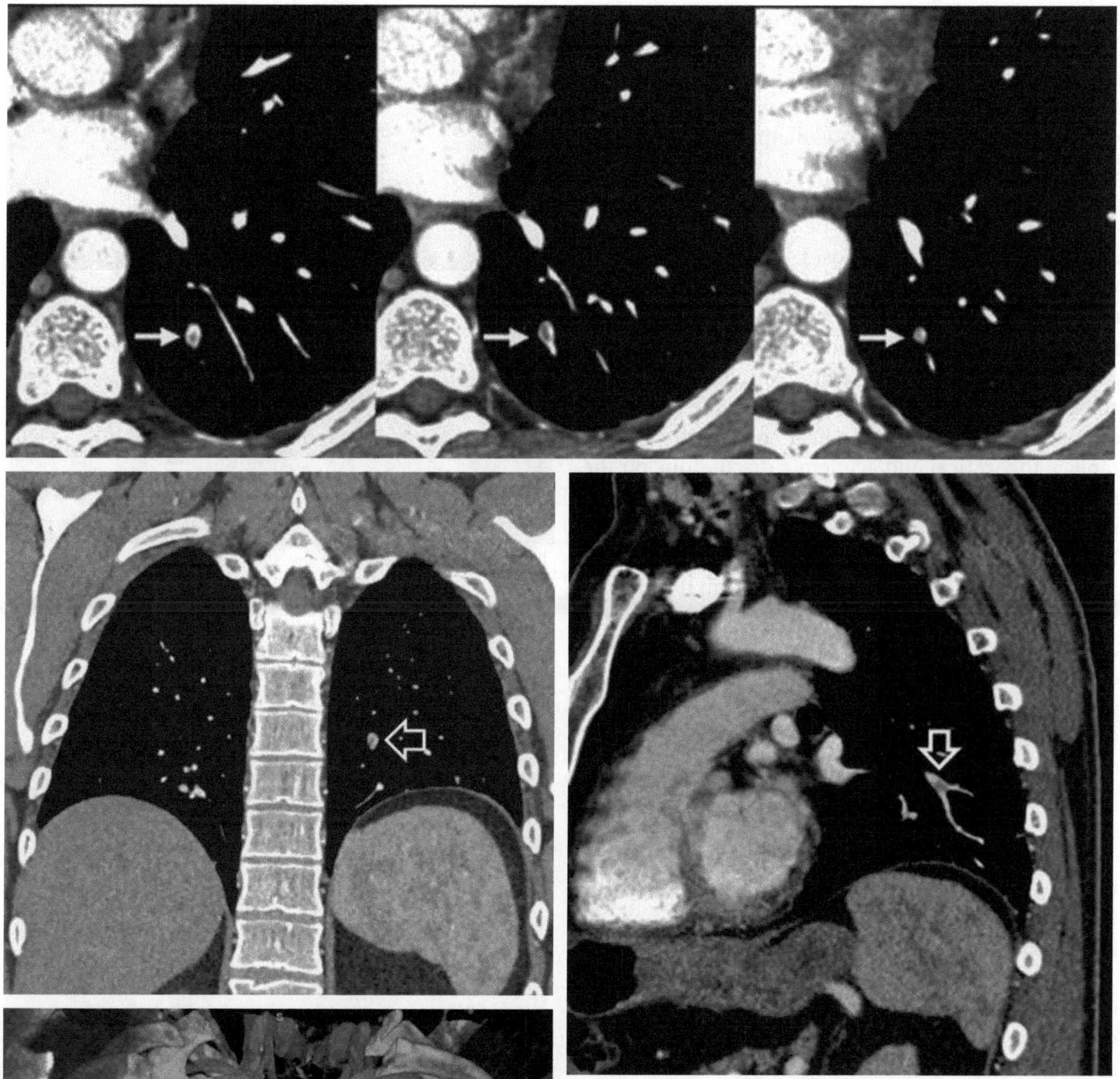

a b c

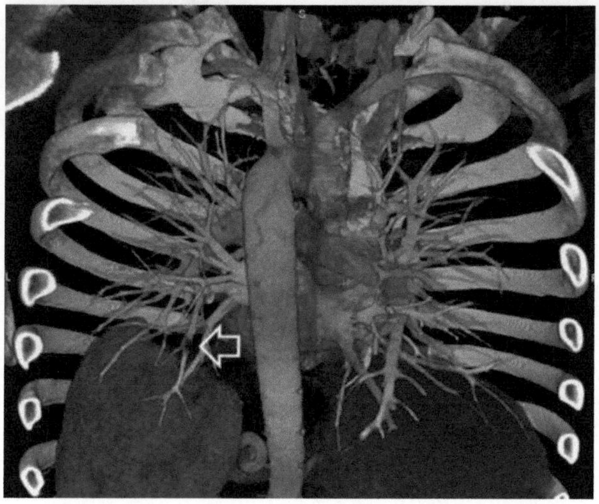

d

Fig. 8.6a–d. Contrast-enhanced 16-slice CT examination with 0.75-mm collimation in a patient with mild pleuritic chest pain. Isolated peripheral pulmonary embolus (*arrows*) in a subsegmental pulmonary artery in segment 9 of the left lung is visualized on three consecutive axial sections (**a**) and on coronal (**b**) and oblique-sagittal (**c**) multiplanar reformats. Volume-rendered display seen from posterior shows isolated peripheral filling defect (**d**) within otherwise normal pulmonary vascular tree that after a negative or low-probability V-Q scan [24]. Thus even single-slice CT is a reliable imaging tool for excluding clinically relevant PE, so that it appears that anticoagulation can be safely withheld when the CT scan is normal and of good diagnostic quality [24, 84].

With MDCT technology, past limitations of CT for the diagnosis of PE should be effectively overcome and, for all practical purposes, CT has become established as the first-line modality for imaging patients with suspected PE. CT has become an attractive means for a safe, highly accurate and cost-effective diagnosis of pulmonary embolism. The lack of a clinically available gold standard for the diagnosis of PE suggests that the medical community should replace theoretical and academic discussions on the relative value of different imaging modalities, with more realistic approaches based on patient outcome. Retrospective and prospective studies [4, 19, 24, 25, 50, 54, 68, 84, 87] have demonstrated the high negative predictive value for a normal MDCT pulmonary angiography study. Once it is accepted by the medical community that a negative CT safely excludes the presence of pulmonary embolism, we believe use of CT for PE diagnosis will be unanimously embraced as the reference modality.

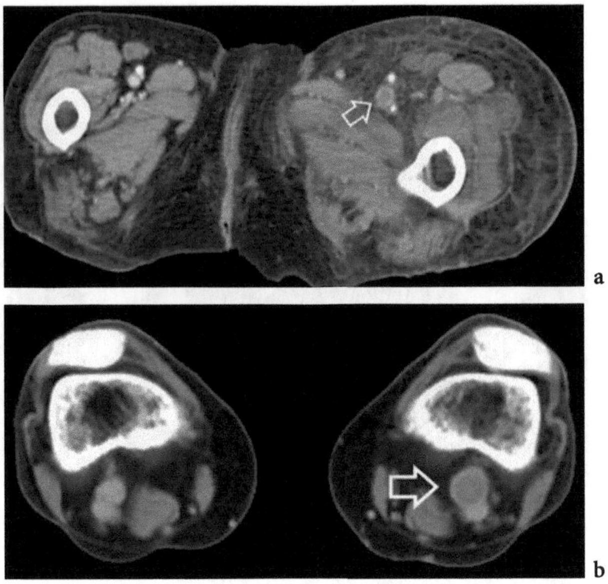

Fig. 8.7 Examples of deep venous thrombosis diagnosed by combined multidetector-row CT pulmonary angiography and venography. Thrombi are delineated as filling defects, seen in the left femoral (**a**) and popliteal (**b**) veins.

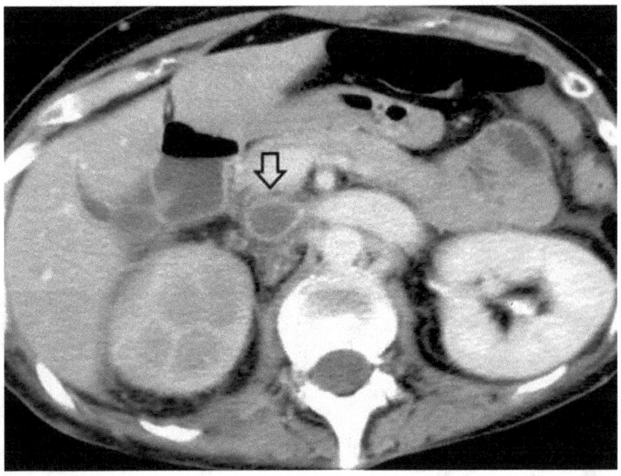

Fig. 8.8a,b. Extensive residual deep venous thrombosis in the inferior vena cava (*arrow*) of a young female patient with acute pulmonary embolism. Compromise of the right renal vein by thrombotic material causes venostasis in the right kidney with differing contrast media attenuation in the right as compared to the left kidney. Thrombosis in the abdominal venous system as noted in this case may be difficult to evaluate with sonography due to extensive abdominal gas but is clearly visualized with CT venography.

8.2 Multidetector-Row CT for Imaging Deep Venous Thrombosis

Combined MDCT venography and pulmonary angiography is a diagnostic test that screens for pulmonary embolism and DVT using a single contrast-medium infusion. This technique has been proposed as a cost-effective means for excluding lower-extremity venous thrombosis in patients undergoing CT pulmonary angiography [45]. Key advantages comprise that no additional contrast media needs to be injected to evaluate both the pulmonary vessels and the deep venous system. Meanwhile use of CT for this purpose seems to be clinically established [7, 12, 20, 46, 97]. We use the volume-covering capabilities, which have become available with MDCT, for a comprehensive diagnosis of PE and DVT in patients without known source of emboli (Figs. 8.7, 8.8, 8.9). In a patient with acute pulmonary embolism who is bound for the intensive care unit, a comprehensive diagnosis of the extent of thromboembolic disease, the source of emboli, and potential residual thrombosis can be diagnosed in a single session by using this approach. CT may even be advantageous over Doppler sonography and conventional venography, since extensive residual thrombosis in the abdominal and pelvic venous system (Fig. 8.8) or in other anatomical regions not accessible by ultrasound (Fig. 8.9) may be better visualized by use of CT. In the vast majority of patients who receive a combined thoracic and venous MDCT examination, the scan either confirms the suspected diagnosis or reveals relevant alternative or additional disease.

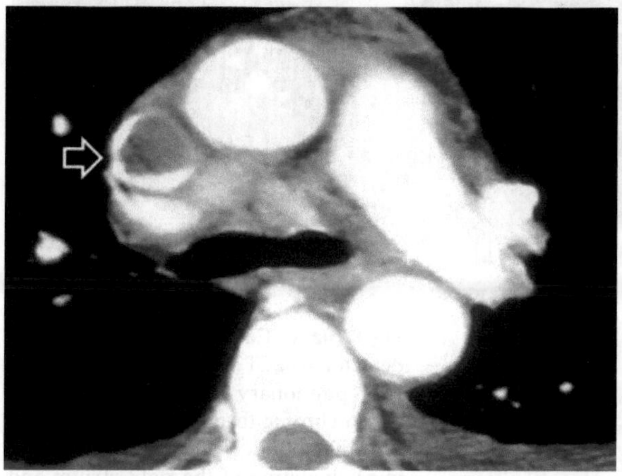

Fig. 8.9 A case of thrombosis in the superior vena cava (*arrow*) is noted in this contrast-enhanced multidetector-row CT angiography of the thoracic vasculature. CT venography enables enhanced possibilities of detecting thrombus in atypical locations.

8.3 Multidetector-Row CT for Evaluating Pulmonary Hypertension

Pulmonary hypertension (PH) of the precapillary pulmonary circulation is a diagnostic challenge. The host of potential underlying disorders includes idiopathic disease, recurrent embolism, and structural lung changes among other more readily identifiable causes [17]. CT has traditionally been an important tool in the diagnostic algorithm of PH, allowing for an accurate assessment of both pathogenesis and extent of the disease. HRCT is the gold standard to evaluate a patient with suspected PH for structural lung changes that may cause increased pre- or postcapillary pressure within the lung vessels. Mosaic attenuation on HRCT, combined with distal pruning of pulmonary arteries, is a sign of impaired pulmonary perfusion due to recurrent peripheral embolism as the underlying cause (Fig. 8.10). Contrast-enhanced CT allows for direct visualization of chronic thromboembolic changes and helps to determine whether the disease is amenable to surgical thrombendarterectomy (Figs. 8.10, 8.11). If neither structural lung changes nor signs of thromboembolism are found in the absence of other identifiable etiologies for PH, such as congenital heart disease or tumor embolism, a diagnosis of primary pulmonary hypertension is usually considered. Since the differential diagnosis of PH includes diseases with both focal and diffuse character, the entire pathology frequently cannot be appreciated with a single CT technique. Thick-collimation, single-slice CT may not suffice to assess interstitial changes. If only HRCT is performed, focal pathology such as thromboembolism is easily missed due to the high-frequency reconstruction algorithms and because scans are acquired at only every 10–20 mm. If single-slice CT is used for evaluation of patients with suspected PH, it is therefore often necessary to perform both a contrast-enhanced spiral acquisition and HRCT for a comprehensive assessment of the underlying pathology. Now a single breath-held, thin-collimation MDCT acquisition generates a set of raw-data that provides all options for image reconstruction, addressing multiple diagnostic problems by performing a single contrast-enhanced scan [75] (Figs. 8.10, 8.11, 8.12). In patients with suspected PH, we routinely perform a thin-slice reconstruction of the entire chest, which can detect pulmonary emboli with high accuracy. In addition, from the same set of raw data, 5-mm contiguous lung sections and HRCT sections at every 1 cm are routinely performed. Thus, from a single set of raw data, a comprehensive analysis of gross and diffuse lung changes and of thromboembolic disease becomes feasible.

8.4 Multidetector-Row CT Imaging of Systemic Arterial Supply to the Lung

Disorders of the systemic arterial supply to the lung are a not-infrequent cause of massive hemoptysis [9]. Systemic arterialization of the lung parenchyma is most often congenital, in which case an aberrant systemic artery supplies the parenchyma involved in congenital pulmonary venolobar syndrome or bronchopulmonary sequestration [13] (Fig. 8.13). Often these congenital conditions go unnoticed until hemoptysis occurs, leading to diagnostic workup and detection of the disorder.

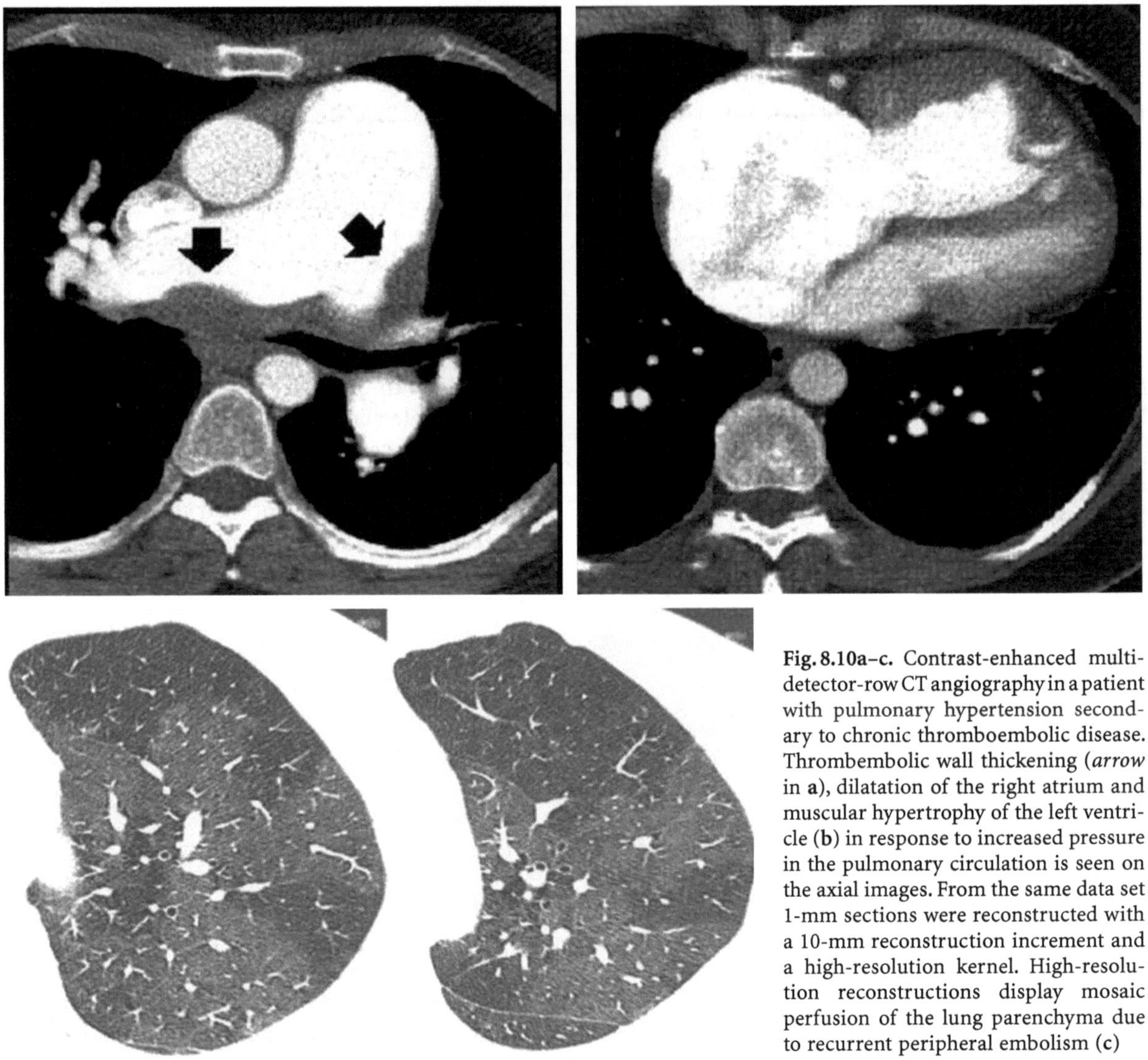

a b c

Fig. 8.10a–c. Contrast-enhanced multidetector-row CT angiography in a patient with pulmonary hypertension secondary to chronic thromboembolic disease. Thrombembolic wall thickening (*arrow* in **a**), dilatation of the right atrium and muscular hypertrophy of the left ventricle (**b**) in response to increased pressure in the pulmonary circulation is seen on the axial images. From the same data set 1-mm sections were reconstructed with a 10-mm reconstruction increment and a high-resolution kernel. High-resolution reconstructions display mosaic perfusion of the lung parenchyma due to recurrent peripheral embolism (**c**)

Bronchial arterial embolization, as a treatment for massive and recurrent hemoptysis, was first described in 1973 by Remy et al. and has since been established as a safe and effective procedure for treatment of this condition [49, 62]. The planning and successful performance of this treatment depends on exact knowledge of the pulmonary vascular anatomy and the location of the hemorrhage. Computed tomography is readily available at most institutions, allowing for a fast diagnosis, even in patients with acute hemoptysis. Thin-section MDCT of the thorax is capable of providing high-resolution images and CT angiograms in a single session. This enables evaluation of structural changes of the lung parenchyma as well as of pulmonary vessels [75], which makes this technology very suitable for comprehensive imaging of disorders of the systemic arterial supply of the lung.

Chronic inflammatory disease can result in acquired systemic arterialization of the lungs, by causing anastomoses between pulmonary and systemic arteries. Most often the anastomoses develop between bronchial and pulmonary arteries within the lung parenchyma, but inflammatory processes in the lung may also cause transpleural anastomoses between pulmonary and systemic nonbronchial arteries. This can occur when an inflammatory process causes pleural adhesion, resulting in neovascularization from regional systemic arteries [51, 91]. Chronic vascular obstruction by inflammatory disorders (e.g., Takayasu's arteritis) or chronic throm-

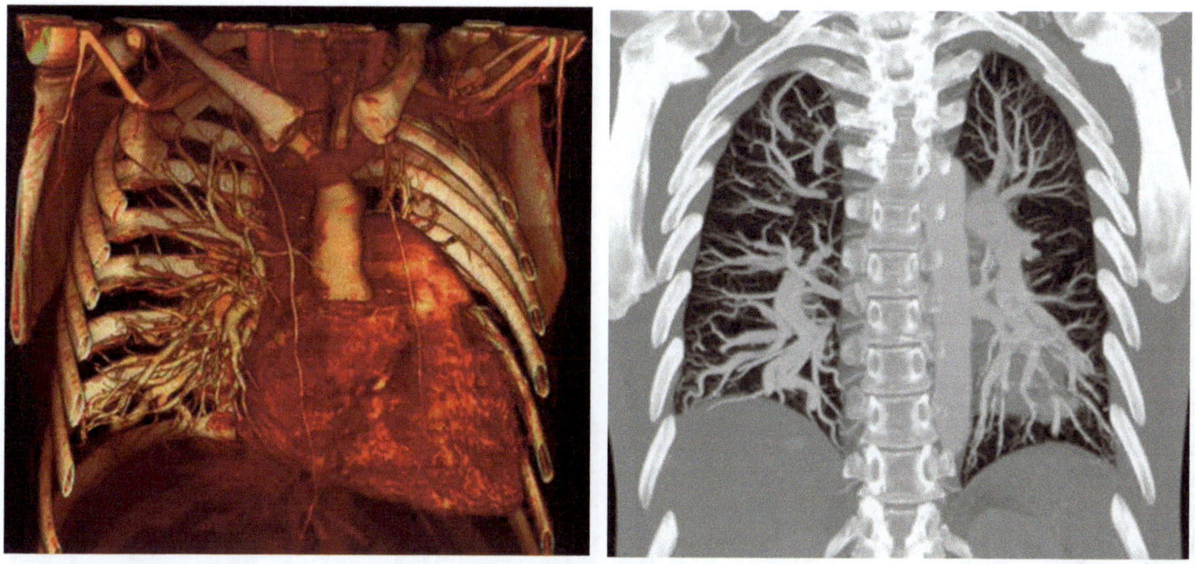

a b

Fig. 8.11a,b. Patient with long-standing idiopathic pulmonary hypertension. Maximum-intensity projection (**a**) and volume rendering (**b**) of a contrast-enhanced 16-slice CT data-set, acquired in less than 10 s, demonstrates tortuous, cork-screw like pulmonary arteries with distal pruning as hallmarks of the disease

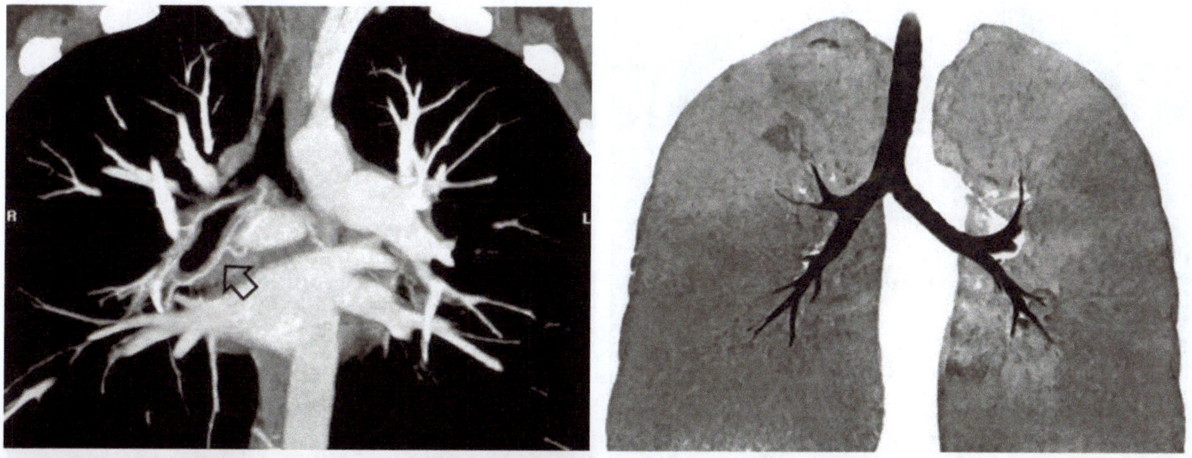

a b

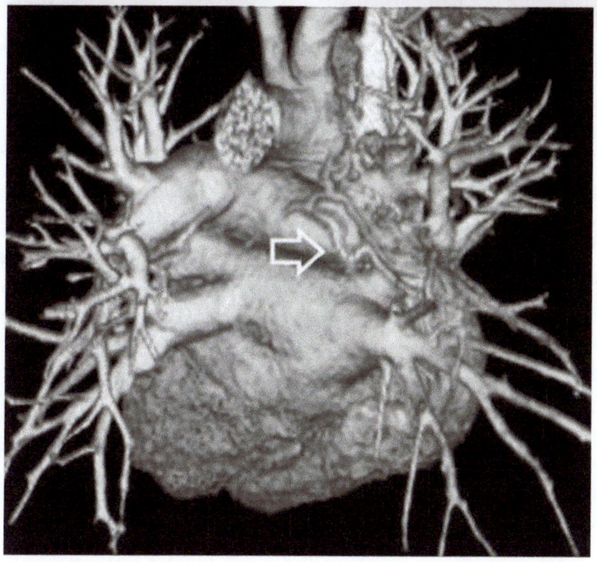

c

Fig. 8.12a–c. Sixteen-slice MDCT angiogram in a patient with long-standing thromboembolic disease. The pulmonary arteries in the right lower lobe are most affected by recurrent thromboembolism and appear obliterated on coronal maximum intensity projections (**a**). Diminished lung perfusion in the affected lower lobes of the lung with maintained perfusion in the upper lobes is demonstrated on coronal minimum intensity projections (**b**) with normal-sized pulmonary veins returning to the left atrium. Blood flow to the right lower lobe is maintained via the bronchial arteries, which are hypertrophied (*arrow* in **a** and **c**) and have formed collaterals bypassing occluded and obliterated pulmonary arteries

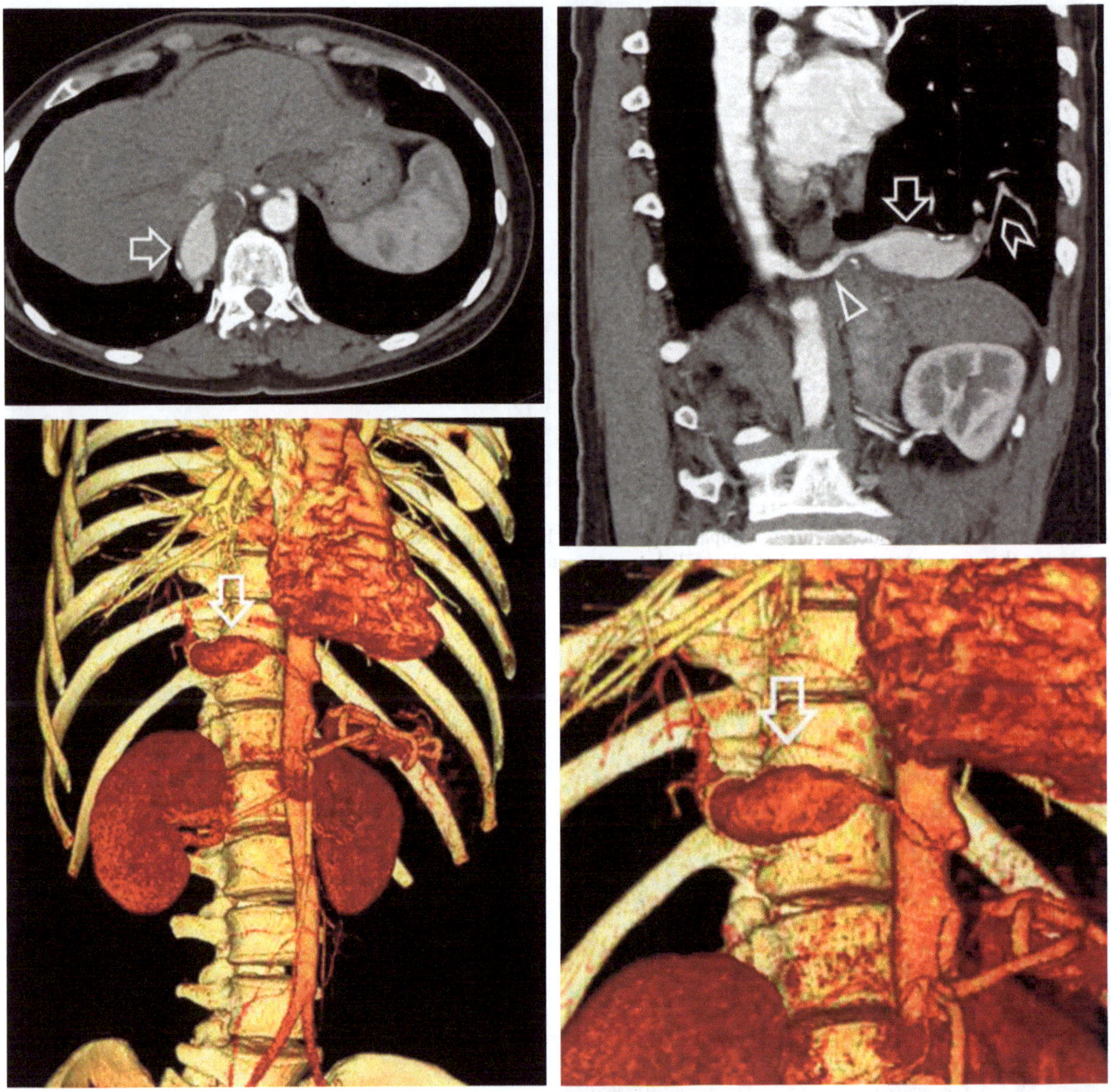

a b c d

Fig. 8.13a–d. High-resolution, contrast-enhanced 16-slice MDCT shows aneurismal dilatation (*large arrows*) of a systemic feeding artery, originating from the aorta cranial to the celiac trunk, supplying a bronchopulmonary sequestration. The feeding artery (*small arrow* in **b**) and the venous drainage (*double arrow* in **b**) are clearly displayed by high-resolution MDCT angiography, facilitating therapeutic planning such as coil-embolization of the vascular anomaly

boembolic changes of the pulmonary arteries can also cause anastomoses between the bronchial and pulmonary arterial systems, resulting in collateralization of the stenosed or obstructed pulmonary arterial bed by the systemic bronchial component of the dual pulmonary blood supply, with subsequent hypertrophy of the bronchial arteries [5, 38, 96] (Fig. 8.12).

8.5 Multidetector-Row CT Imaging of Malignancies of the Pulmonary Circulation

In the evaluation of thoracic malignancy, MDCT angiography of the pulmonary circulation has its premier role in the pre- and posttherapeutic evaluation of the vascular status of tumors of the chest. The correct staging of malignancies of the lung and of the mediastinum, foremost of bronchogenic carcinoma, is a cardinal prerequisite for appropriate tumor management. MDCT imaging, with its high special resolution and its capability of scanning the entire thorax within a short breath-hold in the most dyspneic of patients, has established itself as the modality of choice for this indication. Contrast-enhanced MDCT pulmonary angiography of the pulmonary circulation enables determination of the exact location and extent of tumor mass with respect to pulmonary vessels, and tumor vascularity can be assessed (Figs. 8.14, 8.15, 8.16). Over the course of therapy of bronchogenic carcinoma, therapeutic effects can be accurately monitored by follow up volumetric MDCT scans. The major role of CT angiography is to determine the anatomical relation of tumor mass and pulmonary vasculature before and during therapy, that way also providing crucial information about the risk of hemorrhage, which is an apparent threat when tumor mass is located in the immediate proximity of vessels or when invasion of vessels has already oc-

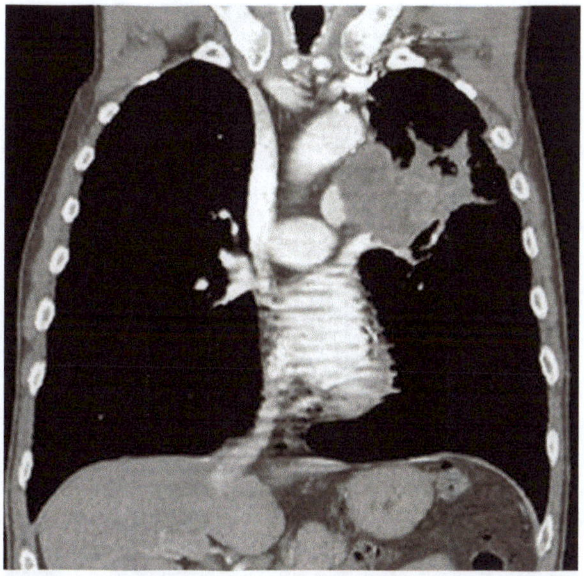

Fig. 8.14 Bronchogenic carcinoma. Contrast-enhanced 2D coronal myocardial perfusion reserve image demonstrates a large aggressive mass which involves the mediastinum, particularly the left superior pulmonary vein

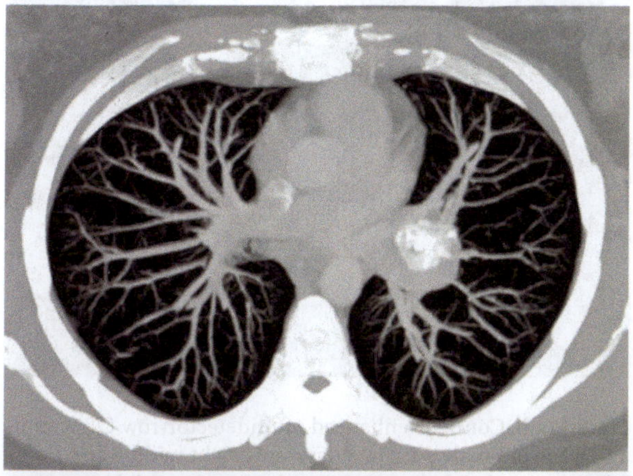

a

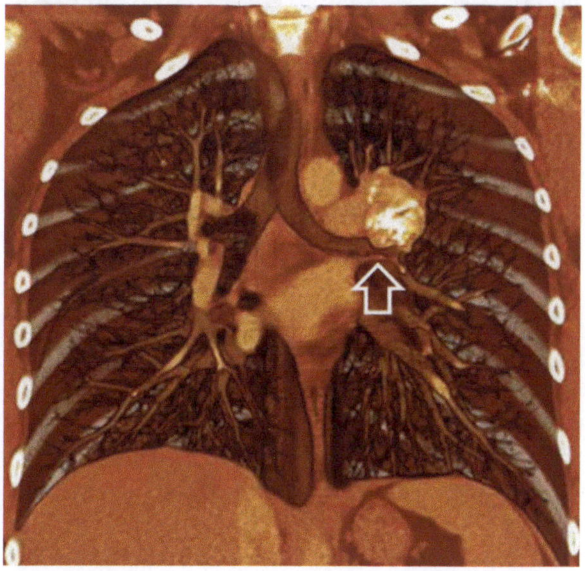

b

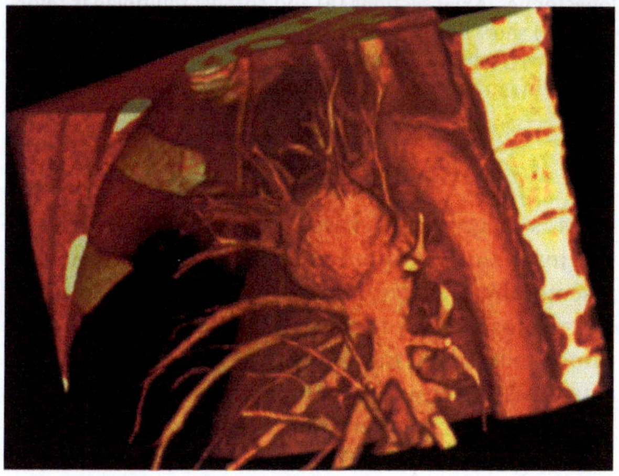

c

Fig. 8.15a–c Metastasis from an abdominal neuroendocrine tumor to the left hilum assessed with contrast-enhanced multidetector-row CT. Axial maximum-intensity projection (**a**) and volume-rendered displays seen from anterior (**b**) and oblique posterior (**c**) perspectives. The heterogeneously calcified soft tissue mass is in immediate spatial relationship with the left main pulmonary artery. A focal polypoid lesion within the left upper lobe bronchus represents endobronchial extension of tumor (*arrow* in **b**)

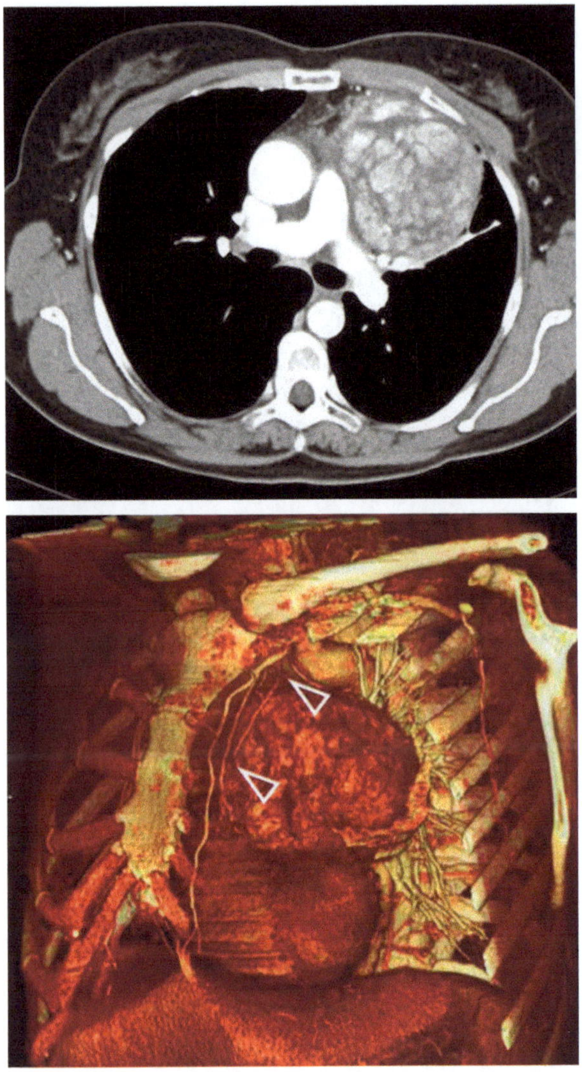

a

b

Fig. 8.16a,b. Invasive thymoma. Contrast-enhanced image (**a**) shows an intensely enhancing nodular mediastinal mass with adjacent atelectasis. Color-enhanced, 3D volume-rendered image (**b**) elucidates the vascular supply of this tumor by malignant neovasculature arising from the left internal thoracic artery (*arrows* in **b**)

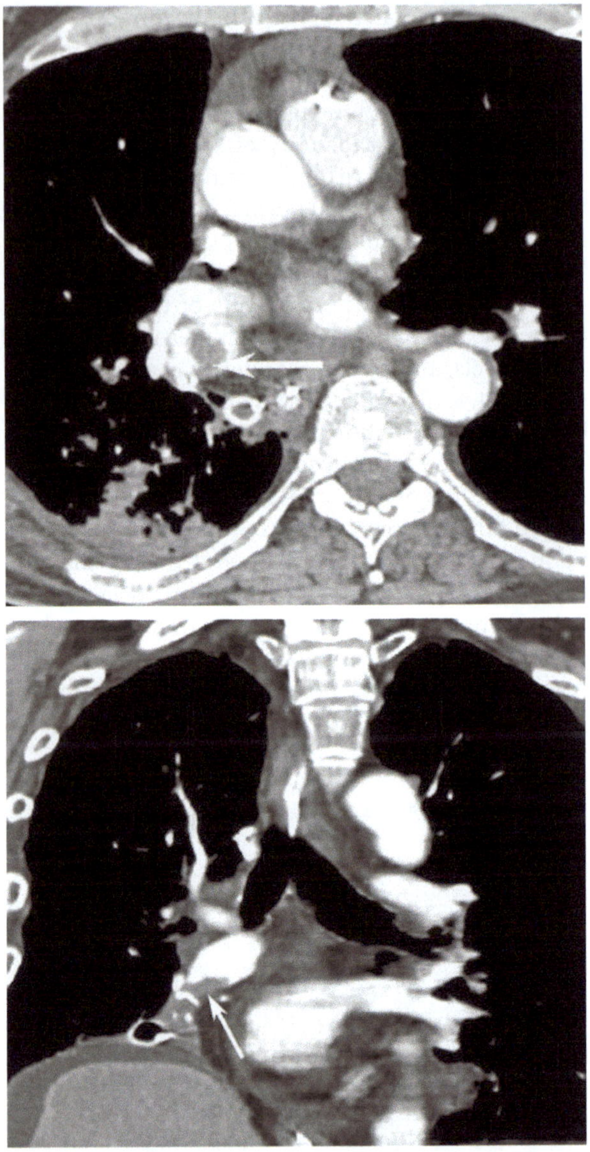

a

b

Fig. 8.17a,b. Contrast-enhanced multidetector-row CT scan in a 54-year-old male patient 5 days post right middle and lower lobectomies. Axial sections (**a**) and coronal multiplanar reformats (**b**) show filling defects in the stump of the right pulmonary artery, representing thrombus formation arising from the suture line in contrast to pulmonary embolism

curred [39]. Visualization of the pulmonary vessels also plays a crucial role for surgical planning, since the appropriate surgical approach is determined by the relation of the tumor to vital anatomy such as the main bronchi and the central pulmonary vessels (Figs. 8.14, 8.15, 8.16). This way, CT guides the decision of whether a more radical surgical approach becomes necessary, if tumor invasion of central structures is diagnosed. Centrally located tumors that do not invade or surround adjacent vessels are usually resected by a sleeve lobectomy and an end-to-end anastomosis of the main stem bronchus. If, however, tumor invasion of more centrally located pulmonary arteries is determined, angioplastic pulmonary artery reconstruction or pneumonectomy is indicated [78]. Postsurgical complications such as arterial strictures and bronchoarterial fistulas following pulmonary artery reconstruction, or clot (Fig. 8.17) in the pulmonary artery stump after lobectomy can be readily identified on follow-up CT angiograms.

Autochthonous malignancies of the pulmonary vasculature are rare neoplasms of the vessel wall, i.e., pulmonary artery sarcomas [57] (Fig. 8.18). The etiology of these tumors is obscure. Histopathologically, most pulmonary artery sarcomas are leiomyosarcomas or "undifferentiated spindle cell sarcomas." Histopathological classification, however, does not seem to be useful clinically or prognostically. Most pulmonary artery sarcomas arise from the dorsal area of the pulmonary trunk, although the tumors also may arise from the right (Fig. 8.18) and left pulmonary arteries, the pulmonary valve, and the right ventricular outflow tract. Because of its rarity and insidious growth characteristics, pulmonary artery sarcoma is often mistaken for pulmonary embolism, resulting in inappropriate therapy such as prolonged anticoagulation or thrombolysis. Symptoms and signs such as weight loss, fever, anemia, and digital clubbing may be subtle clues to diagnosis. Other characteristics, such as the absence of risk factors for DVT, high sedimentation rate, nodular parenchymal infiltrates on CT scans, and lack of response to anticoagulation should raise the suspicion of a process other than pulmonary embolism. CT angiography for a precise preoperative assessment is crucial for the appropriate exploration of the pulmonary artery to ensure complete resection and reconstruction.

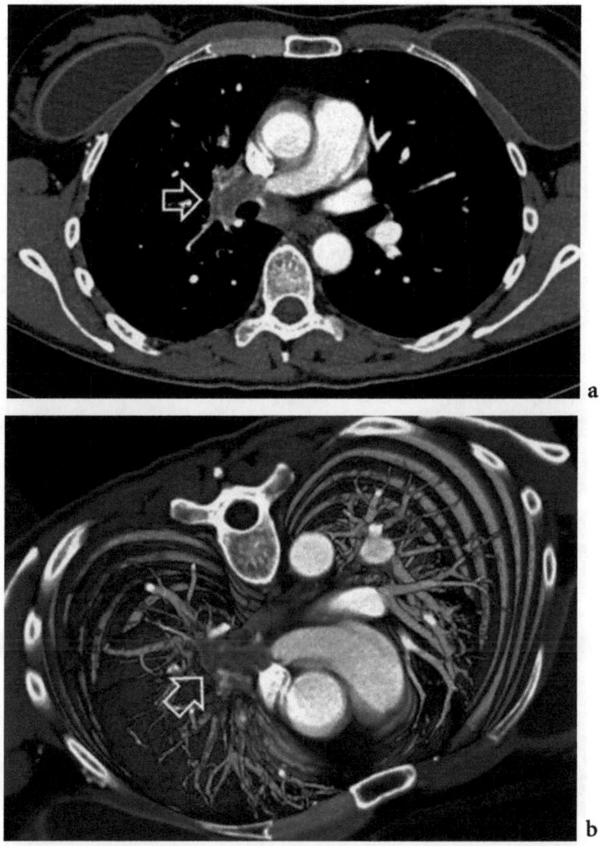

Fig. 8.18a,b. Multidetector-row CT angiography performed in a 52-year-old female patient with dyspnea. Axial sections obtained at the level of the main pulmonary artery (**a**) show an endoluminal filling defect in the right pulmonary artery which was initially felt to be consistent with chronic thromboembolic changes. Surgical exploration after failure of specific treatment established a diagnosis of pulmonary artery sarcoma. 3D volume rendering of the MDCT data set (**b**) may be better suited for appreciating the mass-like nature of the right pulmonary artery lesion

8.6 Multidetector-Row CT Imaging of Congenital Abnormalities of the Pulmonary Circulation

8.6.1 Anomalous Origin of the Left Pulmonary Artery from the Right – "Pulmonary Artery Sling"

Anomalous origin of the left pulmonary artery is usually diagnosed in infancy because of the effect of the aberrant artery on the airway and often the associated tracheal or bronchial stenosis due to complete cartilage rings [43] (Fig. 8.19). This can result in obstruction, feeding problems, and respiratory tract infections. Occasionally, the abnormality may be detected as an incidental finding in an asymptomatic adult or in the adult with respiratory complaints. The aberrant left pulmonary artery originates from the right pulmonary artery and travels across the midline posterior to the distal trachea or right main bronchus, where it turns abruptly to the left, passing between the esophagus and trachea to its destination in the left hilum. This anomalous artery has been called a *sling* (Fig. 8.19). MDCT is well suited for imaging this and other congenital abnormalities. The high acquisition speed and high spatial resolution reduce the need for sedation in pediatric patients and facilitate 3D visualization of complicated vascular anatomy for surgical planning even if very low radiation dose settings, adapted to pediatric patients, are used (Fig. 8.19).

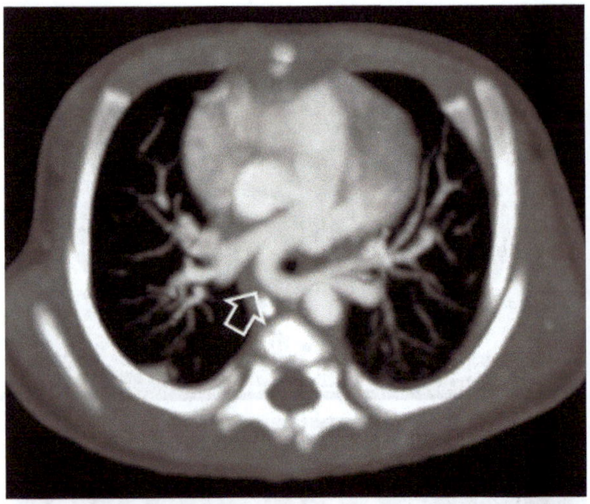

a

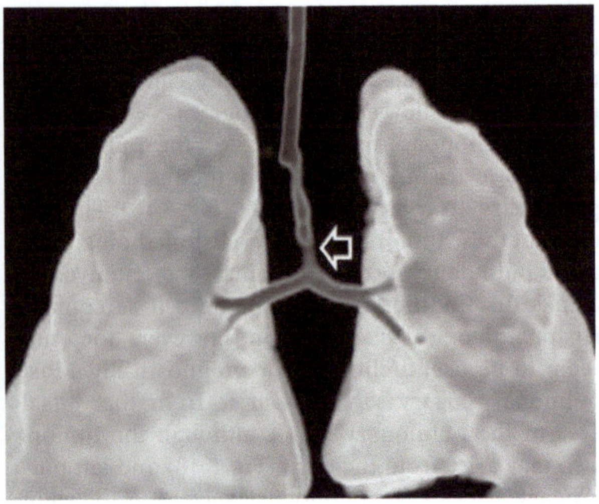

b

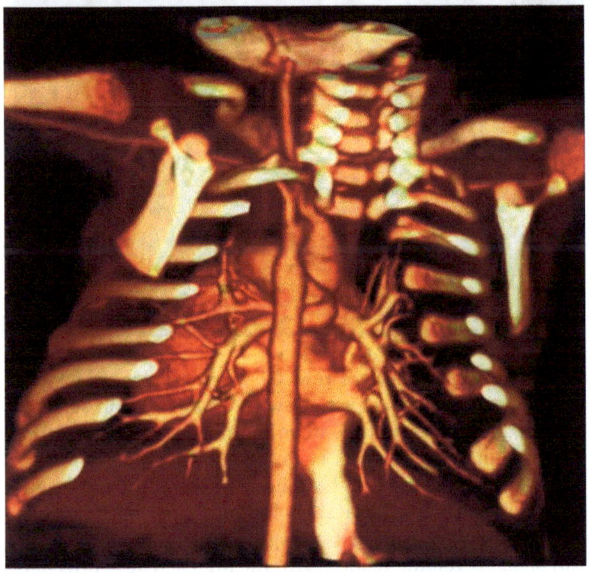

c

Fig. 8.19a–c. Infant presenting with acute shortness of breath. Contrast-enhanced 16-slice MDCT. Axial maximum-intensity projection (**a**) demonstrates the left pulmonary artery taking an aberrant course posterior to the trachea (*arrow* in **a**), forming a pulmonary artery "sling" compressing the trachea. 3D volume-rendered displays of the airways (**b**) and of the thoracic vessels (**c**) demonstrate anomalous vessel course and subsequent compression of the trachea (*arrow* in **b**). In this pediatric case, full diagnostic image quality could be achieved with low-dose scanner settings of 80 kV and 70 mAs (CT data by courtesy of Dr. Roman Fischbach, University of Muenster)

8.6.2 Pulmonary Arteriovenous Malformation

Pulmonary arteriovenous malformation can occur in isolation, be multiple, or be part of a systemic process where arteriovenous communications occur in the skin, mucous membranes, and other organs (hereditary hemorrhagic telangiectasia or Rendu-Osler-Weber disease [83]). CT has proved useful and highly sensitive for the detection of pulmonary arteriovenous malformation and is accepted as the method of choice for routine detection of this vascular abnormality. Apart from detection, CT angiography is also crucial for pretherapeutic evaluation of the angioarchitecture of pulmonary arteriovenous malformations, especially for assessing the number and configuration of feeding and draining vessels connected to the aneurysmal sac (Fig. 8.20). The therapy of choice consists of embolization of the vascular nidus, and the number, course, and orientation of the feeding arteries are the most important factors that determine the technical difficulty and success rate of this procedure. With single-slice CT it often became necessary to obtain a thick-collimation scan of the entire chest for detection of arteriovenous malformations and a high-resolution scan for dedicated evaluation of the angioarchitecture of detected lesions. With the introduction of MDCT technology, acquisition of a single contrast-enhanced scan suffices for both lesion detection and accurate characterization for therapeutic planning (Fig. 8.20).

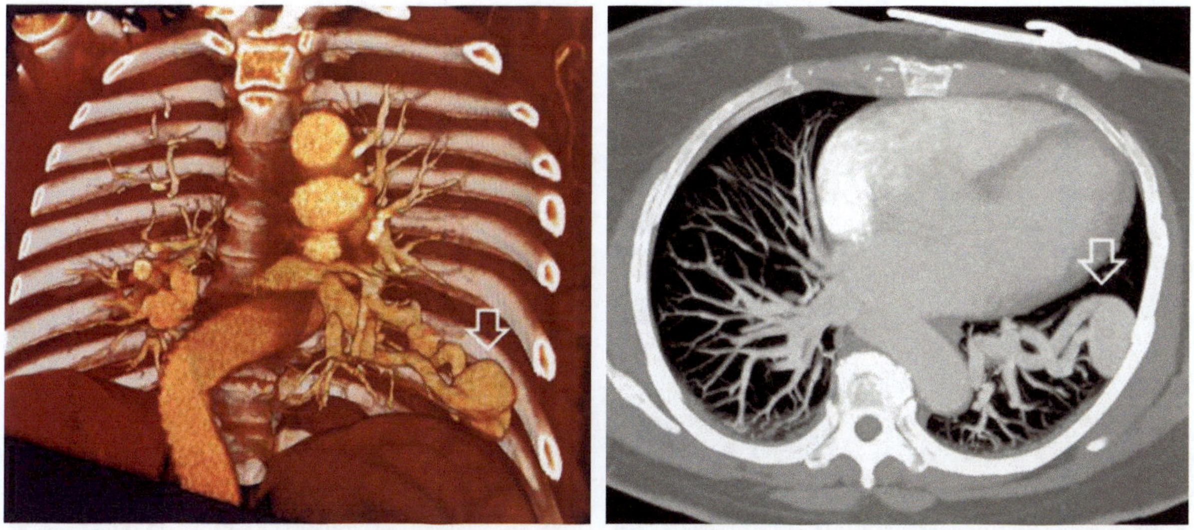

a b

Fig. 8.20a,b. Volume rendering (**a**) and maximum-intensity projection (**b**) of a left lower lobe pulmonary arteriovenous malformation evaluated with contrast-enhanced 16-slice multidetector-row CT angiography. The simple angioarchitecture of the arteriovenous malformation consists of a single feeding artery and a single draining vein, both connected to the aneurysmal sac

8.7 Limitations of CT for Imaging of the Pulmonary Circulation

8.7.1 Contrast Media Injection

Despite ever-advancing CT technology, there are still several factors that can render CT angiography of the pulmonary circulation inconclusive. The most common reasons for nondiagnostic CT studies comprise poor contrast opacification of pulmonary vessels, patient motion, and increased image noise due to excessive patient obesity.

Especially, the advent of MDCT necessitates an extensive revision of contrast-material injection protocols. Faster scan acquisition times allow scan acquisition during maximal contrast opacification of pulmonary vessels [73] but pose an increased challenge for correct timing of the contrast bolus. Strategies that have the potential to improve the delivery of contrast media for high and consistent vascular enhancement during CT pulmonary angiography include use of a test bolus or automated bolus triggering techniques [41]. Saline chasing [32, 33] has been used for effective utilization of contrast media and reduction of streak artifacts arising from dense contrast material in the superior vena cava. Use of multiphasic injection protocols has proven beneficial for general CT angiography [1, 14] but has not been sufficiently evaluated for the pulmonary circulation.

8.7.2 Artifacts and Diagnostic Pitfalls

Another limitation that in some instances results in suboptimal diagnostic quality of CT pulmonary angiography is motion artifacts due to patient respiration or transmitted cardiac pulsation. The short breath-hold times that became feasible with MDCT should facilitate investigation of dyspneic patients [68] and reduce occurrence of respiratory motion artifacts. Similarly, artifacts arising from transmitted cardiac pulsation appear amenable to decreased temporal resolution with fast CT acquisition techniques [73]. ECG synchronization of CT scan acquisition allows for effective reduction of cardiac pulsation artifacts that might interfere with the unambiguous evaluation of cardiac structures, the thoracic aorta, and pulmonary structures [15, 72] (Fig. 8.21). However, the spatial resolution that could be achieved e.g., with retrospectively ECG gated technique using the previous generation of 4-slice MDCT scanners was limited by the relatively long scan duration inherent to data oversampling, [16]. Thus, high-resolution acquisition could only be achieved for relatively small volumes, e.g., the coronary arterial tree, but not for extended

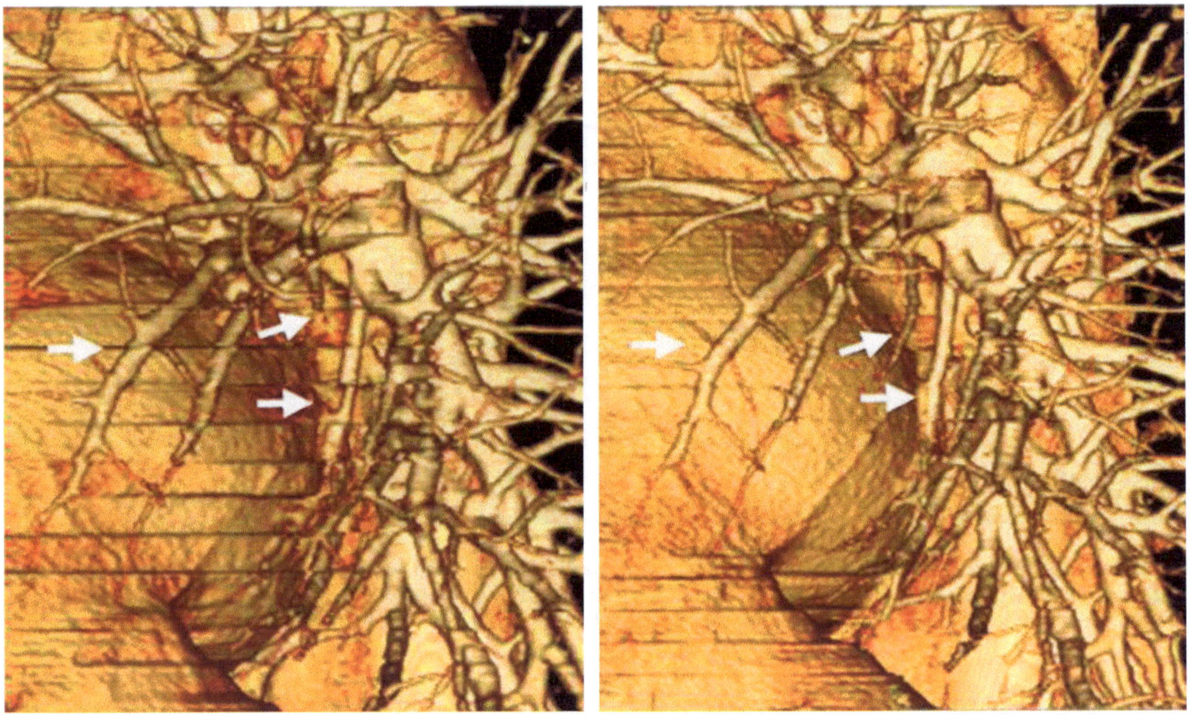

Fig. 8.21 Contrast-enhanced, retrospectively ECG-gated 16-clice CT pulmonary angiography study in a patient with suspected PE. Volume-rendered visualization of paracardiac pulmonary vessels in the left lower lobe. Image reconstruction during systole (*left panel*) results in severe stair-stepping artifacts along the course of the pulmonary vessels (*arrows* in *left panel*) due to transmitted cardiac motion. Image reconstruction of the same data set during the diastolic phase of the cardiac cycle (*right panel*) significantly reduces cardiac pulsation artifacts and enables almost motion-free analysis of paracardiac pulmonary vessels (*arrows* in *right panel*)

coverage of the entire chest. The advent of 16-slice scanners now effectively eliminates these previous trade-offs. With 16-slice MDCT, it is now possible to cover the entire thorax with submillimeter resolution in a single breath-hold with retrospective ECG gating, effectively eliminating transmitted pulsation artifacts (Fig. 8.21; Tables 8.1, 8.2). This way, potential sources of diagnostic pitfalls arising from cardiac motion can be effectively avoided.

8.7.3 Radiation Dose

Use of high-resolution multidetector-CT protocols was shown to improve visualization of pulmonary arteries [21] and the detection of small subsegmental emboli [76]. In suspected PE, establishing an unequivocal diagnosis as to the presence or absence of emboli or other disease based on a high-quality MDCT examination may reduce the overall radiation burden of patients, since further workup with other tests that involve ionizing radiation may be less frequently required. However, if a 4-slice MDCT protocol with 4×1-mm collimation is chosen to replace a single-detector CT protocol based on a 1×5-mm collimation, the increase in radiation dose ranges between 30% [75] and 100% [47]. A similar increase in radiation dose, however, is not to be expected with the introduction of 16-slice multidetector-CT technology with submillimeter resolution capabilities. The addition of detector elements should improve tube output utilization compared with current 4-slice CT scanners and reduce the ratio of excess radiation dose that does not contribute to actual image generation [15]. Also, sophisticated technical devices move into clinical practice that modulate and adapt tube output relative to the geometry and X-ray attenuation of the scanned object, i.e., the patient [22, 36, 37]. Substantial dose savings can thus be realized without compromising on diagnostic quality [27]. The most important factor, however, for ensuring responsible utilization of MDCT's technical prowess is the increased radiation awareness that we currently observe among technologists and radiologists. It has been shown that diagnostic quality of chest CT is not compromised if tube output is adjusted to the body type of the individual patient [94]. Also, with MDCT radiologists are increasingly adapting to the concept of volume imaging and adjust their expectations with regard to the image quality in the individual axial slice that they require for establishing a diagnosis.

8.7.4 Data Management

MDCT increases our diagnostic capabilities; however, the massive amount of data that is generated by this technique puts significant strain on any image-analysis and archiving system. A high-resolution, 16-slice MDCT study in a patient with suspected pulmonary embolism routinely results in 500–600 individual axial images. However, different from focal lung disease, which can be accurately diagnosed by use of maximum-intensity projection reconstructions that beneficially "condense" large-volume MDCT data sets [29], a diagnosis of pulmonary embolism is usually most beneficially established based on individual axial sections. Interpretation of such a study is only feasible by use of digital workstations that allow viewing in "scroll-through" or "cine" mode. Development of dedicated computer-aided detection algorithms [76] may be helpful in the future for the identification of pulmonary emboli in large-volume MDCT data sets. Also, extensive storage capacities are essential for successful routine performance of MDCT in a busy clinical environment. Adapting this environment to the new demands which are generated by the introduction of ever-faster scanning techniques is not a trivial task. New modalities for data transfer, data archiving, and image interpretation will have to be devised in order to make full use of the vast potential of MDCT imaging.

References

1. Bae K, Heiken JP, Brink JA (1998) Aortic and hepatic peak enhancement at CT: effect of contrast medium injection rate – pharmacokinetic analysis and experimental porcine model. Radiology 206:455–464
2. Baile E, King GG, Muller NL, et al. (2000) Spiral computed tomography is comparable to angiography for the diagnosis of pulmonary embolism. Am J Respir Crit Care Med 161:1010–1015
3. Bajc M, Bitzen U, Olsson B et al. (2002) Lung ventilation/perfusion SPECT in the artificially embolized pig. J Nucl Med 43:640–647
4. Blachere H, Latrabe V, Montaudon M et al. (2000) Pulmonary embolism revealed on helical CT angiography: comparison with ventilation-5. perfusion radionuclide lung scanning. AJR Am J Roentgenol 174:1041–1047
5. Boushy SF, North LB, Trics JA (1969) The bronchial arteries in chronic obstructive pulmonary disease. Am J Med 46:506–515
6. Brown MD, Rowe BH, Reeves MJ et al. (2002) The accuracy of the enzyme-linked immunosorbent assay d-dimer test in the diagnosis of pulmonary embolism: a meta-analysis. Ann Emerg Med 40:133–144
7. Cham MD, Yankelevitz DF, Shaham D et al. (2000) Deep venous thrombosis: detection by using indirect CT venography. The Pulmonary Angiography-Indirect Ct Venography Cooperative Group. Radiology 216:744–751
8. Crawford T, Yoon C, Wolfson K et al. (2001) The effect of imaging modality on patient management in the evaluation of pulmonary thromboembolism. J Thorac Imaging 16:163–169
9. Crocco JA, Rooney JJ, Fankushen DS, DiBenedetto RJ, Lyons HA (1968) Massive hemoptysis. Arch Intern Med 121:495–498
10. Diffin D, Leyendecker JR, Johnson SP, Zucker RJ, Grebe PJ (1998) Effect of anatomical distribution of pulmonary emboli on interobserver agreement in the interpretation of pulmonary angiography. AJR Am J Roentgenol 171:1085–1089
11. Dunn KL, Wolf JP, Dorfman DM et al. (2002) Normal d-dimer levels in emergency department patients suspected of acute pulmonary embolism. J Am Coll Cardiol 40:1475
12. Duwe KM, Shiau M, Budorick NE et al. (2000) Evaluation of the lower extremity veins in patients with suspected pulmonary embolism: a retrospective comparison of helical CT venography and sonography. AJR Am J Roentgenol 175:1525–1531
13. Ellis K (1991) Developmental abnormalities in the systemic blood supply to the lungs. AJR Am J Roentgenol 156:669–679
14. Fleischmann D, Rubin GD, Bankier AA, Hittmair K (2000) Improved uniformity of aortic enhancement with customized contrast medium injection protocols at CT angiography. Radiology 214:363–371
15. Flohr T, Prokop M, Becker C et al. (2002) A retrospectively ECG-gated multislice spiral CT scan and reconstruction technique with suppression of heart pulsation artifacts for cardio-thoracic imaging with extended volume coverage. Eur Radiol 12:1497–1503
16. Flohr T, Stierstorfer K, Bruder H et al. (2002) New technical developments in multislice CT. 1. Approaching isotropic resolution with submillimeter 16-slice scanning. Rofo Fortschr Geb Rontgenstr Neuen 17. Bildgeb Verfahr 174:839–845
17. Frazier AA, Galvin JR, Franks TJ, Rosado-De-Christenson ML (2000) From the archives of the AFIP: pulmonary vasculature: hypertension and infarction. Radiographics 20:491–524; quiz 530–531, 532
18. Garg K, Welsh CH, Feyerabend AJ et al. (1998) Pulmonary

embolism: diagnosis with spiral CT and ventilation-perfusion scanning – correlation with pulmonary angiographic results or clinical outcome. Radiology 208:201–208
19. Garg K, Sieler H, Welsh CH et al. (1999) Clinical validity of helical CT being interpreted as negative for pulmonary embolism: implications for patient treatment. AJR Am J Roentgenol 172:1627–1631
20. Garg K, Kemp JL, Wojcik D et al. (2000) Thromboembolic disease: comparison of combined CT pulmonary angiography and venography 21. with bilateral leg sonography in 70 patients. AJR Am J Roentgenol 175:997–1001
21. Ghaye B, Szapiro D, Mastora I et al. (2001) Peripheral pulmonary arteries: how far in the lung does multi-detector row spiral CT allow analysis? Radiology 219:629–636
22. Gies M, Kalender WA, Wolf H, Suess C (1999) Dose reduction in CT by anatomically adapted tube current modulation. I. Simulation studies. Med Phys 26:2235–2247
23. Goodman LR, Curtin JJ, Mewissen MW et al. (1995) Detection of pulmonary embolism in patients with unresolved clinical and scintigraphic diagnosis: helical CT versus angiography. AJR Am J Roentgenol 164:1369–1374
24. Goodman LR, Lipchik RJ, Kuzo RS et al. (2000; Subsequent pulmonary embolism: risk after a negative helical CT pulmonary angiogram – prospective comparison with scintigraphy. Radiology 215:535–542
25. Gottsater A, Berg A, Centergard J et al. (2001) Clinically suspected pulmonary embolism: is it safe to withhold anticoagulation after a negative spiral CT? Eur Radiol 11:65–72
26. Gottschalk A, Stein PD, Goodman LR, Sostman HD (2002) Overview of prospective investigation of pulmonary embolism diagnosis II. Semin Nucl Med 32:173–182
27. Greess H, Nomayr A, Wolf H et al. (2002) Dose reduction in CT examination of children by an attenuation-based on-line modulation of tube current (CARE Dose). Eur Radiol 12:1571–1576
28. Groell R, Peichel KH, Uggowitzer MM et al. (1999) Computed tomography densitometry of the lung: a method to assess perfusion defects in acute pulmonary embolism. Eur J Radiol 32:192–196
29. Gruden JF, Ouanounou S, Tigges S et al. (2002) Incremental benefit of maximum-intensity-projection images on observer detection of small pulmonary nodules revealed by multidetector CT. AJR Am J Roentgenol 179:149–157
30. Gupta A, Frazer CK, Ferguson JM et al. (1999) Acute pulmonary embolism: diagnosis with MR angiography. Radiology 210:353–359
31. Gurney JW (1993) No fooling around: direct visualization of pulmonary embolism. Radiology 188:618–619
32. Haage P, Schmitz-Rode T, Hubner D et al. (2000) Reduction of contrast material dose and artifacts by a saline flush using a double power injector in helical CT of the thorax. AJR Am J Roentgenol 174:1049–1053
33. Hopper KD, Mosher TJ, Kasales CJ et al. (1997) Thoracic spiral CT: delivery of contrast material pushed with injectable saline solution in a power injector. Radiology 205:269–271
34. Hu H, He HD, Foley WD, Fox SH (2000) Four multidetector-row helical CT: image quality and volume coverage speed (in process citation). Radiology 215:55–62
35. Hull R, Raskob GE, Ginsberg JS, et al. (1994) A noninvasive strategy for the treatment of patients with suspected pulmonary embolism. Arch Intern Med 154:289–297
36. Kalender WA, Wolf H, Suess C et al. (1999) Dose reduction in CT by on-line tube current control: principles and validation on phantoms and cadavers. Eur Radiol 9:323–328
37. Kalender WA, Wolf H, Suess C (1999) Dose reduction in CT by anatomically adapted tube current modulation. II. Phantom measurements. Med Phys 26:2248–2253
38. Kauczor HL, Schwickert HC, Mayer E, et al. (1994) Spiral CT of bronchial arteries in chronic thromboembolism. J Comput Assist Tomogr 18:855–861
39. Khanavker B, Stern P, Alberti W, Nakhosteen JA (1991) Complications associated with brachytherapy alone or with laser in lung cancer. Chest 99:1062–1065
40. Khorasani R, Gudas TF, Nikpoor N, Polak JF (1997) Treatment of patients with suspected pulmonary embolism and intermediate-probability lung scans: is diagnostic imaging underused? AJR Am J Roentgenol 169:1355–1357
41. Kirchner J, Kickuth R, Laufer U et al. (2000) Optimized enhancement in helical CT: experiences with a real-time bolus tracking system in 628 patients. Clin Radiol 55:368–373
42. Kruip MJ, Slob MJ, Schijen JH et al. (2002) Use of a clinical decision rule in combination with d-dimer concentration in diagnostic workup of patients with suspected pulmonary embolism: a prospective management study. Arch Intern Med 162:1631–1635
43. Lee KH, Yoon CS, Choe KO et al. (2001) Use of imaging for assessing anatomical relationships of tracheobronchial anomalies associated with left pulmonary artery sling. Pediatr Radiol 31:269–278
44. Leveau P (2002) Diagnostic strategy in pulmonary embolism. National French survey. Presse Med 31:929–932
45. Loud P, Grossman CD, Klippenstein DL, Ray CE (1998) Combined CT venography and pulmonary angiography: a new diagnostic technique for suspected thrombembolic disease. AJR Am J Roentgenol 170:951–954
46. Loud PA, Katz DS, Klippenstein DL et al. (2000) Combined CT venography and pulmonary angiography in suspected thromboembolic disease: diagnostic accuracy for deep venous evaluation. AJR Am J Roentgenol 174:61–65
47. McCollough CH, Zink FE (1999) Performance evaluation of a multi-slice CT system. Med Phys 26:2223–2230
48. Meaney J, Weg JG, Chenevert TL, et al. (1997) Diagnosis of pulmonary embolism with magnetic resonance angiography. N Engl J Med 336:1422–1427
49. Michelle LW, Peter S, Mark JH (2002) Percutaneous embolotherapy for life-threatening hemoptysis. Chest 121:95–102
50. Musset D, Parent F, Meyer G, et al. (2002) Diagnostic strategy for patients with suspected pulmonary embolism: a prospective multicentre outcome study. Lancet 360:1914-1920
51. North LB, Boushy SF, Houk VN (1969) Bronchial and intercostal arteriography in nonneoplastic pulmonary disease. AJR Am J Roentgenol 107:328–342
52. Novelline R, Baltarowich O, Athanasoulis C, Greenfield A, McKusick K (1978) The clinical course of patients with suspected pulmonary embolism and a negative pulmonary angiogram. Radiology 126:561–567
53. Oser RF, Zuckerman DA, Gutierrez FR, Brink JA (1996) Anatomic distribution of pulmonary emboli at pulmonary angiography: implications for cross sectional imaging. Radiology 199:31–35
54. Ost D, Rozenshtein A, Saffran L, Snider A (2001) The nega-

tive predictive value of spiral computed tomography for the diagnosis of pulmonary embolism in patients with nondiagnostic ventilation-perfusion scans. Am J Med 110:16–21
55. Oudkerk M, Beek EJ van, Wielopolski P et al. (2002) Comparison of contrast-enhanced magnetic resonance angiography and conventional pulmonary angiography for the diagnosis of pulmonary embolism: a prospective study. Lancet 359:1643–1647
56. Palmer J, Bitzen U, Jonson B, Bajc M (2001) Comprehensive ventilation/perfusion SPECT. J Nucl Med 42:1288–1294
57. Parish JM, Rosenow EC 3rd, Swensen SJ, Crotty TB (1996) Pulmonary artery sarcoma. Clinical features. Chest 110:1480–1488
58. Patriquin L, Khorasani R, Polak JF (1998) Correlation of diagnostic imaging and subsequent autopsy findings in patients with pulmonary embolism. AJR Am J Roentgenol 171:347–349
59. PIOPED Investigators (1990) Value of the ventilation/perfusion scan in acute pulmonary embolism. JAMA 95:498–502
60. Prologo JD, Glauser J (2002) Variable diagnostic approach to suspected pulmonary embolism in the ED of a major academic tertiary care center. Am J Emerg Med 20:5–9
61. Qanadli SD, Hajjam ME, Mesurolle B et al. (2000) Pulmonary embolism detection: prospective evaluation of dual-section helical CT versus selective pulmonary arteriography in 157 patients. Radiology 217:447–55
62. Remy J, Voisin C, Dupuis C et al. (1974) Treatment of hemoptysis by embolization of the systemic circulation. Ann Radiol (Paris) 17:5–16
63. Remy-Jardin M, Remy J, Wattinne L, Giraud F (1992) Central pulmonary thromboembolism: diagnosis with spiral volumetric CT with the single-breath-hold technique – comparison with pulmonary angiography. Radiology 185:381–387
64. Remy-Jardin M, Remy J, Cauvain O et al. (1995) Diagnosis of central pulmonary embolism with helical CT: role of two-dimensional multiplanar reformations. AJR Am J Roentgenol 165:1131–1138
65. Remy-Jardin M, Remy J, Deschildre F et al. (1996) Diagnosis of pulmonary embolism with spiral CT: comparison with pulmonary angiography and scintigraphy. Radiology 200:699–706
66. Remy-Jardin M, Remy J, Artaud D et al. (1997) Peripheral pulmonary arteries: optimization of the spiral CT acquisition protocol (see Comments). Radiology 204:157–163
67. Remy J, Remy-Jardin M, Artaud D, Fribourg M (1998) Multiplanar and three-dimensional reconstruction techniques in CT: impact on chest diseases. Eur Radiol 8:335–351
68. Remy-Jardin M, Tillie-Leblond I, Szapiro D et al. (2002) CT angiography of pulmonary embolism in patients with underlying respiratory disease: impact of multislice CT on image quality and negative predictive value. Eur Radiol 12:1971–1978
69. Roberts DA, Gefter WB, Hirsch JA et al. (1999) Pulmonary perfusion: respiratory-triggered three-dimensional MR imaging with arterial spin tagging–preliminary results in healthy volunteers. Radiology 212:890–895
70. Schibany N, Fleischmann D, Thallinger C et al. (2001) Equipment availability and diagnostic strategies for suspected pulmonary embolism in Austria. Eur Radiol 11:2287–2294
71. Schluger N, Henschke C, King T et al. (1994) Diagnosis of pulmonary embolism at a large teaching hospital. J Thorac Imaging 9:180–184
72. Schoepf UJ, Becker CR, Bruening RD et al. (1999) Electrocardiographically gated thin-section CT of the lung. Radiology 212:649–654
73. Schoepf UJ, Helmberger T, Holzknecht N et al. (2000) Segmental and subsegmental pulmonary arteries: evaluation with electron-beam versus spiral CT. Radiology 214:433–439
74. Schoepf U, Bruening R, Konschitzky H, et al. (2000) Pulmonary embolism: comprehensive diagnosis using electron-beam computed tomography for detection of emboli and assessment of pulmonary blood flow. Radiology 217:693–700
75. Schoepf U, Bruening RD, Hong C, et al. (2001) Multislice helical CT imaging of focal and diffuse lung disease: comprehensive diagnosis with reconstruction of contiguous and high-resolution CT sections from a single thin-collimation scan. AJR Am J Roentgenol 177:179–184
76. Schoepf U, Das M, Schneider AC, et al. (2002) Computer aided detection (CAD) of segmental and subsegmental pulmonary emboli on 1-mm multidetector-row CT (MDCT) studies. Radiology [Suppl] 225:384
77. Schoepf U, Holzknecht N, Helmberger TK, et al. (2002) Subsegmental pulmonary emboli: improved detection with thin-collimation multidetector-row spiral CT. Radiology 222:483–490
78. Shields TW (1993) Surgical therapy for carcomoma of the lung. Clin Chest Med 14:121–147
79. Stein PD AC, Alavi A et al. (1992) Complications and validity of pulmonary angiography in acute pulmonary embolus. Circulation 85:462–468
80. Stein PD, Gottschalk A (2000) Review of criteria appropriate for a very low probability of pulmonary embolism on ventilation-perfusion lung scans: a position paper. Radiographics 20:99–105
81. Stein PD, Relyea B, Gottschalk A (1996) Evaluation of individual criteria for low probability interpretation of ventilation-perfusion lung scans. J Nucl Med 37:577–581
82. Stein PD, Henry JW, Gottschalk A (1999) Reassessment of pulmonary angiography for the diagnosis of pulmonary embolism: relation of interpreter agreement to the order of the involved pulmonary arterial branch. Radiology 210:689–691
83. Swanson KL, Prakash UB, Stanson AW (1999) Pulmonary arteriovenous fistulas: Mayo Clinic experience, 1982–1997. Mayo Clin Proc 74:671–680
84. Swensen SJ, Sheedy PF 2nd, Ryu JH et al. (2002) Outcomes after withholding anticoagulation from patients with suspected acute pulmonary embolism and negative computed tomographic findings: a cohort study. Mayo Clin Proc 77:130–138
85. Teigen CL, Maus TP, Sheedy PF II, et al. (1995) Pulmonary embolism: diagnosis with contrast-enhanced electron beam CT and comparison with pulmonary angiography. Radiology 194:313–319
86. Tetalman MR, Hoffer PB, Heck LL, Kunzmann A, Gottschalk A (1973) Perfusion lung scan in normal volunteers. Radiology 106:593–594
87. Tillie-Leblond I, Mastora I, Radenne F et al. (2002) Risk of pulmonary embolism after a negative spiral CT angiogram in patients with pulmonary disease: 1-year clinical follow-up study. Radiology 223:461–467

88. Van Erkel AR, Rossum AB van, Bloem JL, Kievit J, Pattynama PNT (1996) Spiral CT angiography for suspected pulmonary embolism: a cost-effectiveness analysis. Radiology 201:29–36
89. Van Rossum AB, Pattynama PM, Mallens WM et al. (1998) Can helical CT replace scintigraphy in the diagnostic process in suspected pulmonary embolism? A retrospective-prospective cohort study focusing on total diagnostic yield. Eur Radiol 8:90–96
90. Van Rossum AB, Erkel AR van, Persijn van, et al. (1998) Accuracy of helical CT for acute pulmonary embolism: ROC analysis of observer performance related to clinical experience. Eur Radiol 8:1160–1164
91. Webb WR, Jacobs RP (1977) Transpleural abdominal systemic artery-pulmonary artery anastomosis in patients with chronic pulmonary infection. AJR Am J Roentgenol 129:233–236
92. Wells PS, Anderson DR, Rodger M et al. (2001) Excluding pulmonary embolism at the bedside without diagnostic imaging: management of patients with suspected pulmonary embolism presenting to the emergency department by using a simple clinical model and d-dimer. Ann Intern Med 135:98–107
93. Wildberger JE, Mahnken AH, Schmitz-Rode T et al. (2001) Individually adapted examination protocols for reduction of radiation exposure in chest CT. Invest Radiol 36:604–611
94. Wildberger JE, Niethammer MU, Klotz E et al. (2001) Multi-slice CT for visualization of pulmonary embolism using perfusion weighted color maps. Rofo Fortschr Geb Rontgenstr Neuen Bildgeb Verfahr 173:289–294
95. Woodard PK (1997) Pulmonary arteries must be seen before they can be assessed. Radiology 204:11–12
96. Yamada I, Shibuya H, Matsubara O et al. (1992) Pulmonary artery disease in Takayasu's arteritis: angiographic findings. AJR Am J Roentgenol 159:263–269
97. Yankelevitz DF, Gamsu G, Shah A et al. (2000) Optimization of combined CT pulmonary angiography with lower extremity CT venography. AJR Am J Roentgenol 174:67–69
98. Zuckerman DA, Sterling KM, Oser RF (1996) Safety of pulmonary angiography in the 1990s. J Vasc Interv Radiol 7:199–205

9 Multidetector-Row CT Angiography of the Coronary Arteries

Christoph R. Becker

CONTENTS

9.1 Introduction

Annually more than 1 million diagnostic cardiac catheter investigations are performed in the United States. Only approximately one-half of all investigations are followed by an interventional procedure. The other patients with symptoms are treated conservatively or by bypass graft surgery. In recent decades coronary angiography has advanced to become a fast and safe investigation. Nevertheless, in particular patients are well aware of the minimal risk and the discomfort of the procedure. Therefore there is need for a noninvasive method to demonstrate the coronary arteries in a way that would allow the triage of patients referred to cardiac catheter.

Initially coronary CT angiography (CTA) performed by electron-beam CT was considered to assess the coronary arteries noninvasively [28]. For the point of temporal resolution with 100 ms exposure time, these CT scanners were ideally suited to image the coronary arteries. However, the spatial resolution and the image noise were considerably higher in these than in any conventional CT scanners, because X-ray-gun power was limited to 130 kVp and 630 mA. In addition the longer scan times necessitate the administration of atropine and high amount of contrast media [1].

C. R. Becker, MD
Associate Professor, Department of Clinical Radiology, University Hospital Grosshadern, University Munich, Marchioninistrasse 15, 81377 Munich, Germany

9.2 Multidetector-Row CT Acquisition Technique

The combination of fast gantry rotation, slow table movement, and multislice helical acquisition for the first time allows conventional CT to image the coronary arteries. With this approach a high number of X-ray-projection data are acquired. For the technique called "retrospective ECG gating," the ECG is recorded simultaneously and the CT images are reconstructed from the slow-motion diastole phase of the heart.

For retrospective ECG gating with multidetector-row CT (MDCT), the pitch factor (detector collimation/table feed per gantry rotation) must not exceed 0.3 to allow for scanning the heart at any heart rate higher than 40 beats/min.

Depending on the clinical question, there are different scan protocols in use for coronary calcium screening, coronary CTA, bypass graft CTA, and pulmonary CT venography. These protocols differ in respect of scan range, duration, slice collimation, X-ray tube current and voltage, contrast-media quantity and flow. A summary of the different protocols for a 4- and 16-detector-row CT scanner is given in Table 9.1.

The exposure time in MDCT with retrospective ECG gating is considerably longer (~200 ms) and the radiation exposure is higher (~10 mSv) than in electron beam CT (~2 mSv). However, image quality is superior in MDCT compared with electron beam CT in respect of higher spatial resolution and lower image noise [3].

In MDCT an attempt has been made to improve temporal resolution by multisector reconstruction. For this technique X-ray-projections of more than

Table 9.1 Four- and sixteen-detector-row CT scan protocols for coronary screening, coronary CT angiography (*CTA*), bypass graft CTA, and pulmonary CT venography (*CTV*)

	Coronary screening		Coronary CTA		Bypass graft CTV		Pulmonary CTV	
Collimation (mm)	4 × 2.5	16 × 0.75	4 × 1	16 × 0.75	4 × 2.5	16 × 0.75	4 × 1	16 × 0.75
Slice thickness (mm)	3	3	1.3	1	3	1	1.3	1
Increment (mm)	1.5	1.5	0.8	0.8	1.5	0.8	0.8	0.8
Effective mAs	100	100	400	500	400	500	200	200
kVp	120	120	120	120	120	120	120	120
Scan range (mm)	12	12	12	12	15	15	15	15
Scan time (s)	20	20	40	20	30	30	20	10
Scan delay (s)	-	-	0	6	3	3	0	6
Iodine concentration (mg/ml)	-	-	300	300	300	300	300	300
Contrast (ml)	-	-	140	90	120	120	80	70
Flow (ml/s)	-	-	3.3	3.3	4	4	4	4
Radiation exposure	1 mSv	1 mSv	4 mSv	5 mSv	5 mSv	6 mSv	2 mSv	2 mSv

Dual injection of contrast media with a saline chaser bolus is recommended

one heartbeat are used to reconstruct an image. This technique requires absolutely consistent data from at least two consecutive heartbeats for successful image reconstruction. Unfortunately, the rhythm of the human heart may change rapidly, in particular under special conditions such as breath holding and the Valsalva maneuver. For this reason, this technique is of limited practical use under clinical conditions.

The redundant radiation occurring during the radiation exposure in the systole can substantially be reduced by a technique called prospective ECG tube-current modulation. On the basis of the ECG signal, the X-ray tube current is switched to its nominal value during the diastole phase and is reduced significantly during the systole phase of the heart, respectively. This technique is most effective in patients with low heart rates. If the heart rate is lower than 60 beats/min, the radiation exposure will be reduced by approximately 50% [22]. The radiation exposure for coronary MDCT is then comparable with what is applied during a typical diagnostic coronary catheter procedure.

Image-retrospective ECG gating always begins with a careful analysis of the ECG trace recorded with the helical scan. The image reconstruction interval is best placed in between the T- and the P-wave of the ECG, corresponding to the mid-diastole interval. The point of time for the least coronary motion may be different for every coronary artery. Least-motion artifacts may result for reconstructing the right coronary artery (RCA), left anterior descending coronary artery (LAD), and left circumflex coronary artery (LCx) at 50%, 55%, and 60% of the RR interval, respectively. Individual adaptation of the point of time for reconstruction seems to further improve image quality. However, the lower the heart rate the easier it is to find the single best interval for all three major branches of the coronary artery tree [17]. With a 16-detector-row CT, near-isotropic spatial resolution of ~0.83 mm^3 can be achieved. The patient room-time is in between 15 and 30 min and image reconstruction and postprocessing can be performed within approximately another 15 min.

In addition, retrospective ECG gating allows for reconstruction of images at any time within the cardiac cycle. Setting the images together that are reconstructed every 10% of the RR interval allows visualization of cardiac function. The functional CT data can be evaluated by software in a similar fashion to magnetic resonance (MR) images, and global as well as regional wall motion can be determined [14]. However, reconstruction of a functional data currently needs at least 20 min postprocessing time, and the currently available ~200 ms exposure time may be not sufficient to reliably assess the cardiac function in the systole phase of the cardiac cycle.

9.3 Patient Preparation

Even in diastole and for morphological assessment of the coronary arteries, reasonably good image quality with ~200 ms exposure time can only be achieved in patients with low heart rates [17]. Therefore, patients should avoid caffeine or any drug such as atropine or nitroglycerin that increases the heart rate prior to a cardiac CTA investigation. Instead, the use of beta-blockers may become necessary for patient preparation aiming at a heart rate of 60 beats/min or less.

To consider a beta-blocker for patient preparation, contraindications (bronchial asthma, atrioventricular (AV) block, severe congestive heart failure, aortic stenosis, etc. [35]) have to be ruled out and informed consent must be obtained from the patient. Where the heart rate of a patient is significantly above 60 beats/min, 50–200 mg of metoprolol tartrate can be administered orally 30–90 min prior to the investigation. Alternatively, 5–20 mg of metoprolol tartrate divided into four doses can be administered intravenously [35] immediately prior to scanning. Monitoring of vital functions, heart rate, and blood pressure is essential during this approach. Indeed, the positive effect of beta-blocker on cardiac MDCT scanning if fourfold: The sedating effect of beta-blocker results in a better patient compliance and less movement during scanning. The patient is exposed to less radiation, because with lower heart rate ECG tube-current modulation works more effectively. Cardiac motion artifacts are substantially reduced and, because of the lower cardiac output with beta-blocker, the contrast enhancement increases.

9.4 Contrast Administration

A timely accurate and homogeneous vascular lumen enhancement is essential for full diagnostic capability of coronary MDCT angiography studies. Higher contrast enhancement is superior to identify small vessels in MDCT. However, dense contrast material in the right atrial cavity may cause streak artifacts arising from the right atrium that may interfere with the RCA. In addition, high enhancement of the coronary arteries may interfere with coronary calcifications and may therefore hinder the delineation of the residual lumen.

A peripheral iodine flow rate of 1–1.4 g/s will result in an enhancement of approximately 250-300 HU in the majority of patients [7] and still allows detection of coronary calcification (Fig. 9.1).

The final vessel enhancement will not only depend on the iodine flow rate but also on the cardiac output of the patient. In patients with low cardiac output, e.g., under beta-blocker medication, the contrast media will accumulate in the cardiac chambers and lead to a higher enhancement than in patients with high

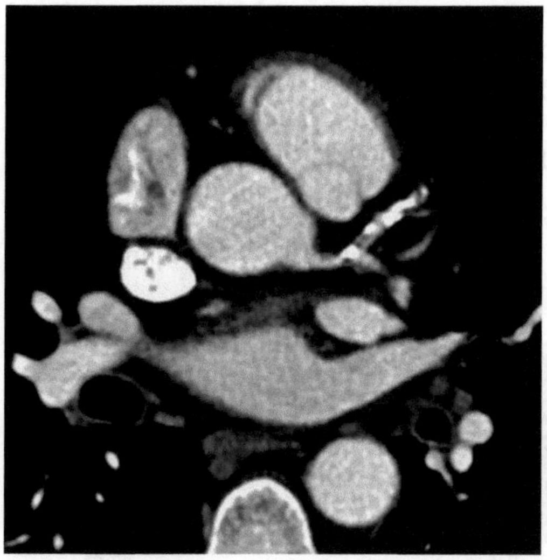

Fig. 9.1. With an iodine flow rate of 1–1.4 g/s, an enhancement in between 250 and 300 HU may be reached. With this enhancement coronary calcifications as well as noncalcified plaques can ideally be delineated.

cardiac output, where the contrast agent will faster be diluted by nonenhanced blood.

The circulation time can be determined by a test bolus of 5 g iodine injected with a 1 g/s iodine flow rate and followed by a saline chaser bolus. A series of scans is acquired at the level of the ascending aorta every other second. The arrival time of the test bolus can be determined by taking the delay time between start of the contrast injection and peak enhancement of the ascending aorta into account.

In a 4-detector-row CT, scanning may start directly at the time of the predetermined peak enhancement of the test bolus. Scanning with a 16-detector-row CT requires an additional delay time to allow the contrast media to reach the left ventricular system and the coronary arteries. In our experience another 6 s should be added to the peak enhancement of the test bolus to allow for complete enhancement of the left ventricular system in a 16-detector-row CT. The contrast media has to be injected for the duration of the scan and the delay time and therefore has to be maintained for 40 s and 26 s in a 4- and 16-detector-row CT, respectively.

With the use of a dual injector with sequential peripheral venous injection of contrast media and saline, the bolus of contrast media with a high viscosity will be kept compact [10], the total amount of contrast media may be reduced [19, 13], and a central venous enhancement profile can be achieved [16]. Reducing the amount and the use of iso-osmolar contrast media may reduce the risk of contrast-induced nephropathy [4]. Changes of heart rate have less frequently been observed during the injection of isoosmolar contrast agent [9]. In a 16-detector-row CT, the sequential injection of contrast media and saline allows for selective enhance the left ventricular cavity (levocardiogram), with washout of dense contrast media in the right atrium (Fig. 9.2) helping to avoid artifacts.

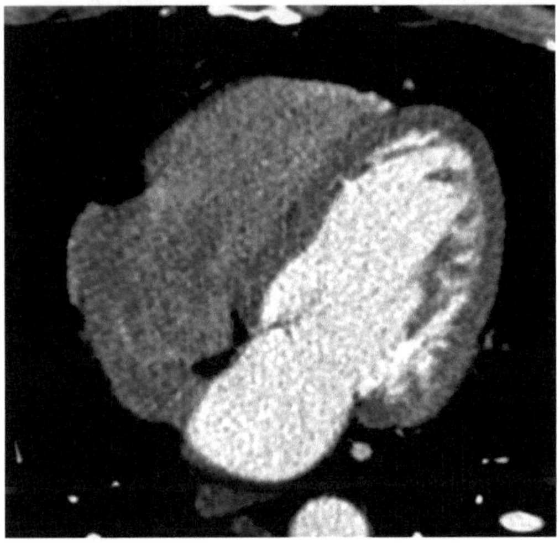

Fig. 9.2 In a 16-row-detector CT, complete and homogeneous enhancement of the left ventricle (levocardiogram) and the coronary arteries can be achieved by a dedicated contrast protocol. The contrast medium has passed the right ventricle and the flush with saline results in a washout of the contrast medium from the right ventricle.

Alternatively, the beginning of the CT scan can be triggered automatically by the arrival of the contrast bolus. A preliminary scan is taken at the level of the aortic root and a region of interest is placed into the ascending aorta. When contrast injection starts, repeated scanning at the same level is performed every second. If the density in the ascending aorta reaches 100 HU, a countdown begins until the acquisition starts. Right at the start of the CT scan acquisition, the patient is instructed to hold their breath. An additional delay time of 4 s and 10 s has to be added in a 4- and 16-detector-row CT, respectively, to allow for an adequate contrast enhancement.

The patients should be instructed to take a deep breath and to avoid the Valsalva maneuver. The Valsalva maneuver increases the intrathoracic pressure, preventing the influx of contrast media through the superior vena cava into the right atrium. Nonenhanced blood from the inferior vena cava entering the right atrium leads to an inhomogeneous enhancement of the cardiac volume during the CTA scan.

9.5 Postprocessing

Primary axial slices are best suited to rule out coronary artery disease (CAD). However, the detection of coronary artery stenoses in axial CT images may be problematic, since every slice displays only a small fragment of the entire coronary artery. Multiplanar reformatting, volume rendering, virtual coronary endoscopy, and shaded surface display have been tested for reconstruction of CTA images to detect coronary artery stenosis. None of this postprocessing proved to be superior to axial slices for this task [41]. Maximum-intensity projection (MIP) postprocessing of CTA images were found to be helpful to follow the course of the coronary arteries and to create angiographic-like projections that may allow for better detection of coronary artery stenoses.

Standardized thin-slab MIP reconstruction may be performed with 5-mm slab thickness and 2.5-mm increments in three different planes similar to standard cardiac catheter projections [23]. MIP along the inter- and atrioventricular groove creates images in similar planes as the right anterior oblique (RAO) and left anterior oblique (LAO) angiographic projections, respectively. The RAO projection is suited to demonstrate the course of the left anterior descending coronary artery (Fig. 9.3), whereas the LAO projection best displays the course of the RCA and LCx (Fig. 9.4). In addition, similar to coronary angiography, an oblique projection can be reconstructed following the long axis of the heart. This projection plane spreads the branches of the LAD and is therefore called the "spider view." The spider view is designed to demonstrate the proximal part of all three major coronary arteries (Fig. 9.5).

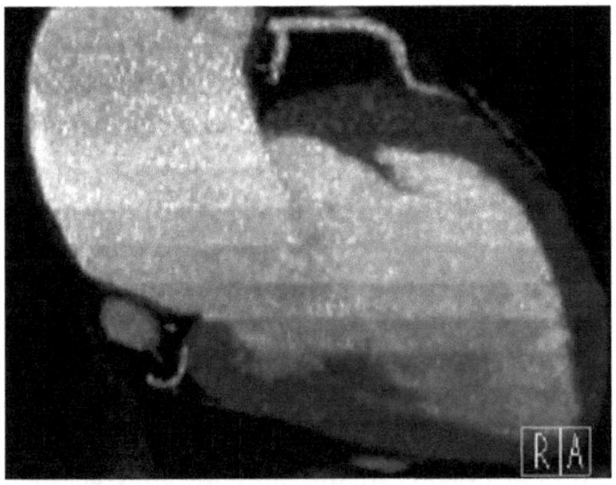

Fig. 9.3 To display the course of the left anterior descending coronary artery, maximum-intensity projections may be performed in right anterior oblique (RAO) projection.

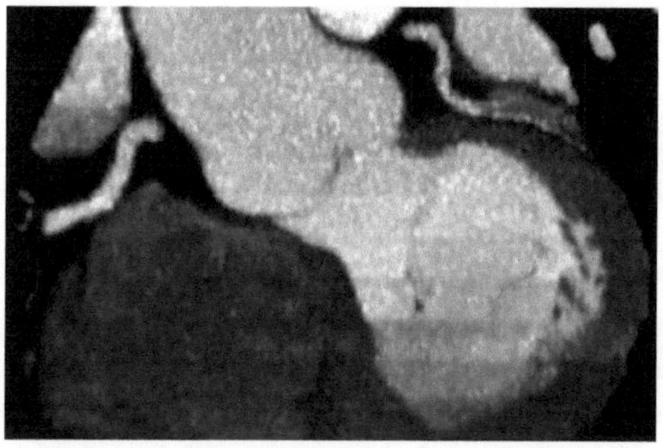

Fig. 9.4 Left anterior oblique (LAO) projections are best suited to display the course of the right and circumflex coronary artery.

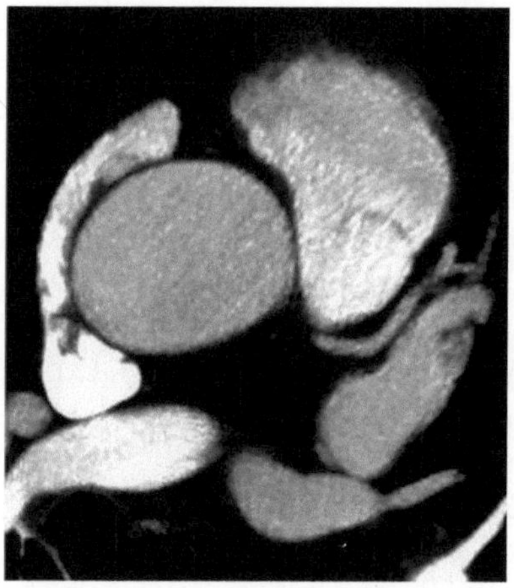

Fig. 9.5 The so-called spider (LAO oblique) displays the course of the left anterior coronary artery and the diagonal branches.

9.6 Evaluation of Coronary CT

For the first run, MIP images may help to identify coronary stenosis. Volume rendering has been found to be helpful to demonstrate the course in the case of coiling and kinking of the coronary arteries, i.e., in hypertensive heart disease, in a coronary fistula, or in case of suspicion of any other coronary anomaly. However, every finding from postprocessed images has to be confirmed in the original axial CT slices.

Image analysis begins with identification of the coronary artery segments in the axial CT slices (Fig. 9.6). Coronary segments can be numbered (Table 9.2) according to the model suggested by the American Heart Association [5].

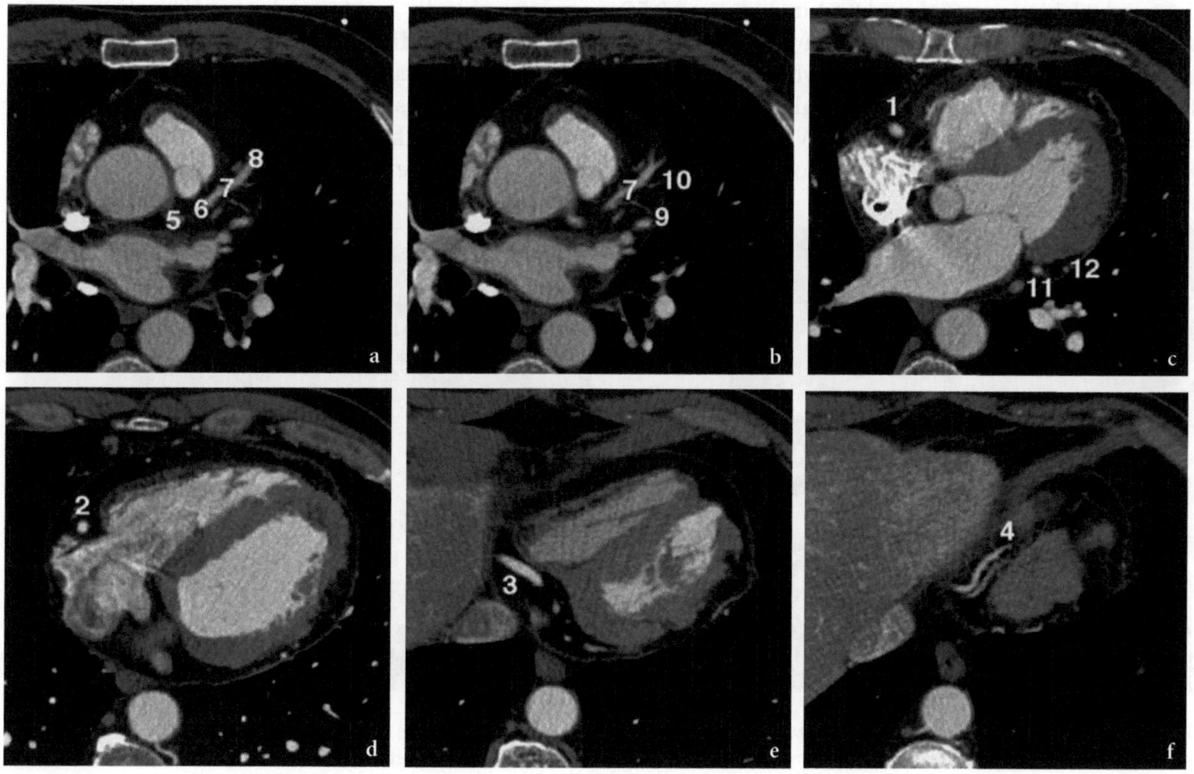

Fig. 9.6 Coronary artery segments are numbered from 1 to 16 according the classification scheme of the AHA.

Table 9.2 Segment numbering according to the AHA scheme [5]

Segment	Name	Abbreviation	Part	Beginning	End
1	Right coronary artery	RCA	Proximal	Ostium	RV
2	Right coronary artery	RCA	Middle	RMD	AM
3	Right coronary artery	RCA	Distal	AM	Crux cordis
4	Posterior descending coronary artery	PDA		Crux cordis	Apex
5	Left main coronary artery	LCA		Ostium	Bifurcation
6	Left anterior descending	LAD	Proximal	Bifurcation	D_1
7	Left anterior descending	LAD	Middle	D_1	D_2
8	Left anterior descending	LAD	Distal	D_2	Apex
9	First diagonal branch	D_1			
10	Second diagonal branch	D_2			
11	Left circumflex coronary artery	LCx	Proximal	Bifurcation	OM
12	Obtuse marginal branch	OM			
13	Left circumflex coronary artery	LCx	Distal	OM	PD
14	Posterolateral branch	PL			
15	Posterior descending branch	PD			

The morphology of calcifications may give a first hint for the presence or absence of significant stenoses in the coronary arteries. From electron beam CT studies, Kajinami et al. reported that the positive predictive value for significant stenosis (≥75%) was 0.04 and 0.17 in none, 0.18 and 0.59 in spotty (Fig. 9.7), 0.32 and 0.87 in long, 0.40 and 0.84 in wide, and 0.56 and 0.96 in diffuse (Fig. 9.8) coronary calcifications, respectively [24]. Therefore, only when small calcifications in the coronary artery wall are present is significant stenosis very unlikely. Where a calcified plaque obscures the lumen of the coronary vessel, a significant stenosis can neither be determined nor ruled out.

A lumen-narrowing scoring system according to Schmermund et al. [36] may be used to describe different grades of coronary artery stenosis in the proximal and middle coronary artery segment: A, angiographically normal segment (0% stenosis); B, nonobstructive disease (1-49% lumen-diameter stenosis); C, significant (50-74%) stenosis; D, high-grade (75-99%) stenosis; E, total occlusion (100% stenosis). The patency of the distal coronary artery segments should be reported as well.

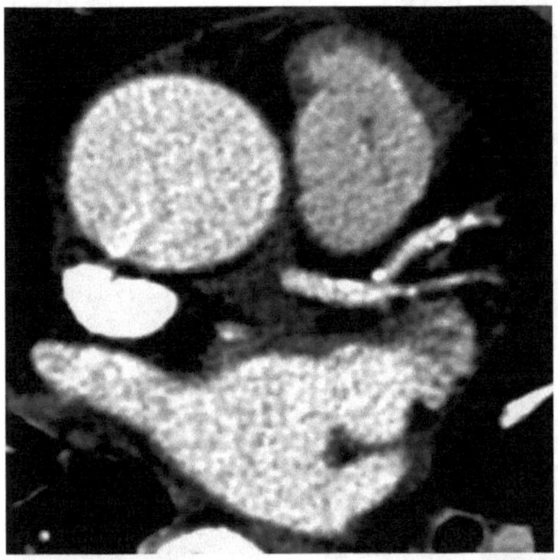

Fig. 9.7 The positive predictive value of spotty coronary calcifications is in between 18% and 59%. Significant coronary stenoses are highly unlikely in the presence of spotty calcifications.

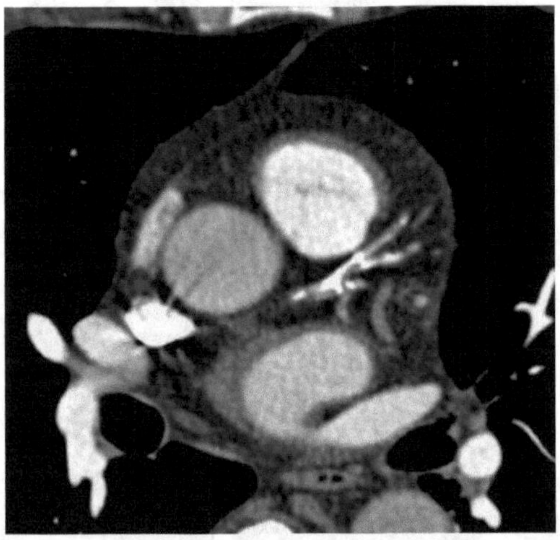

Fig. 9.8 The positive predictive value of diffuse coronary calcifications is between 56% and 96%. In the case of extensive calcifications, coronary artery stenosis can neither be determined correctly nor be ruled out.

9.7 Clinical Application

Initial experiences revealed a number of limitations already known from coronary CTA studies performed with the electron beam CT. Schmermund et al. [36] reported that small vessel diameter may lead to false-positive findings. They also reported that extensive calcifications might interfere with the detection of coronary artery stenoses, resulting in false negative results compared with selective coronary angiography. A reason for this observation may be that standard CT soft tissue reconstruction kernels are leading to a "blooming" of dense material such as coronary stents or calcifications that obscure the vessel lumen and wall changes.

The real nature of CTA is more a cross-sectional display of the wall than the lumen. Because of the limited spatial resolution in CTA and the blooming of calcifications, the definite assessment of the degree of coronary artery stenoses remains still problematic. Therefore, coronary CTA will currently not be suited to determine the progression in patients with known CAD, typical angina, or obvious myocardial ischemia on exercise testing. These patients are better approached by cardiac catheter examination, with the option to perform percutaneous coronary interventions in the same session [29].

It should be considered, when interpreting coronary CTA, that details such as collateral vessels, contrast runoff, and direction of filling of coronary arteries are not visualized by CTA. Finally, the hemodynamic relevance of coronary artery stenoses may not reliably be determined without wall-motion analysis or myocardium perfusion data under rest and exercise. Further limitations have been seen in patients with a body mass index above 30 [41] and absolute arrhythmia [15], leading to a degradation of image quality in CTA by severe image noise and cardiac motion artifacts.

But more than only displaying the lumen of the coronary arteries, MDCT by it cross-sectional nature is well suited to demonstrate changes of the coronary artery wall. Coronary calcifications can easily be assessed even without contrast media and represent an advanced stage of atherosclerosis. However, as different stages of coronary atherosclerosis may be present simultaneously, calcifications may also be associated with more early stages of coronary atherosclerosis. Therefore, the entire extent of coronary atherosclerosis will be underestimated by assessing coronary calcifications alone [42]. With contrast enhancement calcified as well as noncalcified lesions can completely be assessed by MDCT simultaneously.

In patients with an acute coronary syndrome, we have observed noncalcified plaques with irregular border and nonhomogeneous but low (20–40 HU) CT density values [6]. Most likely these soft tissues in the coronary artery corresponds to an intracoronary thrombus formation (Fig. 9.9).

In asymptomatic patients and patients dying for other than cardiac reasons, frequently well-defined noncalcified lesions are found (Fig. 9.10). The density of these plaque may vary in between 50 and 90 HU

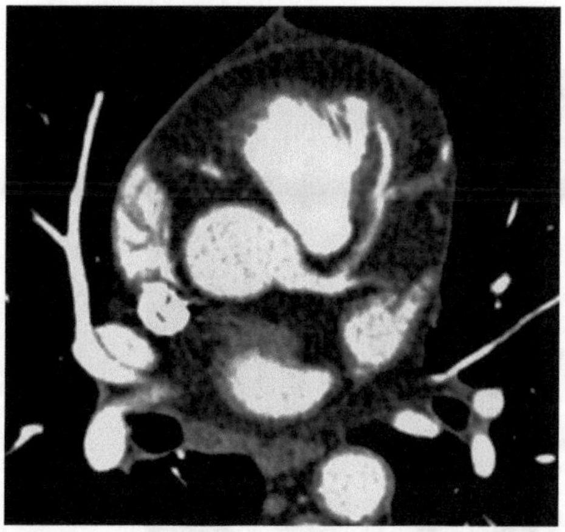

Fig. 9.9 Irregular, inhomogeneous and low dense plaque in the left anterior descending coronary artery in a patient with acute coronary syndrome. The lesion most likely corresponds to a thrombus in the coronary artery.

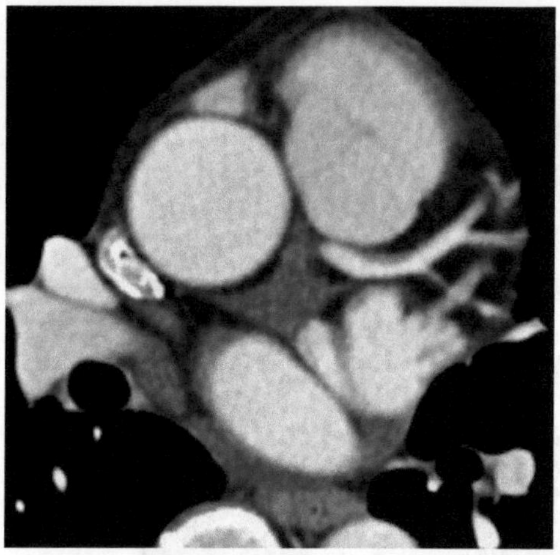

Fig. 9.10 Homogeneous, well-defined noncalcified lesions most likely correspond to coronary atheromas and are found usually in asymptomatic patients.

CT density and may correspond to lipid- or fibrous-rich plaques, respectively [8].

Commonly, spotty calcified lesions may be found in MDCT angiography studies that may be associated with minor wall changes in conventional coronary angiography only [24]. However, it is known that such calcified nodules may also be the source of unheralded plaque rupture and consecutive thrombosis (Fig. 9.11) and may lead to sudden coronary death in very rare cases [40]. In patients with chronic and stable angina, calcified and noncalcified plaques (Fig. 9.12) are commonly found next to each other [26].

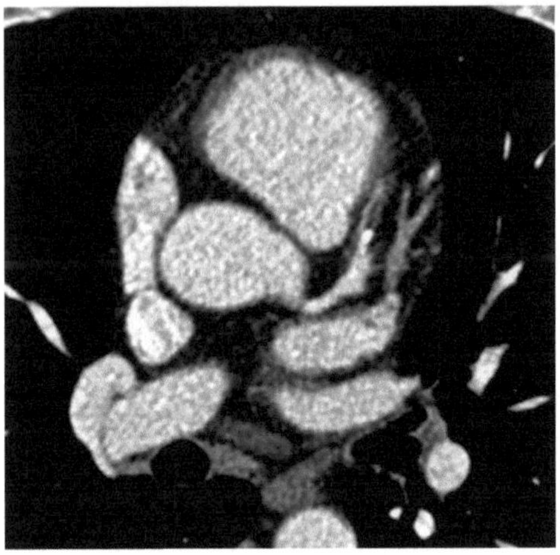

Fig. 9.11 Calcified nodule with consecutive thrombus formation in a patient with unstable angina.

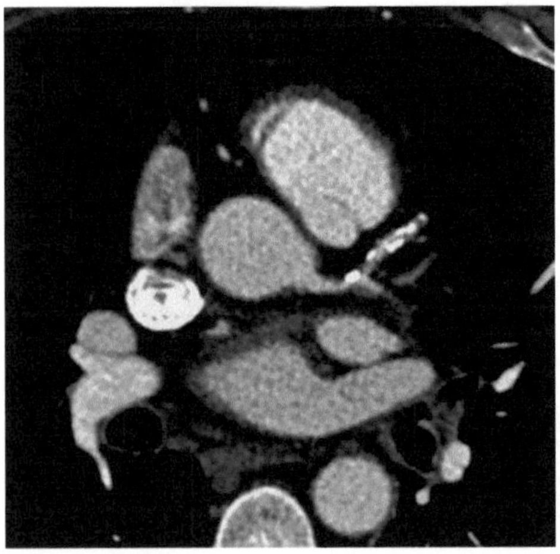

Fig. 9.12 Calcified and noncalcified coronary artery plaques may be present in patients with chronic and stable angina.

Even in contrast-enhanced studies coronary calcifications can easily be detected and quantified because the density of calcium (>350 HU) is beyond the density of contrast media in the coronary artery lumen (250–300 HU) [18]. However, because of partial volume effects it is much more difficult to quantify noncalcified plaques. The optimal quantification algorithm for atherosclerosis determined by MDCT is still under development.

In patients with extensive coronary calcifications, noncalcified plaques are uncommon most likely because the previously described "blooming" artifact prevents their assessment. Therefore and because the coronary artery stenosis cannot be reliably assessed [24] contrast-enhanced MDCT is currently not recommended in patients presenting with extensive coronary calcifications (>100 mg calcium hydroxyapatite or Agatston score >500).

Assessing the myocardium in patients with known history of CAD subendocardial or transmural myocardial infarction scars can frequently be identified as hypodense areas. Every region of the myocardium can be assigned to the territory of the coronary vessel supplying it. The LAD supplies the anterior left ventricular wall with the roof of the left ventricle, the apex, the superior part of the septum and the anterior papillary muscle. The posterior left ventricular wall and the posterior papillary muscle then are supplied by the LCx. The inferior left ventricular wall and the inferior part of the septum finally is supplied by the RCA. Below the mitral valve all three territories can be identified in one axial slice (Fig. 9.13).

With later development of a subendocardial or transmural myocardial infarction may lead to a thinning of the myocardial wall or myocardial aneurysm, respectively. Due to myocardial dysfunction or in atrial fibrillation, thrombus formation is likely to develop in the cardiac chambers and can be detected by CTA (Fig. 9.14) better than by trans-thoracic ultrasound [27].

A late uptake of contrast media after first pass in the myocardium of patients after infarction has already been observed in CT similar to MRI about 17 years ago [27]. It is rather likely that this kind of myocardial enhancement may correspond to interstitial uptake of contrast media within necrotic myocytes, 6 weeks to 3 months after onset. The optimal point of time for scanning may be between 10 and 40 min after first pass of the contrast media [21].

In addition, paracardial findings may frequently be observed in CTA studies and have to be reported.

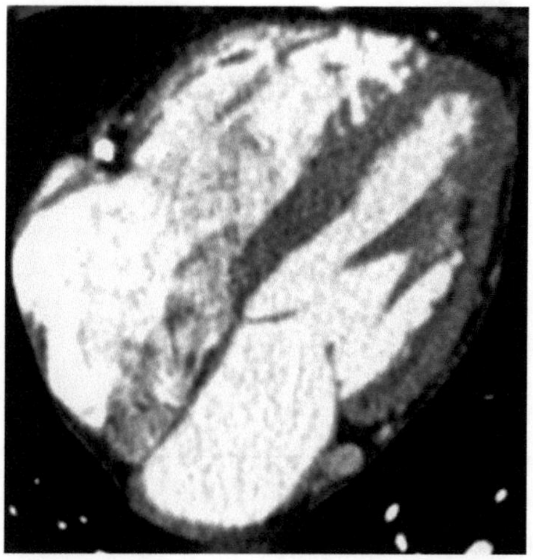

Fig. 9.13 Subendocardial myocardial infarction scar in the posterior wall, including the posterior papillary muscle. This area is supplied by the circumflex coronary artery.

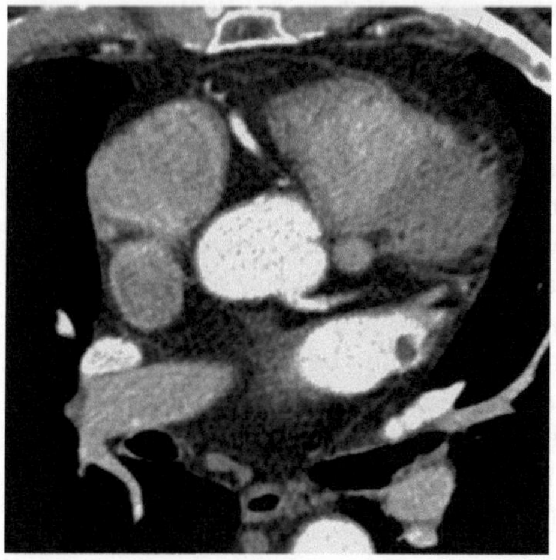

Fig. 9.14 Thrombus in the auricle of the left atrium in a patient with atrial fibrillation.

These findings may include lymph node enlargement, pulmonary nodules and tumors [20], or even, quite commonly, esophageal hernias. These incidental findings should trigger an additional reconstruction with a larger field of view ,or a more dedicated (CT) investigation should then be recommended.

In patients with paroxysmal atrial fibrillation, ablation of ectopic foci is a common interventional procedure. As a possible complication of this intervention, stenosis of the pulmonary vein has been reported. The presence and morphology of these stenoses can easily be assessed by CT [32].

9.8 Comparison with Alternative Investigation Methods

Coronary MDCT has been compared with cardiac catheter by a number of research groups [2, 25, 30, 31, 34]. In summary, comparison with several cardiac catheter studies (Table 9.2) has shown that coronary MDCT angiography has mean sensitivity, specificity, and positive and negative predictive values for detecting significant coronary artery stenoses of 87%, 89%, 77%, and 97%, respectively. However, the findings of a significant stenosis detected by MDCT are neither specific for the site nor the degree of the stenosis as compared to cardiac catheter. All authors agree upon the high negative predictive value of MDCT to rule out CAD. The current limitation is that MDCT has been tested so far in a heterogeneous group of patients with suspected CAD. Further studies are necessary to determine the accuracy of MDCT in a patient cohort with a low-to-moderate pretest probability (Table 9.3) of CAD [11].

Cardiac catheter seems to be unsuited to assess the entire extent of coronary atherosclerosis. Histological and intravascular ultrasound (IVUS) studies have shown that a high atherosclerotic plaque burden can be found even in the absence of high-grade coronary stenoses on conventional coronary angiography. From the clinical standpoint, the correlation between acute cardiac events and high-grade coronary artery stenoses is only poor. Recently it has been reported that 68% of the patients who received coronary angiography by incidence prior to their acute cardiac event did not show any significant coronary artery stenoses [43]. In early stages of CAD, the coronary arteries may undergo a process of positive remodeling that compensates for the coronary wall thickening and keeps the inner lumen of the vessel rather unchanged [12]. The pathomechanism of this phenomenon is still unknown, but the underlying type of CAD may be a fibrous cap atheroma with accumulation of cholesterol. In case of inflammatory processes the fibrous cap of an atheroma may become thinned, putting the plaque on risk for rupture and consecutive thrombosis [40].

The current gold standard to assess coronary atherosclerosis in vivo is intracoronary ultrasound. Schroeder et al. [37] reported that coronary lesions classified as soft, intermediate, and dense in intracoronary ultrasound correspond to coronary artery wall plaques with a density of 14±26 HU, 91±21 HU, and 419±194 HU in MDCT, respectively.

Table 9.3 Comparison between multidetector-row CT angiography and cardiac catheter for detection significant coronary artery stenosis

Author	Channels	Number of patients	Sensitivity (%)	Specificity (%)	Positive predictive value (%)	Negative predictive value (%)	Not assessable (%)
Nieman [30]	4	35	83	90	81	97	30
Achenbach [2]	4	64	85	76	59	98	32
Knez [25]	4	44	78	98	85	96	6
Nieman [31]	16	58	95	86	80	97	0
Ropers [34]	16	77	92	93	79	97	12
Mean			87	89	77	97	18
Sum		278					

Table 9.4 Pretest likelihood of coronary artery disease in symptomatic patients according to age and sex [11].

Age (years)	Nonanginal chest pain (%)		Atypical angina (%)		Typical angina (%)	
	Men	Women	Men	Women	Men	Women
30–39	4	2	34	12	76	26
40–49	13	3	51	22	87	55
50–59	20	7	65	31	93	73
60–69	27	14	72	51	94	86

In general, coronary intervention can hardly be followed by MDCT. Because of their disease, many of these patients have severe calcifications and commonly after angioplasty a coronary stent is implanted that appears like a dense calcification and hinders the detection of an in-stent stenosis. Recently, it has been reported in one case that measuring the contrast-density curve behind the stent enables demonstration of the success of a reintervention [38].

For the morphological assessment of bypass graft patency with MDCT compared with cardiac catheter, Ropers et al. [33] reported a sensitivity and specificity of 97% and 98%. For the detection of bypass graft stenosis, the sensitivity and specificity was significantly lower: 75% and 92%, respectively. Consecutive scanning and administration of a small contrast bolus has already been shown to allow determination of a spiral CT flow index with a single-detector CT. This index agreed with angiographically determined coronary bypass flow in 85% of the grafts investigated [39].

9.9 Conclusion

The newest generation of MDCT now allows for consistently good image quality if regular sinus rhythm is present and the heart rate is in the range between 40 and 60 beats/min. Extensive calcifications and coronary stents may hinder the detection of coronary artery stenosis or restenosis. Coronary atherosclerosis can best be determined and followed by nonenhanced, low-dose MDCT scans. The predictive value of atherosclerotic lesions for cardiac events as detected by MDCT angiography is currently unknown and requires further prospective cohort studies. Because of the high negative predictive value, the MDCT investigation may be justified in symptomatic patients with low-to-moderate pretest probability of CAD. In these patients coronary macroangiopathy in the proximal and middle coronary artery segments can reliably be ruled out and unnecessary cardiac catheter procedures may be avoided. In patients with an acute coronary syndrome, MDCT can demonstrate the site and extent of a coronary thrombus and may be used in the future to guide coronary interventions.

References

1. Achenbach S, Moshage W, Ropers D, Nossen J, Daniel WG (1998) Value of electron-beam computed tomography for the noninvasive detection of high-grade coronary-artery stenosis and occlusion. N Engl J Med 339:1964–1971
2. Achenbach S, Giesler T, Ropers D, et al. (2001) Detection of coronary artery stenoses by contrast-enhanced, retrospectively electrocardiographically-gated, multislice spiral computed tomography. Circulation 103:2535–2538
3. Achenbach S, Giesler T, Ropers D, et al. (2003) Comparison of image quality in contrast-enhanced coronary-artery visualization by electron beam tomography and retrospectively electrocardiogram-gated multislice spiral computed tomography. Invest Radiol 38:119–128
4. Aspelin P, Aubry P, Fransson SG, et al. (2003) Nephrotoxic effects in high-risk patients undergoing angiography. N Engl J Med 348:491–499

5. Austen WG, Edwards JE, Frye RL, et al. (1975) A reporting system on patients evaluated for coronary artery disease. Report of the Ad Hoc Committee for Grading of Coronary Artery Disease, Council on Cardiovascular Surgery, American Heart Association. Circulation 51 [Suppl 4]:5–40
6. Becker CR, Knez A, Ohnesorge B, Schoepf UJ, Reiser MF (2000) Imaging of noncalcified coronary plaques using helical CT with retrospective ECG gating. AJR Am J Roentgenol 175:423–424
7. Becker C, Hong C, Knez A, et al. (2003) Optimal contrast application for cardiac 4-detector-row computer tomography. Invest Radiol 38:690--694
8. Becker C, Nikolaou K, Muders M, et al. (2003) Ex vivo coronary atherosclerotic plaque characterization with multidetector-row CT. Eur Radiol 12 (e-pub ahead of print)
9. Bergstra A, Dijk RB van, Brekke O, et al. (2000) Hemodynamic effects of iodixanol and iohexol during ventriculography in patients with compromised left ventricular function. Catheter Cardiovasc Interv 50:314–321
10. Fleischmann D (2003) Use of high concentration contrast media: principles and rationale vascular district. Eur J Radiol 45:S88–S93
11. Gibbons R, Chatterjee K, Daley J, et al. (1999) ACC/AHA/ACP-ASIM guidelines for the management of patients with chronic stable angina: a report of the American College of Cardiology/American Heart Association Task Force on Practice Guidelines (Committee on Management of Patients With Chronic Stable Angina). J Am Coll Cardiol 33:2092–2197
12. Glagov S, Weisenberg E, Zarins C, Stankunavicius R, Kolettis G (1987) Compensatory enlargement of human atherosclerotic coronary arteries. N Engl J Med 316:1371–1375
13. Haage P, Schmitz-Rode T, Hubner D, Piroth W, Gunther RW (2000) Reduction of contrast material dose and artifacts by a saline flush using a double power injector in helical CT of the thorax. AJR Am J Roentgenol 174:1049–1053
14. Halliburton SS, Petersilka M, Schvartzman PR, Obuchowski N, White RD (2003) Evaluation of left ventricular dysfunction using multiphasic reconstructions of coronary multislice computed tomography data in patients with chronic ischemic heart disease: validation against cine magnetic resonance imaging. Int J Cardiovasc Imaging 19:73–83
15. Herzog C, Abolmaali N, Balzer JO, et al. (2002) Heart-rate-adapted image reconstruction in multidetector-row cardiac CT: influence of physiological and technical prerequisite on image quality. Eur Radiol 12:2670–2678
16. Hittmair K, Fleischmann D (2001) Accuracy of predicting and controlling time-dependent aortic enhancement from a test bolus injection. J Comput Assist Tomogr 25:287–294
17. Hong C, Becker CR, Huber A, et al. (2001) ECG-gated reconstructed multidetector row CT coronary angiography: effect of varying trigger delay on image quality. Radiology 220:712–717
18. Hong C, Becker C, Schoepf UJ, et al. (2002) Absolute quantification of coronary artery calcium in nonenhanced and contrast enhanced multidetector-row CT studies. Radiology 223:474–480
19. Hopper KD, Mosher TJ, Kasales CJ, et al. (1997) Thoracic spiral CT: delivery of contrast material pushed with injectable saline solution in a power injector. Radiology 205:269–271
20. Horton KM, Post WS, Blumenthal RS, Fishman EK (2002) Prevalence of significant noncardiac findings on electron-beam computed tomography coronary artery calcium screening examinations. Circulation 106:532–534
21. Huber D, Lapray J, Hessel S (1981) In vivo evaluation of experimental myocardial infarcts by ungated computed tomography. AJR 136:469–473
22. Jakobs TF, Becker CR, Ohnesorge B, et al. (2002) Multislice helical CT of the heart with retrospective ECG gating: reduction of radiation exposure by ECG-controlled tube current modulation. Eur Radiol 12:1081–1086
23. Johnson M (1996) Principles and practice of coronary angiography. In: Skorton D, Schelbert H, Wolf G, Brundage B (eds) Marcus cardiac imaginng: a companion to Braunwald´s heart disease, vol 1. Saunders, Philadelphia, pp 220–250
24. Kajinami K, Seki H, Takekoshi N, Mabuchi H (1997) Coronary calcification and coronary atherosclerosis: site by site comparative morphologic study of electron beam computed tomography and coronary angiography. J Am Coll Cardiol 29:1549–1556
25. Knez A, Becker C, Leber A, et al. (2001) Usefullness of multislice spiral computed tomography angiography for determination of coronary artery stenoses. Am J Cardiol 88:1191–1194
26. Leber AW, Knez A, White CW, et al. (2003) Composition of coronary atherosclerotic plaques in patients with acute myocardial infarction and stable angina pectoris determined by contrast-enhanced multislice computed tomography. Am J Cardiol 91:714–718
27. Masuda Y, Yoshida H, Morooka N, Watanabe S, Inagaki Y (1984) The usefulness of X-ray computed tomography for the diagnosis of myocardial infarction. Circulation 70:217–225
28. Moshage WE, Achenbach S, Seese B, Bachmann K, Kirchgeorg M (1995) Coronary artery stenoses: three-dimensional imaging with electrocardiographically triggered, contrast agent-enhanced, electron-beam CT. Radiology 196:707–714
29. Nakanishi T, Ito K, Imazu M, Yamakido M (1997) Evaluation of coronary artery stenoses using electron-beam CT and multiplanar reformation. J Comput Assist Tomogr 21:121–127
30. Nieman K, Oudkerk M, Rensing B, et al. (2001) Coronary angiography with multislice computed computed tomography. Lancet 357:599–603
31. Nieman K, Cademartiri F, Lemos PA, et al. (2002) Reliable noninvasive coronary angiography with fast submillimeter multislice spiral computed tomography. Circulation 106:2051–2054
32. Purerfellner H, Cihal R, Aichinger J, Martinek M, Nesser HJ (2003) Pulmonary vein stenosis by ostial irrigated-tip ablation: incidence, time course, and prediction. J Cardiovasc Electrophysiol 14:158–164
33. Ropers D, Ulzheimer S, Wenkel E, et al. (2001) Investigation of aortocoronary artery bypass grafts by multislice spiral computed tomography with electrocardiographic-gated image reconstruction. Am J Cardiol 88:792–795
34. Ropers D, Baum U, Pohle K, et al. (2003) Detection of coronary artery stenoses with thin-slice multidetector row spiral computed tomography and multiplanar reconstruction. Circulation 107:664–666
35. Ryan T, Anderson J, Antman E, et al. (1996) ACC/AHA

guidelines for the management of patients with acute myocardial infarction. A report of the American College of Cardiology/American Heart Association Task Force on Practice Guidelines (Committee on Management of Acute Myocardial Infarction). J Am Coll Cardiol 28:1328–1428
36. Schmermund A, Rensing BJ, Sheedy PF, Bell MR, Rumberger JA (1998) Intravenous electron-beam computed tomographic coronary angiography for segmental analysis of coronary artery stenosis. Am J Cardiol 31:1547–1554
37. Schroeder S, Kopp A, Baumbach A, et al. et al. (2001) Noninvasive detection and evalutation of atherosclerotic coronary plaque with multislice computed tomography. J Am Coll Cardiol 37:1430–1435
38. Storto ML, Marano R, Maddestra N, (2002) Images in cardiovascular medicine. Multislice spiral computed tomography for in-stent restenosis. Circulation 105:2005
39. Tello R, Hartnell GG, Costello P, Ecker CP (2002) Coronary artery bypass graft flow: qualitative evaluation with cine single-detector row CT and comparison with findings at angiography. Radiology 224:913–918
40. Virmani R, Kolodgie FD, Burke AP, Frab A, Schwartz SM (2000) Lessons from sudden coronary death. A comprehensive morphological classification scheme for atherosclerotic lesions. Arterioscler Thromb Vasc Biol 20:1262–1275
41. Vogl TJ, Abolmaali ND, Diebold T, et al. (2002) Techniques for the detection of coronary atherosclerosis: multidetector row CT coronary angiography. Radiology 223:212–220
42. Wexler L, Brundage B, Crouse J, et al. (1996) Coronary artery calcification: pathophysiology, epidemiology, imaging methods, and clinical implications. A statement for health professionals from the American Heart Association. Circulation 94:1175–1192
43. Ziada K, Kapadia S, Tuzcu E, Nissen S (1999) The current status of intravascular ultrasound imaging. Curr Probl Cardiol 24:541–566

10 Abdominal Aorta

Lorenzo Bonomo, Roberto Iezzi, and Biagio Merlino

CONTENTS

10.1 Introduction

Since its advent in 1998, multidetector-row CT (MDCT) has brought significant advantages with respect to single detector-row CT (SSCT): the simultaneous acquisition of more sections during a complete rotation of the gantry, together with its increased rotational speed (0.5 s and less), determined a decrease in the acquisition time, allowing the analysis of large anatomical volumes, with better spatial and temporal resolution of images (they are isotropic images, reconstructed, at each level, with the same spatial resolution of initial section in order to have an optimized 3D resolution), rationalizing the use of contrast medium. The low temperature made the use of the X-ray tube extremely successful with a decrease in operating costs. Among its many advantages we have to include also a shorter data reconstruction time (2 images per second versus 5–8 and more per second) and a better scanning interface with the workstation for transmission of data [6, 47–49].

For these many assets, MDCT gave its best results in other fields already accessible with SSCT angiography (SSCTA; for example, the study of abdominal aorta diseases), widening the clinical information on CT angiography, whereas SSCTA showed technical limitations (suspected mesenteric ischemia, the evaluation of coronary arteries, and lower-extremity arteries [17, 38]).

MDCTA enabled a detailed analysis of the abdominal aorta, made possible for the shorter acquisition time, and the study of the entire aortoiliac system during a single breath-hold. The high spatial resolution, together with fast acquisition and superior 3D reconstructions, allowed a better evaluation of the abdominal aorta and visceral branches during their flow, with an accurate definition and diagnosis of the steno-occlusive pathology.

MDCT angiography represents today the reference point in the study of the abdominal aorta, both in dilative or steno-occlusive pathologies and in the follow-up of the aortic stent-graft placement.

10.2 Technical Requirements

CT angiography consists of a rapid volumetric acquisition of images during a bolus injection of contrast medium, with scanning during the maximum arterial enhancement. The technical requirements for a CT angiography examination are based on: fast acquisition (allowing performance of the acquisition during a single breath-hold in order to reduce motion artifacts with an increased temporal resolution) of large volumes (aiming at including all vascular structures being examined); optimal contrast and spatial resolution, either on the x- or z- axis (in order to evaluate small-caliber vessels, with a trans-

L. Bonomo, MD, Professor; B. Merlino, MD
Department of Radiology, Policlinico Agostino Gemelli, Università Cattolica del Sacro Cuore, L. go F. Vito, 1, 00168 Rome, Italy
R. Iezzi, MD
Department of Radiology, University of Chieti, "SS. Annunziata" Hospital, via dei Vestini, 66031 Chieti Scalo, Italy

versal flow with respect to the level of acquisition, and to obtain isotropic images that optimize the 3D resolution at all levels); adequate contrast-medium injection protocol; and excellent two- and three-dimensional reconstructions (that allow visualization of vascular structures in angiography-equivalent planes other than the axial).

10.3 Contrast-Medium Injection

In CT angiography, contrast-medium administration must be performed at high flow rate (3–5 ml/s) to gain a better contrast resolution, reducing the partial volume enhancement in the evaluation of small horizontal vessels (renal arteries). On the other hand, high flow rates reduce both the injection time and the intravascular contrast medium plateau, with consequent injection of larger amounts of contrast medium to set off this effect (variable between 100 and 150 ml) [38].

In CT angiography, scanning should start when the examined structures have reached an ideal level of opacification and the duration of contrast-medium administration should equal the acquisition time. Hence, it is necessary to optimize the opacification of vascular structures being examined, defining exactly the start delay [20, 48]. Keeping in mind these two factors, it is necessary to know, for each patient, the duration of the contrast-medium administration, which depends on intrinsic and extrinsic factors (such as volume and concentration of contrast medium employed, flow rate, and site of injection).

It is possible to determine the circulation time with a test bolus [28, 56] or by using semiautomatic software (bolus-tracking software) [37, 53] which enables the practitioner to follow a real-time enhancement curve of a specific vascular structure during contrast-medium administration. The main advantage of such semiautomatic systems, with respect to the test bolus, is represented by a single injection of contrast media, with the reduction of its total amount and with the absence of or very little opacification of the excretory system, and venous and parenchymal structures during the following helical acquisition. In our institution bolus tracking is routinely used for the abovementioned advantages.

A very important achievement in CT angiography is the optimal contrast-medium dynamic. Rubin and others demonstrated that, with faster acquisition, hence with the introduction of faster scanners (multislice CT, MSCT), it is possible to reduce the amount of contrast medium injected, by about 20–40%, with obvious benefits mainly to patients with poor renal function. The amount of contrast medium injected, the injection flow rate, and the injection time are correlated to define the enhancement curve. The ideal enhancement curve in CT angiography should be denoted by a long, high, invariable plateau through which it is possible to reach a homogeneous enhancement of all vascular structures being examined. The intravenous injection of contrast media not only determines an initial arterial flow, but also a reflow. In fact, according to the pharmacokinetics of contrast media, the uniphasic injection at the constant flow determines a variable arterial enhancement, with a constant increase in vascular attenuation and a poor enhancement at the beginning and at the end of the acquisition [3, 4].

According to more recent studies, a more homogeneous curve can be obtained with a biphasic or multiphasic injection, with an initial small bolus of contrast medium injected at high flow rate followed by a larger volume at lower flow rate [5, 20, 21].

However, according to our experience, with an adequate start delay, a uniphasic injection of contrast medium at a relatively low flow rate also enables an adequate enhancement of the abdominal aorta, the iliac axis, and the common femoral arteries included in the acquisition volume. Most likely the use of biphasic injection protocol could be appropriate in the evaluation study of larger volumes of acquisition.

In some institutions, immediately after the bolus injection of contrast media, a flush of about 40 ml of saline solution is injected at the same flow rate of the contrast medium, similar to what is routinely performed in magnetic resonance angiography (MRA). This bolus of saline ensures the flow of contrast agent in the vascular system, increasing and lengthening (5–8 s) the peak enhancement, with a consequent reduction of the amount of injected contrast agent [39].

With the reduction of volume of contrast medium, achieved through the use of high-concentration (370 mg I/ml and more) contrast agents, the routine use of saline flush is mandatory. Highly concentrated contrast agents enable the reduction of volumes of contrast media injected, achieving superior quantitative and qualitative results in terms of arterial enhancement, when compared with larger volumes of contrast media injected at lower flow rate [19].

Our injection protocol consists of a single intravenous bolus injection of 120 ml of nonionic contrast medium (300 mg I/ml), with a 20-gauge i.v. cannula into an antecubital vein of the arm, at a flow rate of 3 ml/s.

10.4 Technical Parameters of Acquisition

With the advent of MDCT, new technical and methodological problems have had to be overcome, such as the optimization of the protocol of tests, the printing operation, and the filing process of enormous quantities of images obtained with a single test (data explosion), as well as the need to employ new visualizing and reporting modalities (dedicated workstation) [48]. The acquisition protocol must be chosen according to the clinical condition of the patient.

10.4.1 Dilatative and Steno-occlusive Diseases

In our experience, a precontrast acquisition must always be performed, aiming at:

- The visualization of parietal calcification of the abdominal aorta and of visceral, iliac, and femoral vessels
- The analysis of the thrombus, to exclude the presence of an intraplaque hemorrhage (unstable thrombus)
- The selection of contrast-enhanced volume of acquisition and the placement of the region of interest (ROI). (in this case, bolus tracking software is used).

The precontrast acquisition is performed with a low-resolution protocol, with a 2.5-mm collimation, a gantry rotation time of 0.5 s, a reconstruction interval of 5 mm, an acquisition time of about 12 s, with a field of view (FOV) of approximately 240 mm, and a volume of interest from D12 to the symphysis pubis.

Postcontrast acquisition generally requires a high-resolution protocol, with a 1-mm collimation, a pitch of 6, a gantry rotation time of 0.5 s, a slice thickness of 1.25 mm, and a reconstruction interval of 1 mm.

The volume of interest extends from the celiac trunk to the common femoral artery, with an average acquisition time of 25 s.

In cases of suspected inflammatory aneurysm, it is necessary to complete the examination with delayed scans (start delay of 60 s) using the same technical parameters of the arterial phase, in order to evaluate the presence of arterial wall and to determine the relationship of this inflammatory tissue with the other retroperitoneal structures.

10.4.2 Aortic Endoprosthesis Follow-up

Our acquisition protocol in the study of patients treated with an aortic prosthesis includes an initial precontrast acquisition, a postcontrast arterial phase, and then a delayed acquisition, about 60 s after the initial injection, with the same technical parameter mentioned above. The delayed acquisition aims at the study of the endoprosthesis alone, to better exclude the presence of reperfusions of the aneurysmal sac (endoleak), which represents a serious complication of the procedure, since it may contribute to the enlargement of the aneurysmal sac and a great chance for an aneurysmal rupture. CT angiography is the examination of choice for the follow-up of such patients and it provides a high sensitivity for the detection of endoleaks [26]. The precontrast acquisition identifies the volumetric acquisition of the following arterial phase, and it also helps in the evaluation of postcontrast data sets in order to detect small leaks and differentiate these from parietal thrombocalcific appositions and/or metallic portions of prosthesis [34, 43]. In addition to this [44], in a recent comparative study of different acquisition protocols (first protocol: precontrast scanning + arterial phase; second protocol: arterial phase + delayed phase; third protocol: precontrast + arterial phase + delayed phase) showed that, in 33 patients with endoleaks, (positive group) and 40 patients with any leaks or aneurysmal sac enlargement (negative group), only precontrast acquisitions allowed exclusion of the presence of leaks in 20% of patients belonging to the negative group, for which the biphasic protocol (arterial phase + delayed phase) provided incomplete information. The delayed phase, on the other hand, is mandatory in the detection of low-flow leaks [24].

10.5 2D and 3D Reconstructions

Data sets acquired with correct contrast-medium administration may be processed to DCT images without increasing the X-ray exposure to the patient. Although transverse images remain the main reference point in the evaluation of a CT angiography study, the potential to reconstruct and visualize 3D images has many advantages. Data processing is different in each process, and the clinical importance of each is also different [30].

10.5.1 Multiplanar Reformations

Multiplanar reformations (MPR) are 2D reconstructions with no depth, fast to acquire with software available on any CT scanner in which the volumetric acquisition is reconstructed arbitrarily (coronal, sagittal, or oblique). The quality of these images depends on the spatial resolution along the *z*-axis, since a low spatial resolution means poor quality with stair-step artifacts. With the advent of MDCT and the use of isotropic images, the quality of these reconstructions became excellent without artifacts. A more complex application allows, furthermore, curved reconstructions in which the arteries are free from any superimposition (curved planar reformations, CPR).

With this application it is possible to visualize, clearly and also lengthwise, the stenosis, the calcification around the vessel, and it is possible to evaluate the patency of intraluminal stent. The main limitation of these reconstructions is represented by the impossibility of performing any measurement on curved multiplanar reformations.

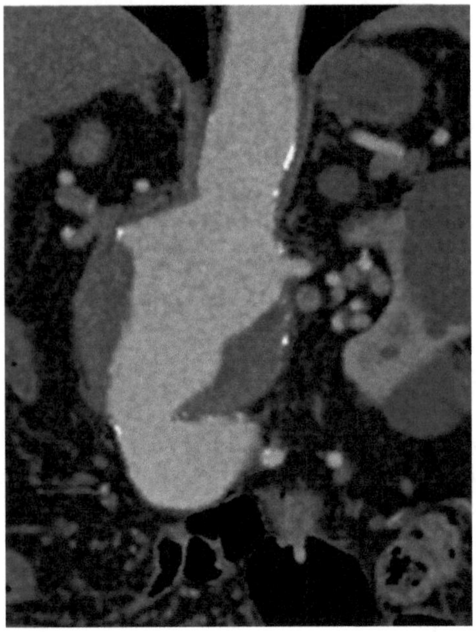

Fig. 10.1 Multiplanar reformation (MPR) image: patient with abdominal aortic aneurysm involving the ostium of renal arteries. MPR image allows representation of lumen and thrombus in planes other than the transverse.

10.5.2 Maximum-Intensity Projection

The algorithm for maximum-intensity projection (MIP) reconstructions evaluates each voxel along a traced line, from a defined perspective, with volumetric data acquired previously. The maximum value of each one of them is codified on a 2D image very similar to a traditional angiographic image, without depth and unable to separate vessels and superimpositions of structures. This reconstructed algorithm allows a good evaluation of calcifications, stents, and small-caliber vessels, but it requires an editing process to remove structures superimposed to vessels and in particular bones. Manual editing needs a long processing time to obtain diagnostic reconstructions and, in some cases, it is impossible to completely eliminate bony structures superimposed on the vessels, thus making vessels difficult to evaluate. The availability of appropriate software to perform the automatic editing undoubtedly represents an advantage for time-saving in processing medical reports; however, the complex evaluation of dimensions, shape, intensity, location, and proximity relationships performed by the human eye are difficult to computerize. Therefore, the algorithms developed to date (2004) are not always good for all applications and often the editing process becomes semiautomatic, requiring the contribution of an expert operator [10, 18]. Further technological improvements will overcome these limitations, shortening to a few seconds the total processing time of images.

10.5.3 Volume-Rendering Techniques

In volume-rendering techniques (VRT), each voxel is evaluated according to its opacity and its brightness in order to establish a histogram of intensity. The

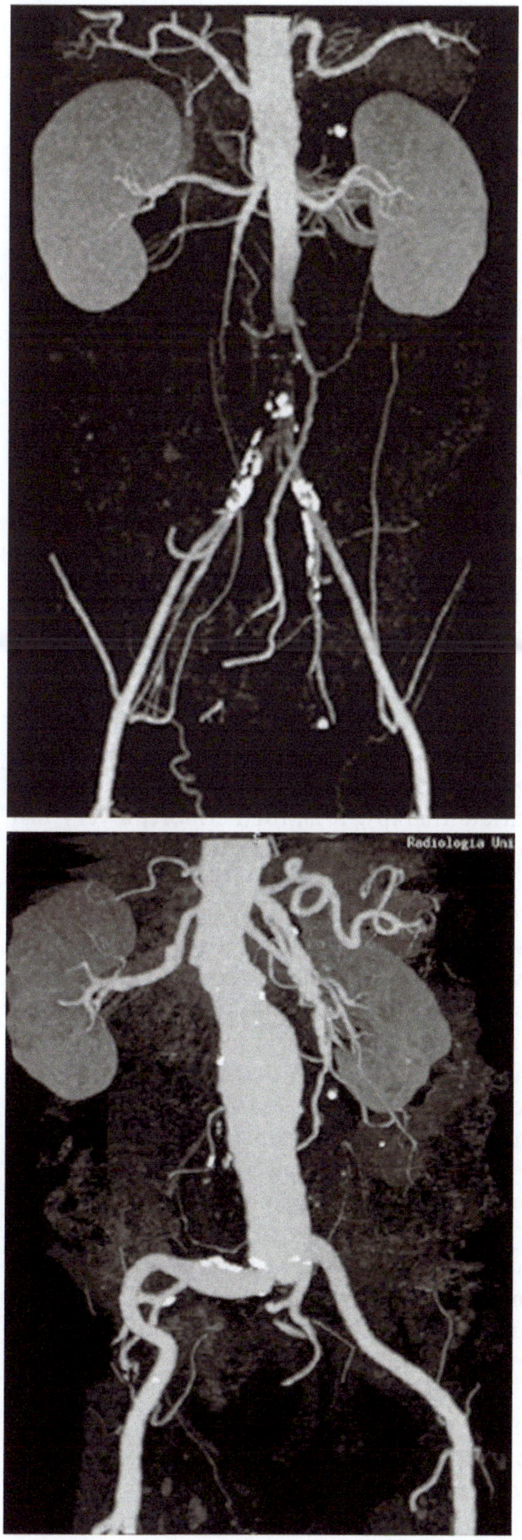

a
b

Fig. 10.2a,b Maximum-intensity projection (MIP) images: **a** patient with aortoiliac obstruction; **b** patient with infrarenal abdominal aortic aneurysm extending to the aortic bifurcation. MIP images allow angiography-like images with good evaluation of calcifications and small-caliber vessels.

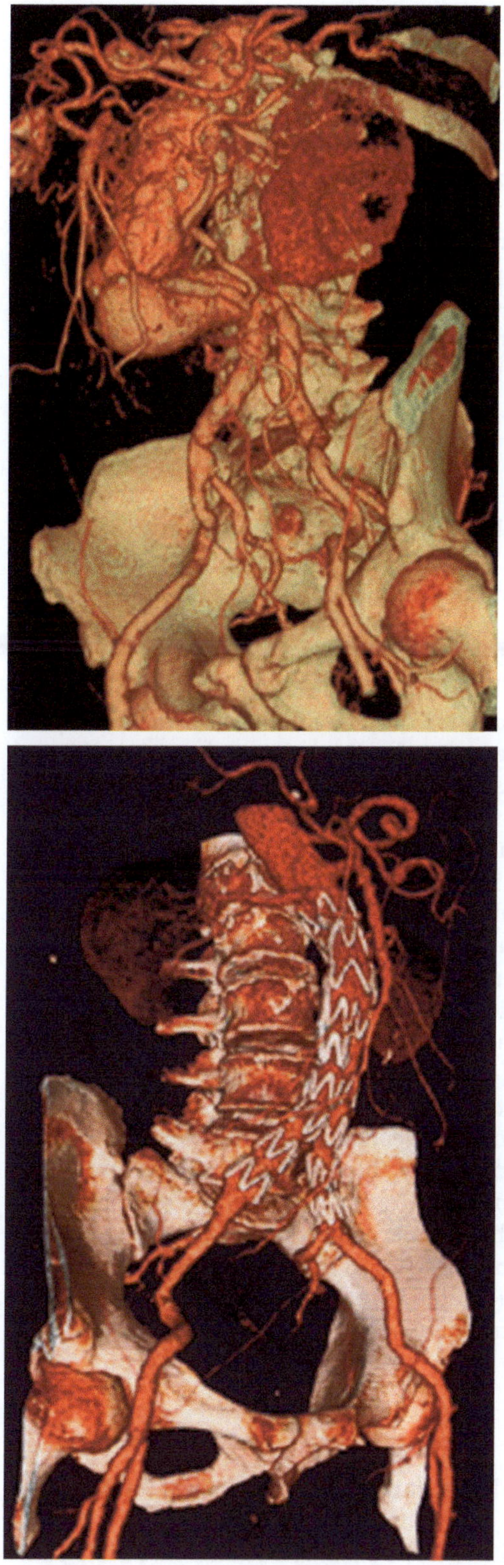
a
b

Fig. 10.3a,b Volume-rendered (VR) images: **a** patient with infrarenal abdominal aortic aneurysm involving the aortic bifurcation; **b** follow-up examination after endovascular treatment with a stent graft.

related attenuation value of each voxel is recorded on the final image, using a gray scale, and this is the opacity or semitransparent representation of a volume, and not of a surface. These reconstructions allow representation and differentiation of superimposing skeletal and vascular structures without any editing process.

Their main advantages consist of the speed of acquisition and a good visualization of vascular structures. Such a reconstructed algorithm, in order to have reasonably fast images, requires a very complex workstation not available everywhere.

10.6 Image Evaluation and Management

The combined evaluation of transverse and postprocessed images (MPR, MIP, VRT) allows an overall evaluation of the vascular pathology with respect to the level of stenosis and wall anomalies (plaques or calcifications), the characteristics of the aneurysm, and presence of collateral vessels and incidental findings. The main limitations are represented by the great number of native images obtained with a single acquisition and the time required for postprocessing the data set. The evaluation of a CT angiography study must be performed on dedicated workstations on which it is possible to evaluate transverse images in cine-mode according to which the radiologist interactively chooses the reconstruction that better clears away any possible diagnostic doubt [45]. With digital subtraction angiography (DSA), the evaluation of vascular structures is done by standard projections, while, on the contrary, with CT angiography this limitation is overcome by a real-time visualization of the volume of acquisition; hence the vascular structures are evaluated from all points of view [42]. At the end of the review process, for iconographic purposes, only a few summarizing reconstructions will be printed.

10.7 Clinical Evaluation of Aneurysmal Pathology

Abdominal aortic aneurysm is an irreversible pathological dilatation of the normal aortic lumen which involves one or more segments, with a diameter at least 1.5 × greater than the normal proximal aortic tract. The incidence of abdominal aortic aneurysms is estimated to be 20-40 cases every 100,000 persons each year; these aneurysms are also responsible for 1.7% of deaths of persons between the age of 65 and 74 years. The natural history of abdominal aortic aneurysms is represented by its progressive enlargement (4 mm each year) until its rupture, which may result in a very high incidence of death (80-90%) [9]. The bigger the aneurysmal sac, the greater the chances of its rupture, varying from 8%, in cases of a diameter smaller than 4 cm, to more than 45% if the aneurysm is bigger than 7 cm [7, 13]. Abdominal aortic aneurysms may be classified according to their morphology (fusiform or saccular), their location (supra- or infrarenal), their dimensions, and their etiology (atherosclerotic, congenital, inflammatory, infectious or mycotic, luetic or degenerative).

CT angiography represents the standard of reference in the evaluation of aneurysmal pathology and in the selection of patients who may take advantage of an endovascular percutaneous stent graft, positioned percutaneously in the abdominal aorta. CT angiography is, indeed, able to provide information on the anatomy of the vessel, the type of the pathology and it extension, and the presence of complications with the possibility to choose accordingly the appropriate therapy. It is, furthermore, a very fast test, widely available in the territory and easily reproducible.

Recently, the development of endovascular techniques introduced and developed a new and less invasive technique, providing extremely encouraging results, as an alternative to traditional vascular surgical repair. Surgery has a mortality risk of 1.4-6.5%, which may increase to 5.7-31% in patients with other concurrent pathologies [16, 29]. Endovascular treatment has a 2.7% intraoperative mortality risk and it reduces the risk of bleeding, the hospitalization time, and the patient's posttreatment recovery [59].

A successful endovascular treatment, without intra- and posttreatment complications and with aneurysmal sac exclusion, is strictly related to an accurate selection of patients, enrolling only cases in which the procedure can be easy and effective.

The guidelines for this technique are constantly developing, as a result of the increasing experience of the operators and the availability of new and more versatile models of endoprostheses, which are easier to use. The clinical criteria for the choice of patients consider a less invasive procedure, which may be applied in patients at high risk for open surgery or patients with "hostile abdomen" caused by previous repeated laparotomy.

10.7.1 Pretreatment Evaluation

In the evaluation of abdominal aortic aneurysms, CT angiography allows selection of patient candidates for endovascular treatment and defining of the characteristics of the device suitable for a specific patient to optimize the procedure outcome.

In the evaluation of abdominal aortic aneurysms, it is necessary first of all to define:

- Nature (atherosclerotic or inflammatory)
- Location (whether it involves the renal artery origin)
- Size of the aneurysmal sac (essential in the follow-up of patients who do not require any treatment and to monitor the endovascular treatment)
- Length (whether it involves the carrefour and the iliac arteries)

Furthermore, it is necessary to evaluate:

- The presence of a parietal thrombotic apposition
- The maximum thickness of the thrombus
- The CT characteristics of the thrombus (stable or unstable thrombus)

The transverse image in Fig. 10.5, for example, shows an abdominal aorta aneurysm with eccentric thrombus on the rear left side of the wall, where it is possible to see a hyperdense, half-moon-shaped component, which is the evidence of unstable thrombus. The aneurysm with unstable thrombus has greater incidence of rupture.

When choosing the endovascular treatment, some anatomical criteria always need to be taken into account in order to have a safe attachment of

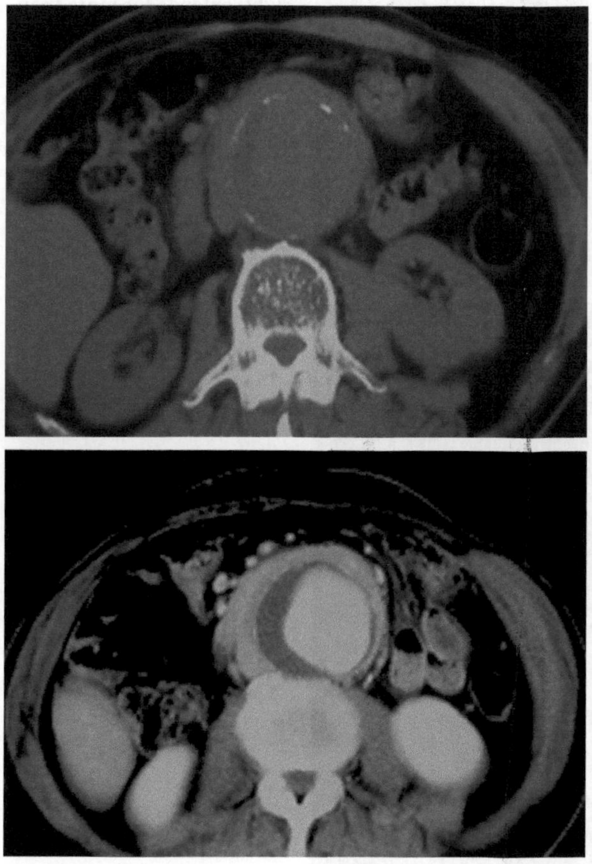

a b

Fig. 10.4a,b Precontrast (**a**) and postcontrast (**b**) transverse images. Aneurysmal dilatation of the abdominal aorta with enhancing periaortic soft tissue, typical of an inflammatory aneurysm.

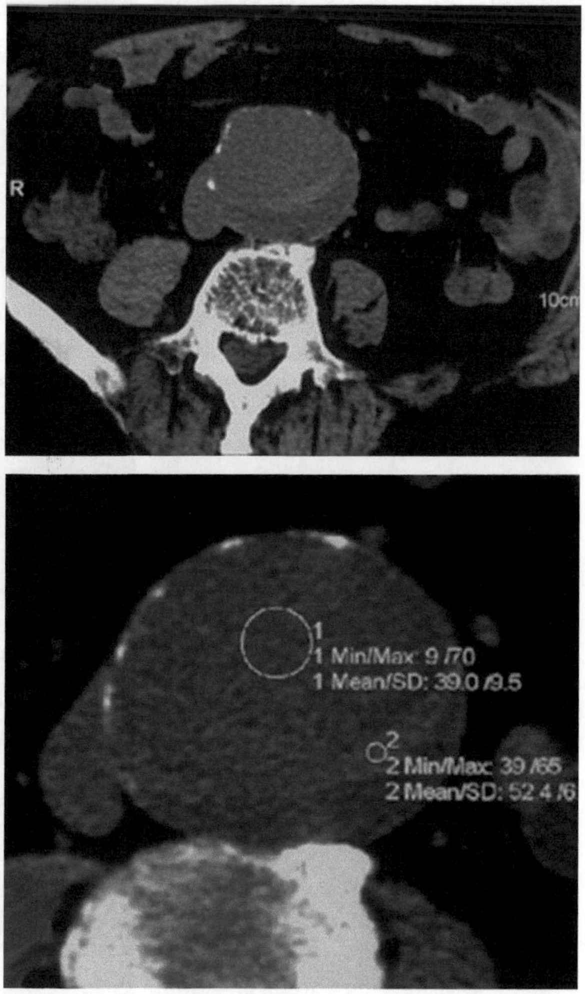

a b

Fig. 10.5a,b Transverse images: aneurysm of the abdominal aorta with unstable thrombus.

the prosthesis. The quality of the proximal neck of the abdominal aortic aneurysm (that is the distance from the caudal renal artery to the proximal boundary of the aneurysm) is the limiting factor. A fundamental requirement, to ensure an adequate proximal attachment of the prosthesis, is a proximal neck with the following characteristics:

- Length of about 1.5 cm
- Straight or with an angle less than 55°
- Without any parietal thrombotic appositions and/or concentric calcifications
- A maximum diameter smaller than 32 mm [1]

The information on the proximal neck has to be acquired both from transverse images and reconstructed images, through which it is possible to better evaluate its course, whether it is straight or angled (Fig. 10.6)

CT angiography must also provide anatomical information on the iliac arteries, which must not:

- Have a more than 90° tortuosity (Fig. 10.7)
- Have circumferential calcifications
- Have a vessel diameter smaller than 8 mm., to allow the passage of large-caliber endoprosthesis catheters [35, 40, 41]

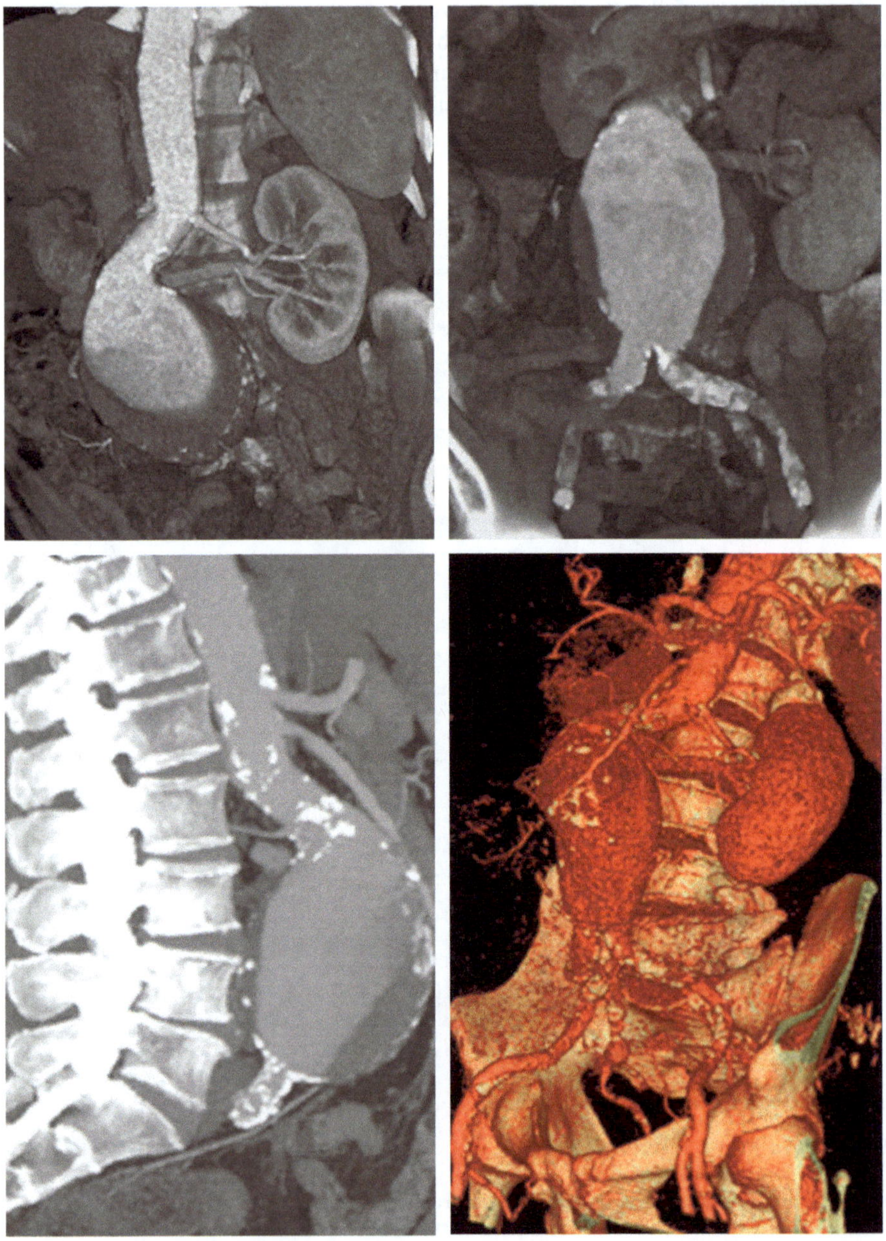

a c b d

Fig. 10.6a–d MPR (**a, b, c**) and VR (**d**) reconstructions. Infrarenal abdominal aortic aneurysm distally extending to the aortic bifurcation without involvement of iliac arteries. The proximal neck, slightly angulated (<55°) anterolaterally to the right, extends for more than 15 mm.

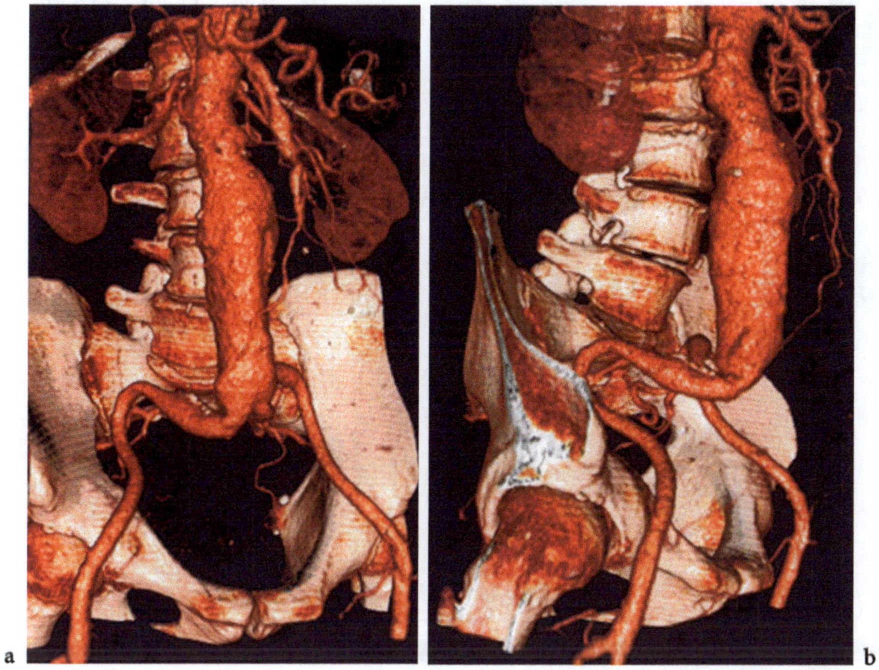

Fig. 10.7a,b VR images: infrarenal abdominal aortic aneurysm extending to the aortic bifurcation. Iliac arteries tortuosity does not indicate positioning of an aortic stent graft.

To choose an endovascular treatment, it is also necessary to consider:

- The presence, number and caliber of lumbar arteries which arise from the aneurysmal sac
- The patency of the celiac trunk and mesenteric arteries (superior and inferior)
- Whether hypogastric arteries are involved in the aneurysmal sac or not
- The patency of hypogastric arteries, not only for their function in the rich grid of collateral circulation with intestinal branches, but also as final branches of the muscular vasculature
- The presence of possible vascular anatomical variants (for example the presence of retroaortic left renal vein)

10.7.2 Aortic Endoprosthesis Follow-up

A successful procedure depends on the reduction of aneurysmal sac, with total exclusion of the thrombus and thrombosis of the excluded lumen. CT is the standard of reference in the follow-up of aortic endoprosthesis, being effective and specific in the detection of the presence, in the follow-up, of aortic endoprosthesis and periprosthesis leaks, with a sensitivity and specificity in detecting periprosthesis leaks of, respectively, 92% and 90%, as compared to 63% and 77% of DSA [32].

CT angiography not only diagnoses the presence of endoleaks, but it also detects its location, etiology, and length, taking into account any possible interrelated complications. The presence of leaks and the enlargement of the aneurysmal sac indicate an incomplete exclusion of the aneurysm [43].

CT angiography in the follow-up of these patients must be performed, according to our protocol, 1 month, 6 months, and 1 year after aortic endoprosthesis positioning. In the follow up after aortic endoprosthesis positioning, the following aspects must be evaluated:

- The patency and integrity of the prosthesis and the maximum axial diameter of the patency of aneurysmal sac. A prosthesis occlusion, caused by the presence of kinking, angulation, or thrombosis, are relatively rare events [8, 14, 34]. Figure 10.8 shows a case of complete occlusion of the left iliac branch in a patient with an aorto-biiliac stent-graft. Small changes of the prosthesis shape are acceptable, while serious twisting or kinking of branches may cause the failure of the procedure. With the reduction of the axial diameter of the aneurysm, as the result of a successful procedure, we may also encounter a reduction of the length, with possible kinking formation [11,

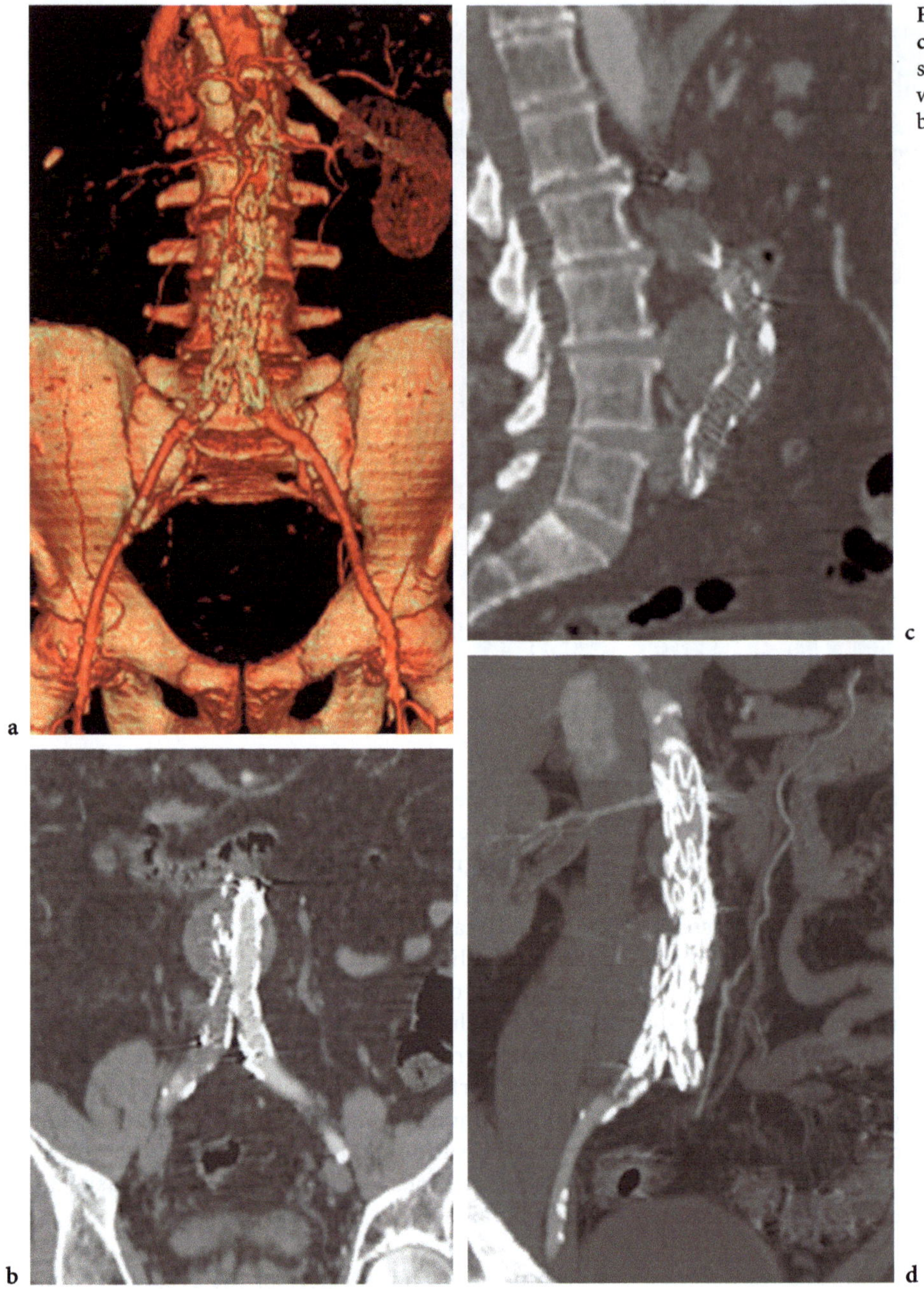

Fig. 10.8a,b VR (a), MPR (b, c), and MIP (d) images. Patient submitted to aortic stenting with occlusion of the right iliac branch.

25, 58]. Kinking of the prosthesis could also be the consequence of its sinking at the proximal attachment site, with consequent caudal migration [27]. Angulation of the prosthesis may determine a stenosis, thrombosis, or detachment of an iliac branch with consequent reduction of either the inflow or outflow, with increased possibility of intrastent parietal thrombotic appositions, which can be manifest in about 3–19% of cases [8] and needs therefore to be monitored. These complications are better evaluated on 3D than on transverse images.

- The presence of endoleaks means the persistence of flow within the aneurysmal sac excluded from the endoprosthesis [25]. This is the most frequent complication occurring according to several with a frequency ranging between 2 and 45% [12, 22, 23, 25, 32]. The presence of endoleaks means that the attempt to exclude the aneurysmal sac failed, but it does not necessarily imply that the procedure itself failed. In fact, although the presence of endoleaks may cause the enlargement of the aneurysmal sac with possible caudal migration of the prosthesis or rupture of the aneurysm in

12–44% of patients [31], a spontaneous solution may also occur. Endoleaks are the most frequent cause of conversion to open surgery [55], which has a mortality rate of about 24% (6 times higher than the mortality rate of surgery as first treatment). Endoleaks can be classified according to temporal criteria (primary or secondary) to their etiology (types I, II, III, IV, and V) or according to their location [12, 25].

A primary leak appears within 30 days of treatment, documented or shown on the intraoperative angiographic examination performed at the end of the procedure or during the first CT angiography follow-up study. A primary leak is usually a result of incorrect positioning of the stent-graft, of presence of an angled short neck (less than 1.5 cm), or of thrombocalcific apposition, which prevents a safe fastening of the proximal portion of the prosthesis. Secondary leaks, which tend to come out approximately 1 month after positioning of the prosthesis, may be related to caudal migration, only partial exclusion of the aneurysm in the distal tract, incomplete overlap of main body and iliac branch, and damaged prosthesis.

In contrast, according to their etiology, endoleaks are classified into:

- Type I, incomplete attachment of the proximal and the distal tract of the prosthesis, caused by technical or anatomical problems
- Type II, regressed flow in the aneurysmal sac caused by secondary arteries, such as the inferior mesenteric artery, lumbar arteries, and hypogastric arteries
- Type III, caused by holes in the prosthesis or detachment of its various sections
- Type IV, porosity of the prosthesis
- Type V, or endotension, in case of impossibility to demonstrate residual flow, but with evidence of persistent pressure in the aneurysmal sac, demonstrated by an increase in the diameter of the aneurysm [22]

We may also classify endoleaks as proximal, middle, and distal according to their site [1, 15, 25].

Proximal and distal endoleaks are related to an incomplete attachment of the prosthesis to the aortic walls or to its migration [14], whereas middle endoleaks are related to prosthesis defects or to regressed flow of vessels in the aneurysmal sac.

Transverse images in Fig. 10.9 of a follow-up study in a patient with an aorto-biiliac stent-graft show, in the arterial phase, reperfusion of the aneurysmal sac near the side walls extending caudally along the branches as far as their distal ends. This finding, also evident on reconstructed images, shows a type I distal leak, as an incomplete attachment of distal portions of the prosthesis, caused by dilatation of the common iliac arteries, as confirmed by angiography.

In the transverse image of Fig. 10.10, on the other hand, the reperfusion of the aneurysmal sac is located near the left anterolateral wall, close to the origin of the inferior mesenteric artery, as demonstrated on the 3D reconstruction. This finding is also related to a leak with aneurysmal sac reperfusion and regressed flow from the inferior mesenteric artery: type II leak.

In Fig. 10.11 it is also possible to see, either on axial or reconstructed images, reperfusion of the aneurysmal sac in a patient with an aortic endoprosthesis entering from the left side of the main body. In this case the reperfusion is located near the anterior wall of the right iliac branch, with cranial limits placed at the main juncture point of the prosthesis. The location of the leak, its relationship with the prosthetic branch, and the absence of secondary arteries that could justify it, suggest a type III leak, caused by detachment of the prosthesis segments.

The prosthesis is positioned to evaluate and document its possible caudal migration caused by:

- Incorrect positioning of the proximal portion (reduction of the radial strength of the prosthesis and inadequate contact between the proximal neck and the proximal portion of the prosthesis, mainly if this appears to be too short, angled, or with excessive parietal thrombocalcific apposition) [33, 50, 51]
- Modification of the morphology of the aneurysm (for instance dilatation of proximal neck)

The caudal migration of the prosthesis determines a leak with an enlargement of the diameter of the aneurysmal sac and consequently an increased risk of rupture of the aneurysm. Figure 10.12 shows an example of caudal migration with damaged prosthesis, 6 months after positioning.

Other postprocedural complications may be classified as local or systemic. Among local vascular problems, it is worthwhile mentioning iliac dissection or artery rupture, caused by large-caliber catheters [50], pseudoaneurysm formation, especially nearby the entrance site [36], and also hematomas, infections, and lymphocyst near the femoral

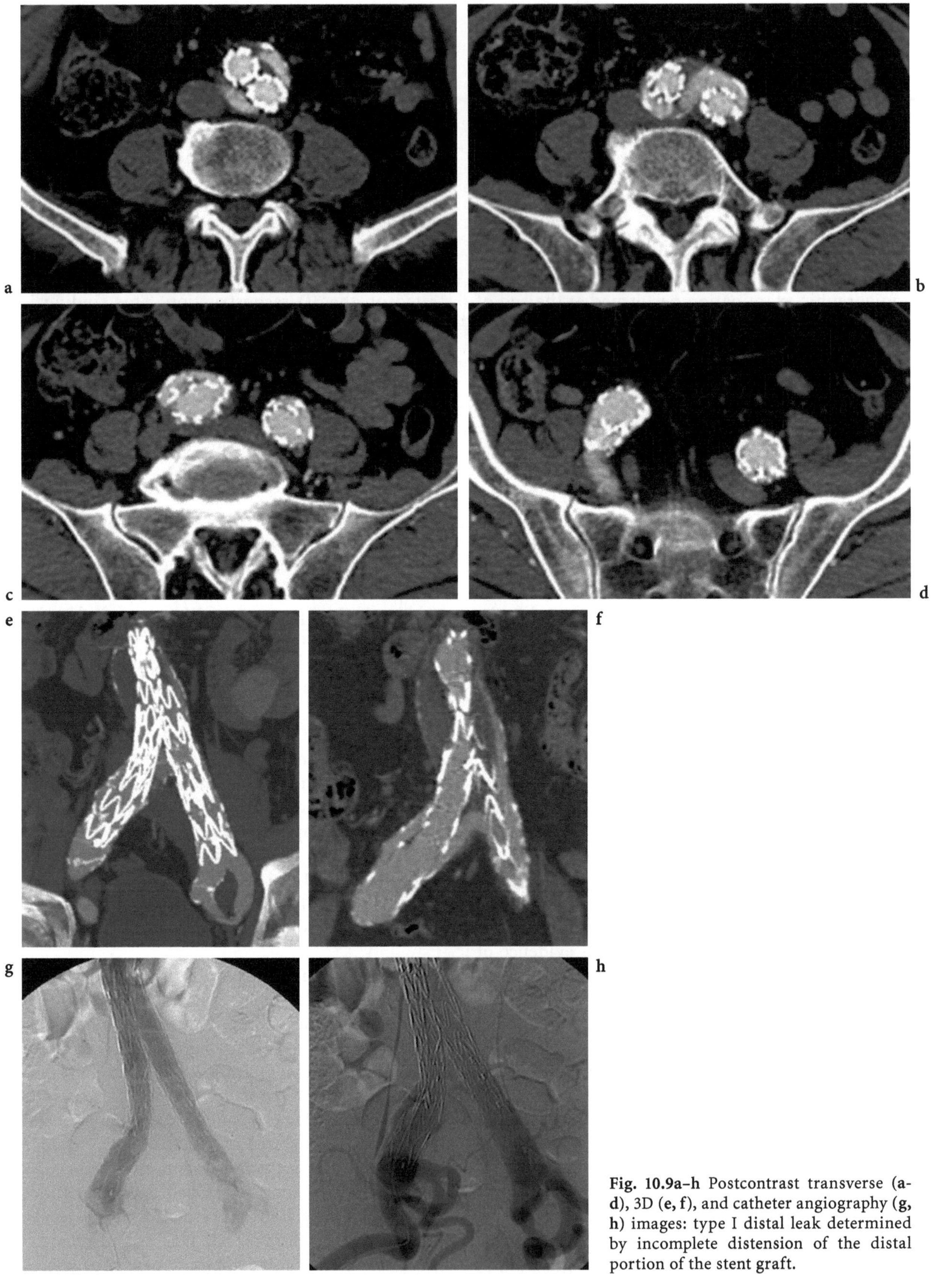

Fig. 10.9a–h Postcontrast transverse (a-d), 3D (e, f), and catheter angiography (g, h) images: type I distal leak determined by incomplete distension of the distal portion of the stent graft.

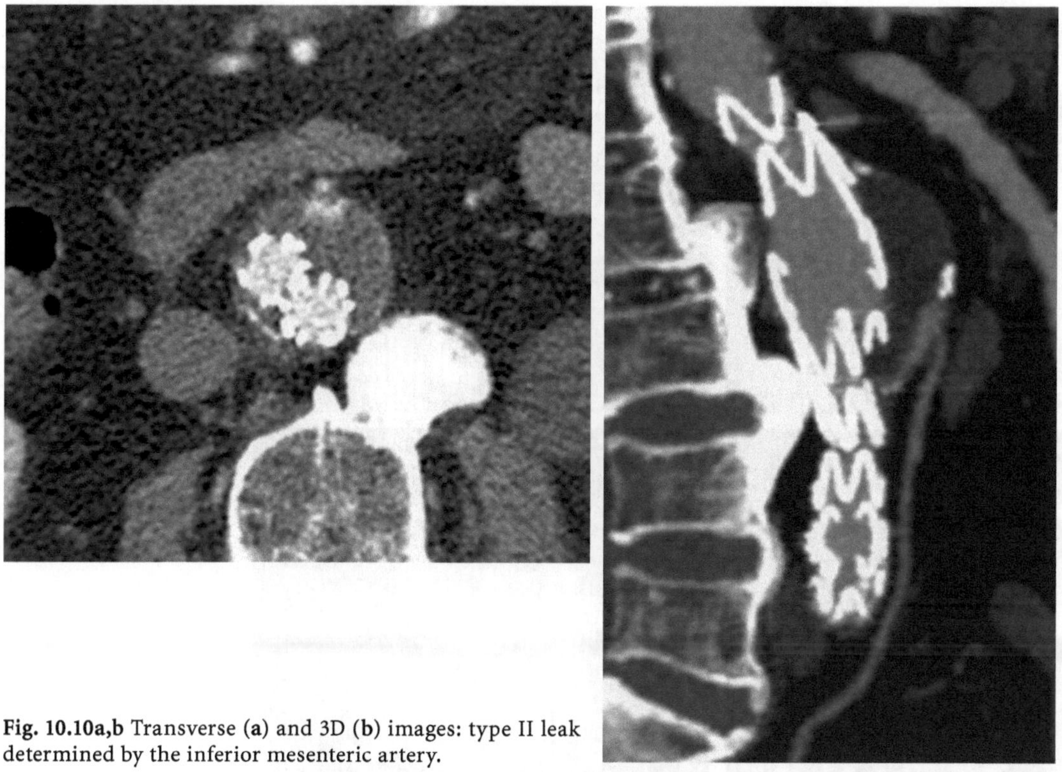
a b

Fig. 10.10a,b Transverse (a) and 3D (b) images: type II leak determined by the inferior mesenteric artery.

incision. Systemic complications are not different from typical postvascular surgery complications: to cardiac and respiratory risks we need to add renal failure, caused by i.v. administration of iodinated contrast medium, renal embolization by the aortic thrombus, renal artery ostium obstruction by the covered portion of the stent, and mesenteric ischemia related to occlusion of the inferior mesenteric and/or hypogastric arteries in patients with steno-occlusive disease of the celiac trunk and superior mesenteric artery [54].

10.8 Clinical Evaluation in Steno-occlusive Disease

Steno-occlusive disease of the abdominal aorta and its visceral branches may be acute or chronic. Acute occlusion is usually caused by an embolism, acute thrombosis of a stenotic artery, or by aortic dissection. Atherosclerosis is by far the most common cause of chronic occlusion.

We may differentiate infrarenal aortic occlusion, which may reach the renal arteries, from distal aortoiliac steno-occlusive disease, which involves the aortic carrefour and the iliac arteries, and from the small-aorta syndrome, which is a focal atherosclerotic stenosis of the distal aorta often affecting, young smoking women and usually associated with inguinal occlusive disease.

The most important steno-occlusive disease of the aortoiliac compartment is the Leriche syndrome, defined as a chronic thrombosis of the aortic bifurcation on a parietal atherosclerotic segmental lesion. The discriminating characteristics of this disease, with respect to other types of aortoiliac arteriosclerosis, is the absence of significant lesions in the peripheral compartment. Leriche syndrome mainly affects men between the age of 45 and 60 years. The main collaterals depend on the epigastric circulation formed by the internal mammary, intercostal and lumbar arteries with the reconstitution of distal external iliac and common femoral arteries [1, 57].With respect to this disease, the major limitation of X-ray angiography is that, although the catheter positioned distal in the abdominal aorta allows to visualize the level of occlusion and the possible patency of visceral branches, it is not possible to adequately evaluate distal arterial compartments because of the cranial origin of major collateral vessels (inter-

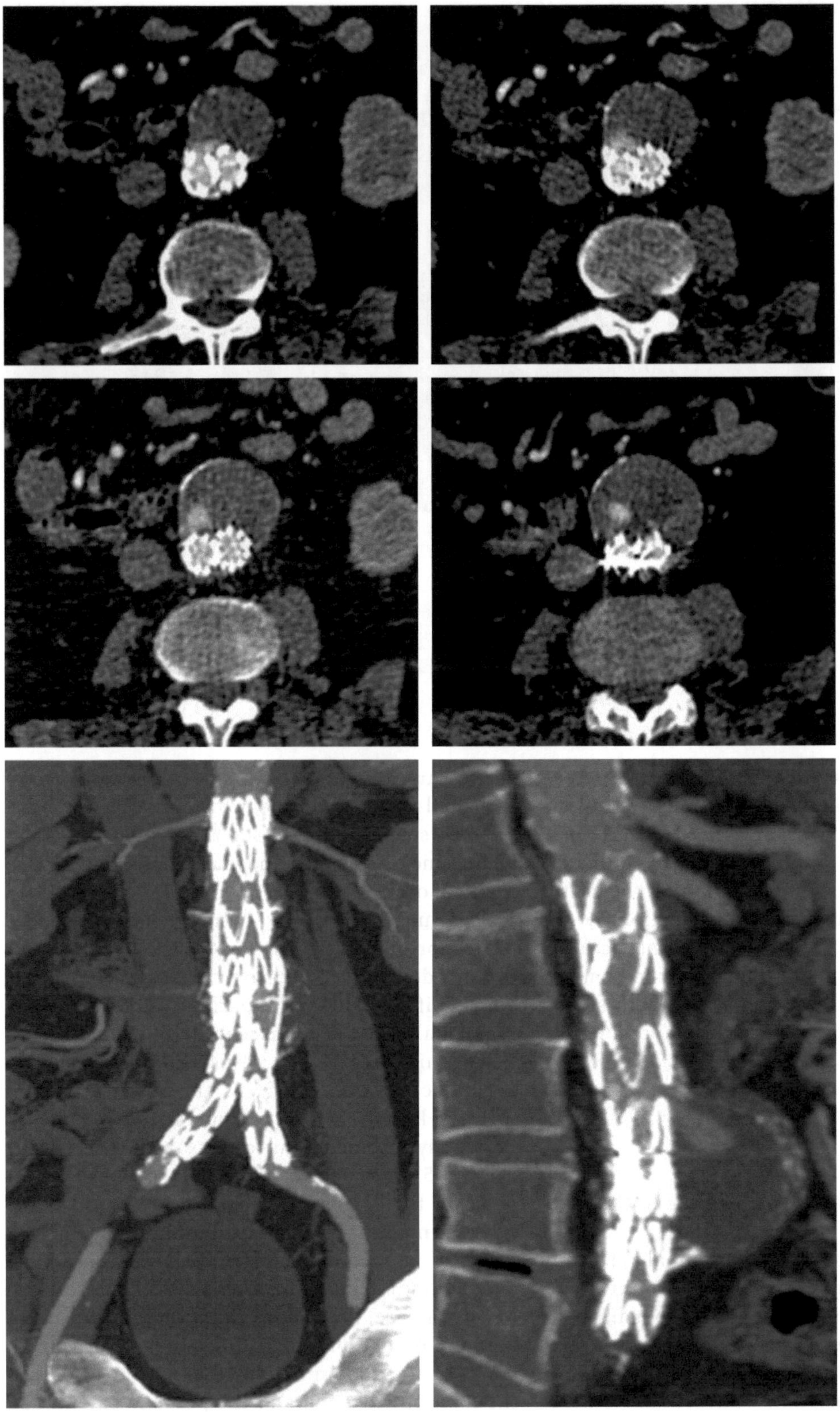

a b c d e f

Fig. 10.11a–f Transverse (**a-d**) and reconstructed (**e-f**) images in patient submitted to bifurcated aortic stenting with release of the main body from the left side: type III leak determined by detachment of stent modules.

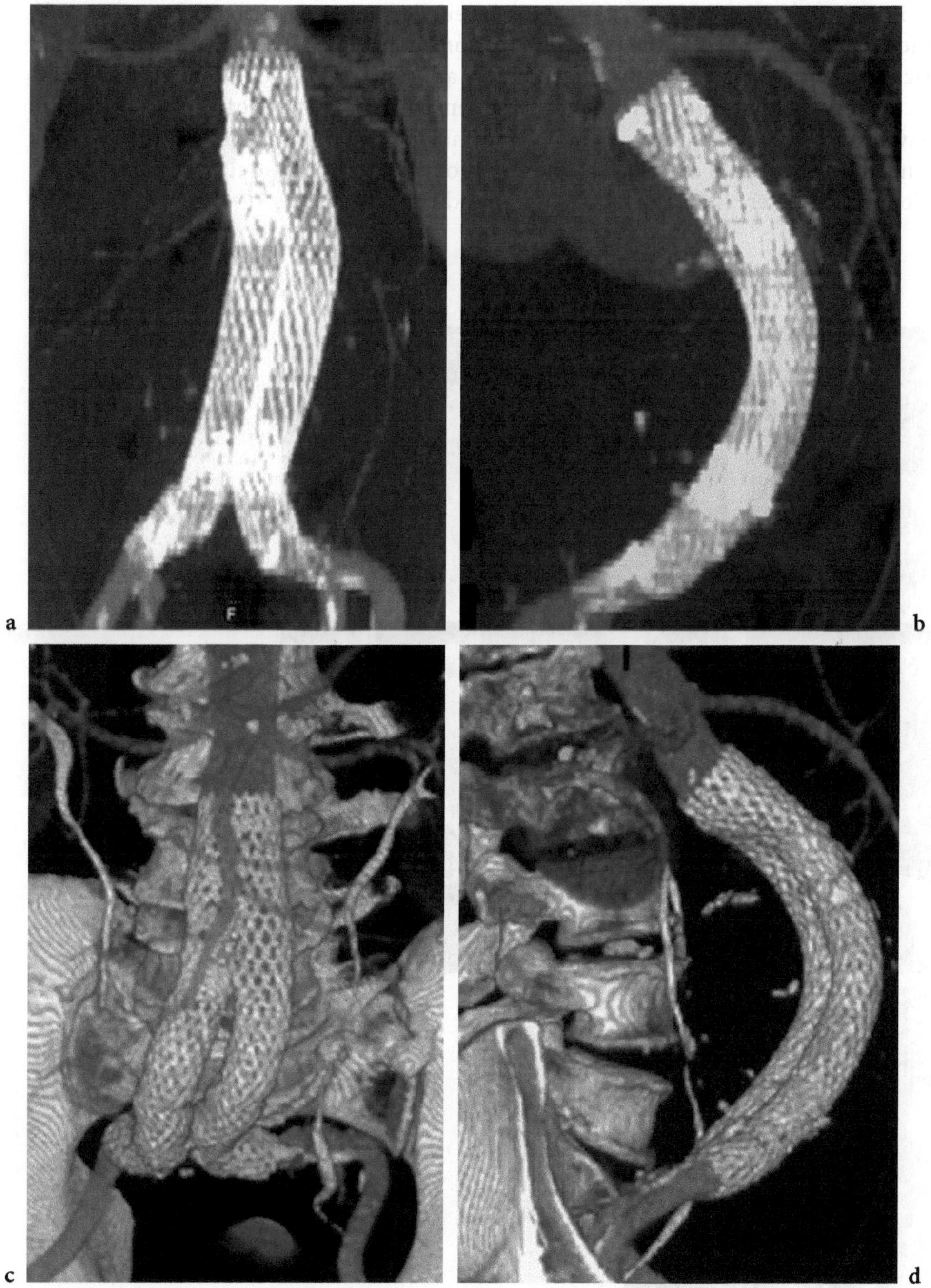

Fig. 10.12a–d Follow-up CT examination performed 1 month after stenting (**a, b**); follow-up examination performed at 6 months (**c, d**): distal migration of the stent.

nal mammary artery and intercostal branches). On the other hand, even if the catheter is placed in the aortic arch, with opacification of upper collateral branches, it is necessary to inject a high quantity of contrast medium to have an adequate visualization of distal compartments of the occluded artery. With MDCT the limitations of catheter angiography may be easily overcome with a relatively small amount of contrast medium, as shown in Fig. 10.13, in which CT angiography, in a patient with Leriche syndrome, enables evaluation of the occlusion of the abdominal aorta, the patency of its visceral branches providing an optimal visualization of collateral and run-off vessels.

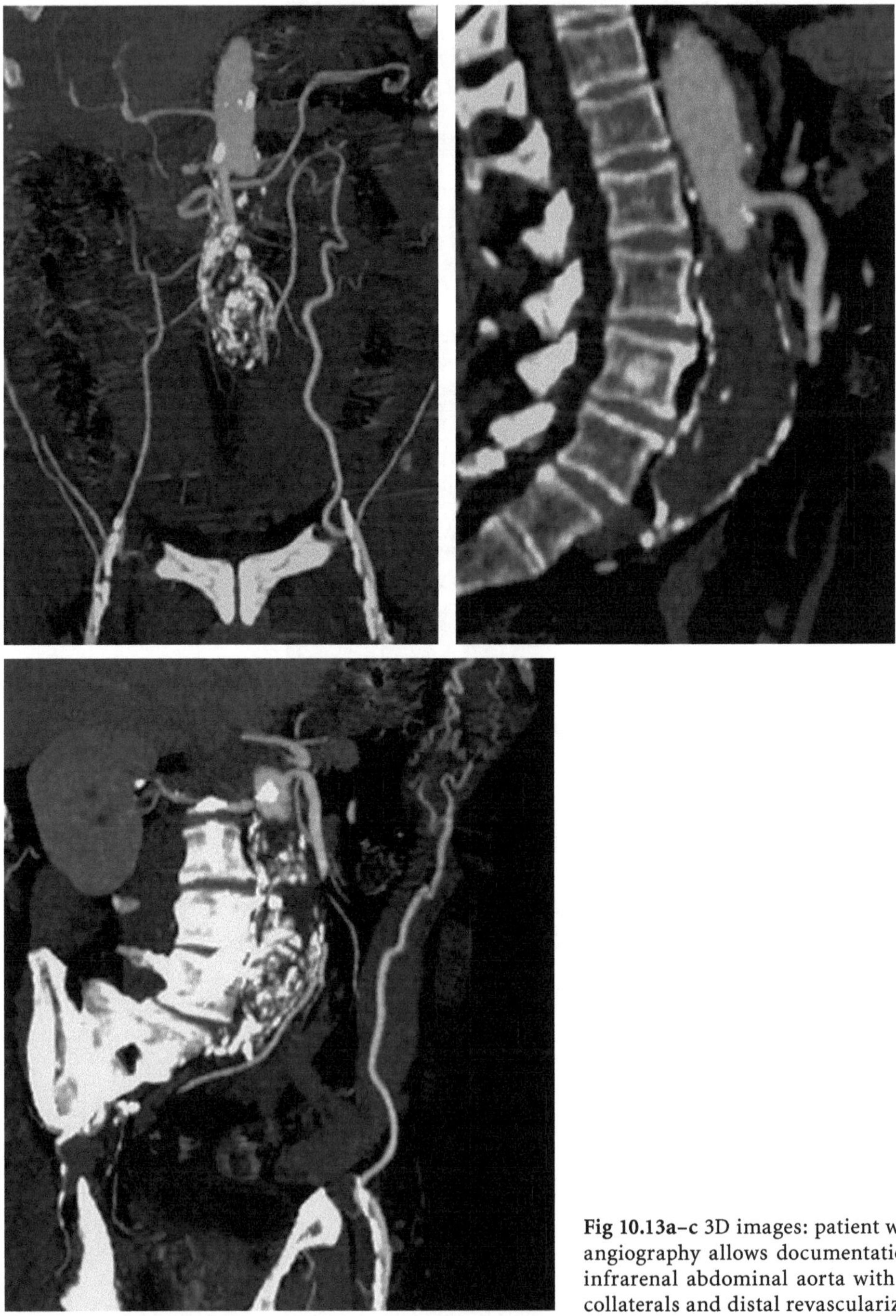

a b c

Fig 10.13a–c 3D images: patient with Leriche syndrome. CT angiography allows documentation of the occlusion of the infrarenal abdominal aorta with excellent visualization of collaterals and distal revascularization.

References

1. Armerding MA, Rubin GD, Beaulieu CF et al. (2000) Aortic aneurysmal disease: assessment of stent-graft treatment-CT versus conventional angiography. Radiology 215:138–146
2. Arnold JR, Greenberg JD, Clements S (2000) Internal mammary artery perfusing the Leriche's syndrome. Ann Thorac Surg 69:1244–1246
3. Bae KT, Heiken JP, Brink JA (1998) Aortic and hepatic contrast medium enhancement at CT. I. Prediction with a computer model. Radiology 207:647–655
4. Bae KT, Heiken JP, Brink JA (1998) Aortic and hepatic contrast medium enhancement at CT. II. Effect of reduced cardiac output in a porcine model. Radiology 207:657–662
5. Bae KT, Tran HQ, Heiken JP (2000) Multiphasic injection method for uniform prolonged vascular enhancement at CT angiography; pharmacokinetic analysis and experimental porcine model. Radiology 216:872–880
6. Blum A, Walter F, Ludig T et al. (2000) Multi-detector TC: principles and new applications. J Radiol 81:1597–1614
7. Blum U, Langer M, Spillner G et al. (1996) Abdominal aortic aneurysms: preliminary technical and clinical results with transfemoral placement of endovascular self-expanding stent-grafts. Radiology 198:25–31
8. Blum U, Krumme B, Flugel P et al. (1997) Treatment of ostial renal-artery stenoses with vascular endoprostheses after unsuccessful balloon angioplasty. N Engl J Med 336:459–465
9. Bosch JL, Kaufman JA, Beinfeld MT et al. (2002) Abdominal aortic aneurysms: cost-effectiveness of elective endovascular and open surgical repair. Radiology 225:337–344
10. Calhoun PS, Kuszyk BS, Heath DG et al. (1999) Three-dimensional volume rendering of spiral CT data: theory and method. Radiographics 19:745–764
11. Chuter TA, Gordon RL, Reilly LM et al. (1999) Abdominal aortic aneurysm in high-risk patients: short- to intermediate-term results of endovascular repair. Radiology 210:361–365
12. Cuypers P, Buth J, Harris PL et al. (1999) Realistic expectations for patients with stent-graft treatment of abdominal aortic aneurysms. Results of a european multicentre registry. Eur J Vasc Endovasc Surg 17:507–516
13. Darling RC, Messina CR, Brewster DC et al. (1977) Autopsy study of unoperated abdominal aortic aneurysm in mean age 65 to 74 years. The case for early resection. Cardiovasc Surg 56:161–163
14. Dorffner R (1999) Helical CT after aortic stent-graft implantation. AJR Am J Roentgenol 172:1690–1691
15. Dorffner R, Thumher S, Polterauer P et al. (1997) Treatment of abdominal aortic aneurysms with transfemoral placement of stent-grafts: complications and secondary radiologic intervention. Radiology 204:79–86
16. Ernst CB (1993) Abdominal aortic aneurysm. N Engl J Med 328:1167–1172
17. Fishman EK (2001) CT angiography: clinical applications in the abdomen. Radiographics [Suppl] 21:3–16
18. Fishman EK, Liang CC, Kuszyk BS et al. (1996) Automated bone editing algorithm for CT angiography: preliminary results. AJR Am J Roentgenol 166:669–672
19. Fleischmann D (2002) Present and future trends in multiple detector-row CT applications: CT angiography. Eur Radiol [Suppl 2] 12:11–16
20. Fleischmann D, Hittmair K (2000) Mathematical analysis of arterial enhancement and optimization of bolus geometry for CT angiography using the discrete fourier transform. J Comput Assist Tomogr 23:474–484
21. Fleischmann D, Rubin GD, Bankier AA et al. (2000) Improved uniformity of aortic enhancement with customized contrast medium injection protocols at CT angiography. Radiology 214:363–371
22. Gilling-Smith G, Brennan J, Harris P et al. (1999) Endotension after endovascular aneurysm repair: definition, classification, and strategies for surveillance and intervention. J Endovasc Surg 6:305–307
23. Golzarian J, Struyven J, Abada HT et al. (1997) Endovascular aortic stent-grafts: transcatheter embolization of persistent perigraft leaks. Radiology 202:731–734
24. Golzarian J, Dussaussois L, Abada HT et al. (1998) Helical CT of aorta after endoluminal stent-graft therapy: value of biphasic acquisition. AJR Am J Roentgenol 171:329–331
25. Gorich J, Rilinger N, Sokiranski R et al. (1999) Leakages after endovascular repair of aortic aneurysm: classification based on findings at CT, angiography, and radiography. Radiology 213:767–772
26. Gorich J, Rilinger N, Sokiranski R et al. (2001) Endoleaks after endovascular repair of aortic aneurysm: are they predictable? Initial results. Radiology 218:477–480
27. Harris P, Brennan J, Martin J et al. (1999) Longitudinal aneurysm shrinkage following endovascular aortic aneurysm repair: a source of intermediate and late complications. J Endovasc Surg 6:11–16
28. Hittmair K, Fleischmann D (2001) Accuracy of predicting and controlling time-dependent aortic enhancement from a test bolus injection. J Comput Assist Tomogr 25:287–294
29. Hollier LH, Reigel MM, Kazmier FJ et al. (1986) Conventional repair of abdominal aortic aneurysm in the high-risk patient: a plea for abandonment of nonresective treatment. J Vasc Surg 3:712–717
30. Hu H (1999) Multi-slice helical CT: scan and reconstruction. Med Phys 26:5–18
31. Lumsden AB, Allen RC, Chaikof EL et al. (1995) Delayed rupture of aortic aneurysms following endovascular stent grafting. Am J Surg 170:174–178
32. Makaroun MS, Deaton DH (2001) Is proximal aortic neck dilatation after endovascular aneurysm exclusion a cause for concern? J Vasc Surg [Suppl 2] 33:39–45
33. Malina M, Ivancev K, Chuter CA et al. (1997) Changing aneurysmal morphology after endovascular grafting: relation to leakage or persistent perfusion. J Endovasc Surg 4:23–30
34. May J, White GH, Harris JP (2001) Endoluminal repair of abdominal aortic aneurysms – state of the art. Eur J Radiol 39:16–21
35. Parodi JC (1995) Endovascular repair of abdominal aortic aneurysm and other arterial lesions. J Vasc Surg 21:549–557
36. Parodi JC, Palmaz JC, Barone HD (1991) Transfemoral intraluminal graft implantation for abdominal aortic aneurysm. Ann Vasc Surg 5:491–499
37. Prokop M (1999) Protocols and future directions in

imaging of renal artery stenosis: CT angiography. J Comput Assist Tomogr [Suppl 1] 23:101–110
38. Prokop M (2000) Multislice CT angiography. Eur of Radiol 36:86–96
39. Prokop M, Schaefer-Prokop C, Galanski M (1997) Spiral CT angiography of the abdomen. Abdominal Imaging 22:143–53
40. Quanadli SD, Mesurolle B, Coggia M et al. (2000) Abdominal aortic aneurysm. AJR Am J Roentgenol 174:181–187
41. Raptopoulos V, Rosen MP, Kent KC et al. (1996) Sequential helical CT angiography of aortoiliac disease. AJR Am J Roentgenol 166:1347–1354
42. Rieker O, Duber C, Pitton M et al. (1997) CT angiography versus intraarterial digital substraction angiography for assessment of aortoiliac occlusive disease. AJR Am J Roentgenol 169:1133–1138
43. Rozenblit A, Marin ML, Veith FJ et al. (1995) Endovascular repair of abdominal aortic aneurysm: value of postoperative follow-up with helical CT. AJR Am J Roentgenol 165:1473–1479
44. Rozenblit A, Patlas M, Rosenbaum AT et al. (2003) Detection of endoleaks after endovascular repair of abdominal aortic aneurysm: value of unenhanced and delay helical CT acquisitions. Radiology 227:426–433
45. Rubin GD (2000) Data explosion: the challenge of multidetector row CT. Eur Radiol 36:74–80
46. Rubin GD, Dake MD, Semba CP (1995) Current status of 3D spiral CT scanning for imaging the vasculature. Radiol Clin North Am 33:51–70
47. Rubin GD, Shiau MC, Schmidt AJ et al. (1999) Computed tomographic angiography: historical perspective and new state-of-art using multi-detector-row helical computed tomography. J Computed Assist Tomogr 23 [Suppl 1]:S83–S90
48. Rubin GD, Shiau MC, Leung AN et al. (2000) Aorta and iliac arteries: single versus multiple detector-row helical CT angiography. Radiology 215:670–676
49. Rydberg J, Buckwalter KA, Caldemeyer KS et al. (2000) Multisection CT: scanning techniques and clinical applications. Radiographics 20:1787–1806
50. Rydberg J, Kopecky KK, Johnson MS et al. (2001) Endovascular repair of abdominal aortic aneurysms: assessment with multislice CT. AJR Am J Roentgenol 177:607–614
51. Rydberg J, Kopecky KK, Lalka SG et al. (2001) Stent grafting of abdominal aortic aneurysms: preand postoperative evaluation with multislice helical CT. J Comput Assist Tomogr 25:580–586
52. Sawhney R, Kerlan RK, Wall SD et al. (2001) Analysis of initial CT findings after endovascular repair of abdominal aortic aneurysm. Radiology 220:157–160
53. Silverman PM, Roberts S, Tefft MC et al. (1995) Helical CT of the liver: clinical application of an automated computer techinique, SmartPrep, for obtained images with optimal contrast enhancement. AJR Am J Roentgenol 165:73–78
54. Thompson MM, Smith J, Naylor AR et al. (1997) Microembolization during endovascular and conventional aneurysm repair. J Vasc Surg 25:179–186
55. Vallabhaneni SR, Harris PL (2001) Lessons learnt from the EUROSTAR registry on endovascular repair of abdominal aneurysm repair. Eur J Radiol 39:34–41
56. Van Hoe L, Marchal G, Baert AL et al. (1995) Determination of scan delay-time in spiral CT-angiography: utility of a test bolus injection. J Comput Assist Tomogr 19:216–220
57. Vogt FM, Goyen M, Debatin JF (2001) Modern diagnostic concepts in dissection and aortic occlusion. Radiology 41:640–652
58. Wolf YG, Hill BB, Lee WA (2001) Eccentric stent graft compression: an indicator of insecure proximal fixation of aortic stent graft. J Vasc Surg 33:481–487
59. Zarins CK White RA, Hodgson KJ et al. (2000) Endoleak as a predictor of outcome after endovascular aneurysm repair: AneuRx multicenter clinical trial. J Vasc Surg 32:90–107

11 Hepatic Vessels

Takamichi Murakami, Masatoshi Hori, Tonsok Kim, Masatomo Kuwabara, Hisashi Abe, Azzam Anwar Khankan, and Hironobu Nakamura

CONTENTS

11.1 Introduction

Dynamic computed tomography (CT) images with a helical CT have been used for detecting and characterizing primary and metastatic hepatic neoplasms [1–3]. Several authors have demonstrated that the dynamic helical CT data with thin-section collimation and three-dimensional (3D) displays could also accurately demonstrate the major visceral arteries [4–7], such as the celiac axis and its branches, and the superior and inferior mesenteric arteries. Therefore, CT angiography is expected to prove extremely valuable for applications such as preoperative planning for hepatic resection, preoperative evaluation and planning for liver transplantation, pretreatment planning for patients considered for hepatic arterial infusion chemotherapy, and pretreatment evaluation of portal vein patency for a variety of reasons [6, 8–13]. CT angiography can also provide supplemental information in patients with cirrhosis, upper gastrointestinal tract bleeding due to varices, or primary extrahepatic neoplasms. However, as approximately 30 s has been needed to cover the entire liver and pancreas with thin-section collimation with a single detector-row helical CT because of its limited speed of scanning [5, 7], it is hard to obtain the arterial or portal venous dominant phase images of large anatomical areas during peak arterial or portal venous enhancement, respectively. Multidetector-row helical CT (MDCT) can acquire multiple CT data sets with each rotation of the X-ray tube [14] and can scan through large anatomical areas much faster than single-detector-row helical CT scanners. This system, therefore, gives us the opportunity to acquire CT images of the upper abdominal area, including liver, with thinner-section collimation within the time period generally regarded as the hepatic arterial or portal venous dominant phase. These images are used to reconstruct 3D CT angiograms, which help in the evaluation of vascular anatomical information and vascular invasion of tumors.

In this article, techniques used for optimization of the scan protocols and postprocessing of CT angiography are addressed. The clinical advantages of CT angiography in evaluating liver disease are also discussed.

11.2 Techniques of Contrast-Medium Administration

Dynamic-study images are useful to reconstruct CT angiograms of each hepatic vessels. However, to perform a good dynamic study, we have to employ optimal parameters such as injection rate, total volume of contrast medium, injection duration, scan time, concentration of contrast medium, and delay time of scan.

T. Murakami, MD, PhD, Associate Professor and Vicechairman; M. Hori, MD, PhD; T. Kim, MD; M. Kuwabara, MD; H. Abe, MD; A. A. Khankan, MD; H. Nakamura, MD, PhD
Department of Radiology, Osaka University Graduate School of Medicine D1, 2-2, Yamadaoka, Suita-City, Osaka 565-0871, Japan

Peak arterial enhancement is mainly affected by total amount of iodine injected during a unit time that is proved by a higher injection rate, higher concentration of contrast medium, injection duration [15–17]. Injection rate affects the maximum arterial enhancement and delay time of peak aortic enhancement after initiation of contrast medium. When we inject contrast medium faster, peak enhancement becomes higher and delay time of peak enhancement becomes shorter [15, 16]. When the same amount of contrast medium and the same injection rate are employed, contrast medium with higher concentration can improve peak arterial enhancement of each region. With the same concentration of contrast medium and the same injection rate, longer injection duration (larger amount of contrast medium) shows higher peak arterial enhancement [17].Injection duration is almost equal to the marked arterial enhanced period, so imaging time should be shorter than the injection duration [17]. MDCT can obtain the image faster, so when we obtain only arterial phase images, we may reduce the total volume of the contrast medium (injection rate times injection duration). However, because of variables such as patient size and cardiovascular status, CT images may show varying degrees of hepatic arterial, portal venous, hepatic venous, and parenchymal enhancement. To compensate for the patient's size, 2–2.5 ml of contrast medium should be administered per kilogram body weight [18]. In our institute, 2 ml/kg of 300 mg I/ml of contrast medium is injected intravenously by power injector at a rate of 4-5 ml/s, or 1.7 ml/kg of 350-370 mg I/ml of contrast medium at a rate of 4 ml/s through a 20-gauge plastic intravenous catheter placed in an antecubital vein. However, when a patient's weight is low, total amount of contrast medium is also small and injection duration (total amount of contrast medium divided by injection rate) becomes short. The scan time of the arterial phase imaging of MDCT is about 20 s, therefore a minimum of 100 ml of contrast medium should be used to keep the injection duration longer than scan time (injection duration is 20 or 25 s at the rate of 5 or 4 ml/s, respectively).

Many investigators have initiated arterial phase imaging with a scan delay of 20-30 s using an injection rate of 4 or 5 ml/s [3, 19]. However, the exact definition and optimal timing of the hepatic arterial dominant phase remains somewhat uncertain and controversial, because it can be influenced by numerous variables such as the patient's size and cardiovascular status.To determine the optimal delay time to start with, test-bolus injection techniques or automatic bolus-tracking techniques can be employed [20]. The scanning time delay is determined using a test bolus (15 ml at 5 ml/s) of 300 mg I/ml of nonionic contrast medium through a 20-gauge intravenous catheter placed in the antecubital vein followed by a series of single-level CT scans at low dose (120 KVp, 10 mA). The scan location is 20 cm below the dome of the liver, and the monitoring scans are acquired every 2 s from 10–40 s. A cursor is placed over the abdominal aorta at this level, and the time interval to peak aortic enhancement is used to determine the scan delay for the early arterial phase images. The time to peak arterial enhancement from initiation of contrast medium is used as delay time of the early arterial phase. As a result of this test injection technique in our study [20], the scanning delays for the arterial phases were quite variable. Therefore, we doubt that a standard scan delay would reliably result in optimal timing for arterial phase set of CT images. If a fully automatic bolus-tracking technique is available, it may be also useful to adjust the timing of arterial-phase CT scan of the liver. In our experience, the scan should be automatically started at least 7-10 s, including the time of voice for breath-hold and table movement, etc., after triggering at a threshold of 100 HU relative enhancement of the abdominal aorta [21].

11.3 Imaging Protocol of MDCT

Scan parameters are different in each grade of MDCT. When 8-channel or 4-channel MDCT units are used, the detector configuration is 8×1.25 or 4×2.5 mm, in which eight or four interspaced helical data sets are collected from eight 1.25-mm detector rows, respectively. A pitch of 10.8 or 6 with the table speed set at 15 mm/rotation is employed. One rotation of the X-ray tube is 0.5 s. The axial images are reconstructed and displayed as 40 slices with5-mm thickness slices for each phase set. Each phase helical CT data is retrospectively reconstructed for multiplanar reconstruction with a standard soft algorithm at 0.63-mm increments with a 0.63-mm thickness in 16-channel MDCT, 0.63-mm increments with a 1.25-mm thickness in 8-channel MDCT or 1.25-mm increments with a 2.5-mm section thickness in 4-channel MDCT. Field of view is 30 cm.

Scanning begins from the dome of the liver (location determined by the scout digital radiograph) and proceeds in a caudal direction, covering a *z*-axis distance of at least 20 cm at an optimal delay time after initiation of injection of contrast medium determined in the way mentioned previously. These CT images constitute the early arterial phase of the double arterial phase imaging. After an interscan delay of 5 s, for table movement, scanning resumes from the dome of the liver in a caudal direction. This constitutes the late arterial phase. The total acquisition time is about 20 s and is accomplished in a single breath-hold. Sixty to seventy seconds after the start of the injection of contrast medium, the portal venous phase is imaged with the same parameter when the contrast medium distributed to the bowel is collecting in the liver. As mentioned above, double arterial phase and portal venous phase images are obtained for liver imaging.

11.4 Postprocessing Techniques of CT Angiography

These CT data are transferred to a computer workstation that can reconstruct 3D CT angiograms. Computer workstations that allow direct interaction with all the CT data for a particular study are used. The quality of 3D CT angiograms depends on the performance of the workstation. Radiologists reconstruct oblique, thick-slab maximum-intensity projection (target MIP) images with 2- to 3-cm-thick slab and volume-rendering images to obtain the CT arteriogram. Radiologists should take an active role in image analysis, because they can best choose the optimal plane and orientation for demonstrating the extent and presence of pathological conditions by using real-time rendering.

As mentioned previously, our preferred 3D rendering techniques for CT angiography are volume rendering [22–24] and target MIP [25] (Fig. 11.1). CT angiography with volume rendering has a number of theoretical advantages over MIP and shaded surface display [24, 26, 27]. The volume-rendered images maintain the original anatomical spatial relationships of the CT data set and have a 3D appearance, facilitating interpretation of vascular interrelationships (Fig. 11.1a, d). Its specific advantages in vascular imaging are more accurate visualization of vessel detail, stenosis, and presence and location of vascular anomalies. Because the MIP algorithm selects only the highest-intensity voxel, the final images fails to depict overlapping vessels (Fig. 11.1b). However, by making target MIP images, we can eliminate overlapping vessels [25] (Fig. 11.1c). Moreover, we also find that MIP rendering is valuable as an adjunct display, especially for depicting smaller vessels within an enhancing organ such as the liver [25] (Fig. 11.1b, e).

Shaded surface renderings do not convey information rendering the relative attenuations of voxels in the original data set. Accordingly, shaded surface renderings do not depict calcification distinct from vascular enhancement, while volume-rendered displays can be interactively optimized by adjusting the window width and window level to make this important distinction [26, 27].

11.5 Visibility Using CT Angiography

When reviewing the two separate sets of hepatic arterial dominant phase (early and late arterial phase) and portal venous phase CT images of the liver in the MDCT protocol, we noted that the small branches of the hepatic arteries often could be visualized without portal venous enhancement during the early arterial phase, and that the peripheral branches of the portal vein could be demonstrated by the contrast medium returning from the splenic vein during the late arterial phase without hepatic venous enhancement.

In a previous study [25], with an initial model of 4-channel MDCT, CT angiography reconstructed from the early arterial phase (CT arteriography) with the MIP technique can show small branches of the hepatic arteries without portal venous enhancement (Fig. 11.1a, c), and the peripheral branches of the portal vein could be demonstrated on CT angiograms reconstructed from the late arterial phase images without the hepatic venous enhancement (CT portography) (Fig. 11.1d, e). CT angiograms reconstructed from the portal venous phase (CT portography and hepatic venography) shows intra- and extrahepatic portal vein enhanced by the contrast medium coming back from the superior and inferior mesenteric, and splenic vein, and the hepatic vein clearly visible (Fig. 11.1f). However, when a patient suffers from portal hypertension, portal and hepatic venous visualization may be obscure.

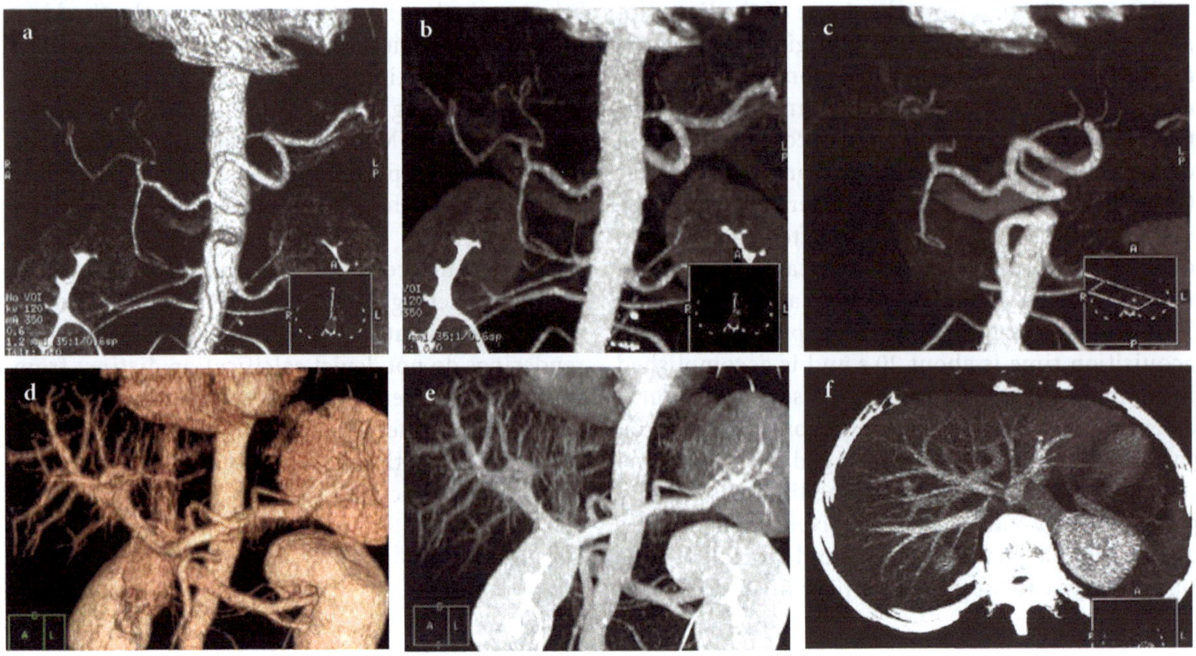

Fig. 11.1a–f Normal hepatic vessels. **a** The volume-rendered CT angiogram reconstructed from the early arterial phase images (CT arteriography) are useful for accurate visualization of arterial detail without overlapping vessels. **b** CT arteriogram with maximum-intensity projection technique (MIP) can show small branches of the hepatic arteries without portal venous enhancement. **c** Target-MIP CT arteriography can eliminate overlapping vessels. **d** The peripheral branches of the portal vein without the hepatic venous enhancement could be demonstrated on a volume-rendered CT angiogram reconstructed from the late arterial phase images (CT portography). **e** A CT portogram with MIP rendering is valuable as an adjunct display, especially for depicting smaller vessels within an enhancing organ such as the liver. **f** CT angiogram reconstructed from the portal venous phase images (CT portohepatic venography) shows the portal vein enhanced by the contrast medium coming back from the superior, inferior mesenteric, and splenic vein, and the hepatic vein very clearly.

11.5.1 Arterial Visualization

With the initial model of 4-channel MDCT, 100% of major arterial trunks (celiac, hepatic, superior mesenteric, left gastric) can be observed, and approximately 90% or more of the small branches of the hepatic arteries (right, middle, and left hepatic; cystic; right gastric; right and left inferior phrenic; and posterior superior, anterior superior, and inferior pancreaticoduodenal) are detected in the early arterial phase [25]. Recently, MDCT with 8- or 16-channel data acquisition has become available, and it enable us to obtain much thinner thick-slice images with faster acquisition time. CT arteriograms from these CT data show small hepatic arterial branches more clearly [28] (Fig. 11.2).

11.5.2 Portal Venous Visualization

The portal vein and its major tributaries (splenic and superior mesenteric veins, etc.) are seen in 100% of CT angiograms. Subsegmental or more peripheral branches of portal vein are seen in about 90% of CT angiograms during the late arterial phase and in about 100% during the portal venous phase [25] (Fig. 11.1d, e). Subsegmental branches of the portal vein were more frequently demonstrated on the late arterial phase than on the portal venous phase because hepatic parenchymal enhancement obscures them.

11.5.3 Hepatic Venous Visualization

The hepatic vein is clearly seen on CT portohepatic venograms (Fig. 11.1f). However, when a patient is suffering from portal hypertension, portal and hepatic venous visualization may be obscure.

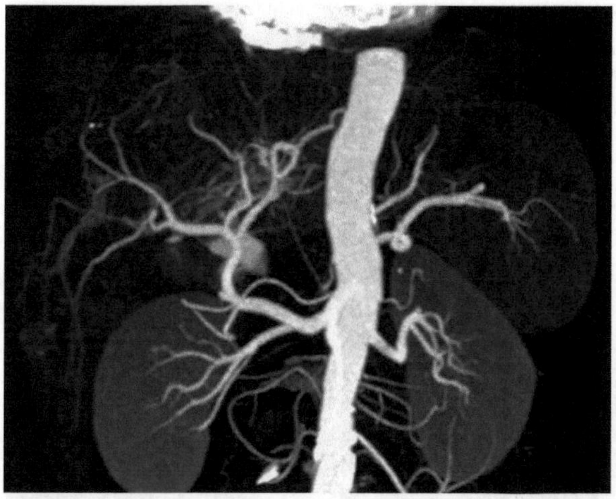

Fig. 11.2 A tumor thrombus of hepatocellular carcinoma. The CT arteriogram from MDCT with 16-channel data acquisition data clearly shows small hepatic arterial branches. The common hepatic artery branching from the superior mesenteric artery and the right phrenic artery branching from the aorta (*arrowheads*) are seen. Thread-and-streak signs indicate the presence of tumor thrombus (*arrow*).

11.6 Clinical Applications of Hepatic CT Angiography

Little attention has been paid for small branches of hepatic artery, such as middle hepatic artery, cystic artery, and right gastric artery, on CT scan. However, it is potentially important to evaluate these small arteries for preoperative evaluation of hepatic resection and liver transplantation including potential recipients and living related donors, and for pre-interventional radiological treatment evaluation of hepatic arterial infusion chemotherapy, transjugular intrahepatic portosystemic shunt placement or transcatheter arterial chemoembolization, etc [8–13]. CT angiography can replace conventional angiography.

11.6.1 Planning Liver Resection for Hepatic Tumors

The imaging technique for CT angiography by using multidetector-row helical CT is also useful for detecting and assessing the extent of hepatic neoplasms. These images help in decision-making about resectability and in surgical planning for hepatic resection. As mentioned previously, the double arterial and portal venous phase CT images and CT angiograms reconstructed from them allow the construction of highly detailed and accurate hepatic arterial, portal venous, and hepatic venous maps that are used as a guide for surgical planning (Fig. 11.1). These vascular maps provide better detail of possible tumoral vascular invasion by displaying the course of the vessels in optimal planes (Figs. 11.3, 11.4). Portal vein or hepatic venous invasion due to tumor thrombus is recognized during CT portography from the late arterial phase images or CT hepatic venography from the portal venous phase images. CT angiography with the volume-rendering technique and target MIP are useful to depict the relationship of the hepatic veins and intrahepatic portal veins to the segmental anatomical structure and to the tumor (Fig. 11.3). These images are critical for surgical planning

11.6.2 Hepatic Arterial Infusion Chemotherapy

CT arteriography can provide important arterial anatomical information before performing hepatic arterial infusion chemotherapy or transcatheter chemoembolization. Some of vascular anatomy can easily be detected on CT angiograms, but not on conventional angiograms. All arteries are enhanced simultaneously on intravenous enhanced CT images, while each artery is searched for to place a catheter using conventional angiography; for example, the inferior phrenic artery arising from the abdominal aorta or the renal artery cannot be demonstrated with celiac angiography (Figs. 11.2, 11.5). When we implant a catheter in the hepatic artery for continuous arterial infusion chemotherapy, it is important to know the hepatic arterial anatomy before the interventional procedure to implant the catheter in a appropriate position for perfusing anticancer drugs to the whole liver, including tumors (Fig. 11.5).

11.6.3 Portal Hypertension Due to Cirrhosis

Dilatation of the main portal vein and the splenic and superior mesenteric vein can also be seen in some cirrhotic patients. The hepatic artery is frequently enlarged and tortuous in advanced cirrhosis and may demonstrate increased flow [29]. Portosystemic shunt vessels such as intrahepatic portal venous shunt (Fig. 11.6), patent paraumbilical veins, dilated coronary veins, gastroesophageal varices, short gas-

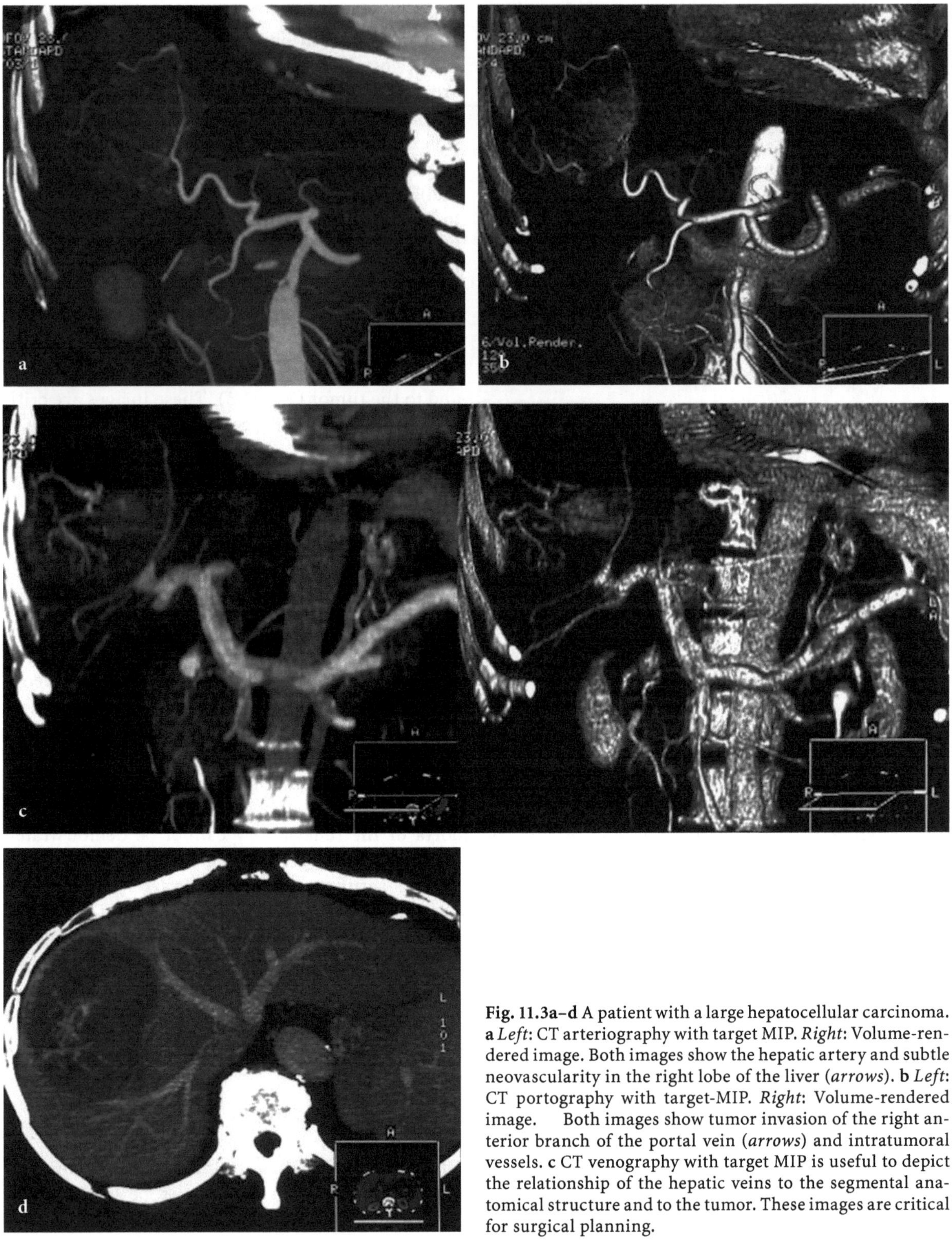

Fig. 11.3a–d A patient with a large hepatocellular carcinoma. **a** *Left*: CT arteriography with target MIP. *Right*: Volume-rendered image. Both images show the hepatic artery and subtle neovascularity in the right lobe of the liver (*arrows*). **b** *Left*: CT portography with target-MIP. *Right*: Volume-rendered image. Both images show tumor invasion of the right anterior branch of the portal vein (*arrows*) and intratumoral vessels. **c** CT venography with target MIP is useful to depict the relationship of the hepatic veins to the segmental anatomical structure and to the tumor. These images are critical for surgical planning.

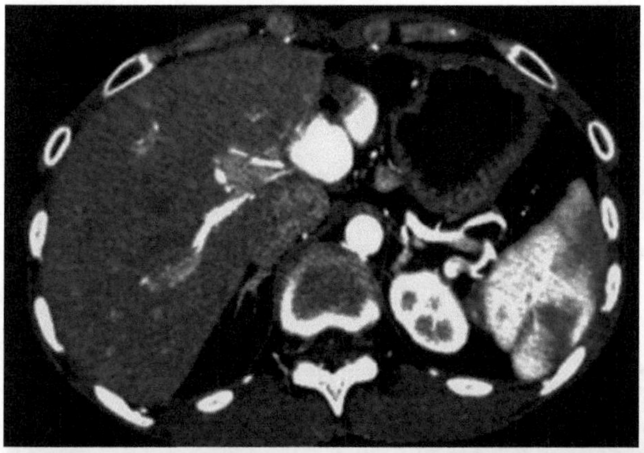

a

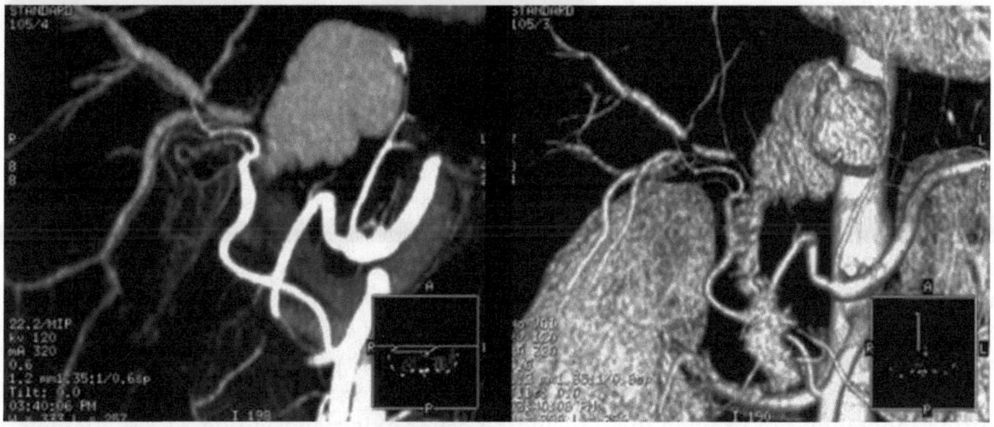

b

Fig. 11.4a,b A patient with gall bladder cancer. **a** The early arterial phase image with drip infusion cholecystography shows suspected encasement bile duct and hepatic artery (*arrows*). **b** *Left*: CT arteriography with target-MIP, *Right*: Volume-rendered image. Right branch of intrahepatic bile duct (*arrows*) and right hepatic arterial encasement (*arrowheads*) are clearly revealed.

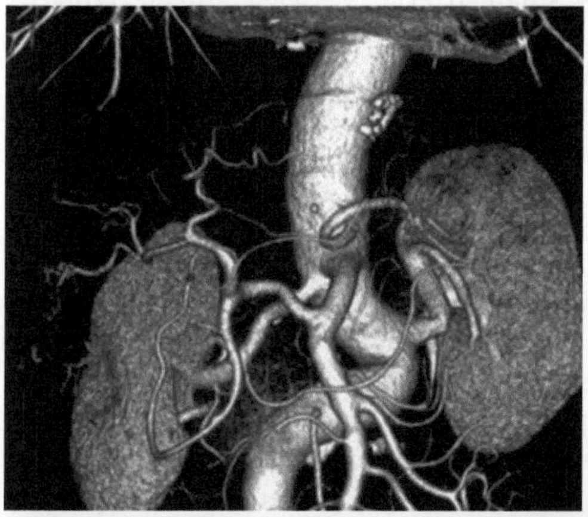

a

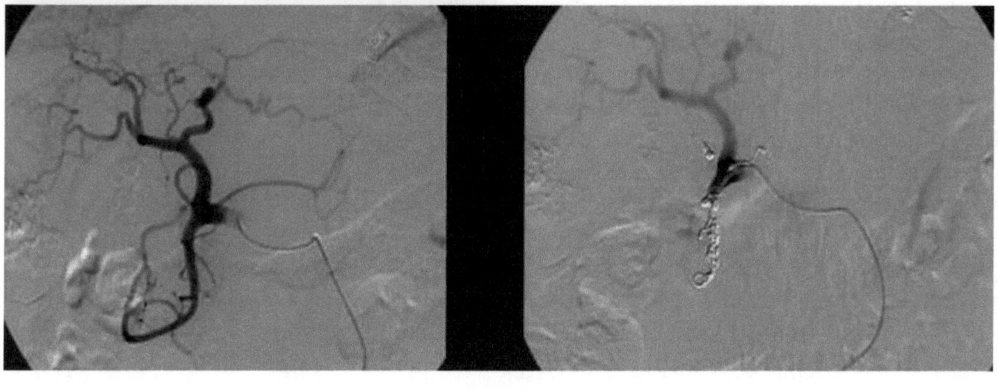

b

Fig. 11.5a,b A case with hepatic arterial infusion chemotherapy. **a** Volume-rendered CT arteriogram shows the entire hepatic trunk arising from superior mesenteric artery. The right gastric artery branching from the common hepatic artery is visible (*arrow*). **b** *Left*: Common hepatic digital subtraction angiogram (*DSA*). *Right*: After implantation of catheter for arterial infusion chemotherapy with embolic coil fixation (*arrow*). DSA shows the same anatomical information about the artery as the CT angiogram

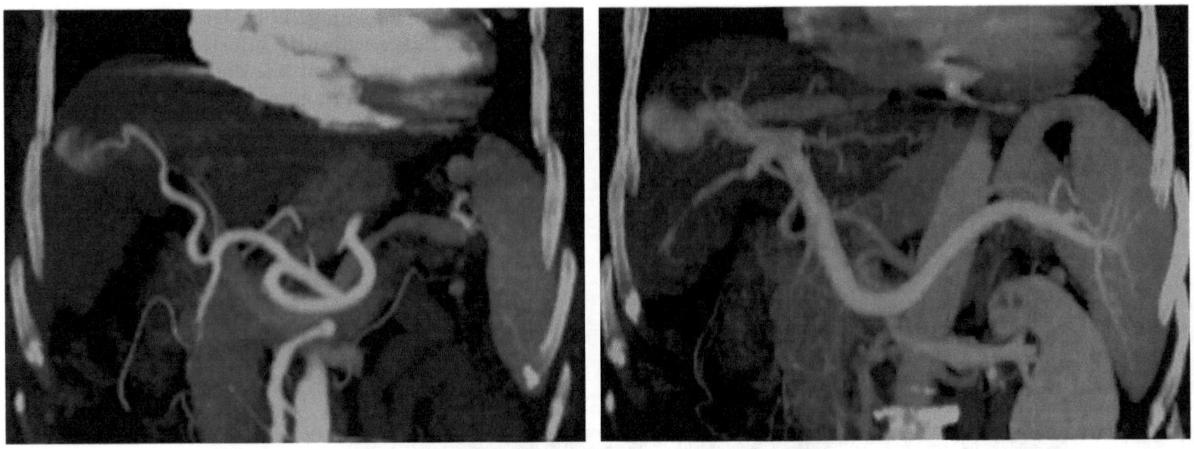

a b

Fig. 11.6a,b Arterioportal-venous fistula in a cirrhotic liver. **a** Target-MIP coronal CT arteriogram shows the hepatic artery filling nidus (*arrow*) and early portal venous enhancement (*arrowhead*). **b** Target-MIP coronal CT portogram shows early hepatic venous enhancement (*arrow*), indicating the presence of arterioportal-venous shunt.

tric varices, retroperitoneal and subcutaneous collateral vessels, and spontaneous splenorenal shunts are also recognized in some cases.

CT portography reconstructed from late arterial or CT portohepatic venography from the portal venous phase images can show the anatomical information of these varices very clearly (Figs. 11.6, 11.7). CT portohepatic venography can provide the anatomical relationship between hepatic and portal veins, which is very useful for procedures of transjugular intrahepatic portosystemic shunt (TIPS). The patency of shunt is also assessed by CT portohepatic venography noninvasively. In- and outflow vessels of gastric varices shown on CT portohepatic venograms is also helpful for interventional procedures of balloon occluded retrograde transvenous obliteration (BRTO) (Fig. 11.6).

11.6.4 Evaluation for Liver Transplantation

Dynamic MDCT with double arterial and portal venous phase imaging of the liver is a very important modality in the evaluation of both recipient and living donors of liver transplantation [12, 30, 31]. As mentioned previously, each phase CT image and CT angiogram reconstructed from these images can provide many kinds of information about the status of the liver parenchyma (i.e., fatty liver), volume of the liver, presence of intra- or extrahepatic disease (i.e., hepatocellular carcinoma or varices) (Figs. 11.2, 11.3, 11.4, 11.7), or anatomical variation (Figs. 11.2, 11.5) and patency of hepatic arterial, portal venous and hepatic venous systems (Fig. 11.8a). They can provide a comprehensive preoperative liver transplant evaluation, supplying the information necessary for both patient selection and surgical planning [12]. It was reported that this noninvasive imaging modality provides significant impact on surgical planning for hepatic transplantation, including celiac axis stenosis (Fig. 11.8a), diameter of inflow small arterial vessel, complete replacement of hepatic arterial supply (Fig. 11.8a), portal vein thrombosis, and splenic artery aneurysm [6]. In a case of liver transplantation with parent-to-child liver donation, the adult typically donates the lateral segment of the left lobe. CT angiography of the adult liver is performed to define the vascular map and to measure liver volumes. On the other hand, in a case of adult-to-adult living-donor transplantation, the right lobe of the donor's liver is usually used. In this case, anatomy of the portal venous system is most important. When a potential donor does not have common a portal trunk of anterior and posterior branches of the right portal vein, transplantation of the right lobe is contraindicated (Fig. 11.9a). Anatomy of the middle hepatic artery and branches of the middle segment and of the middle hepatic and inferior right hepatic vein that drain the right anterior segment are also important, because a decision has to be made whether to ligate or anastomose these vessels at the time of transplantation (Fig. 11.9b, c).

After the liver has been transplanted, CT angiography can also be useful for evaluation of potential transplant complications in either the transplant donor or recipient. The technique is

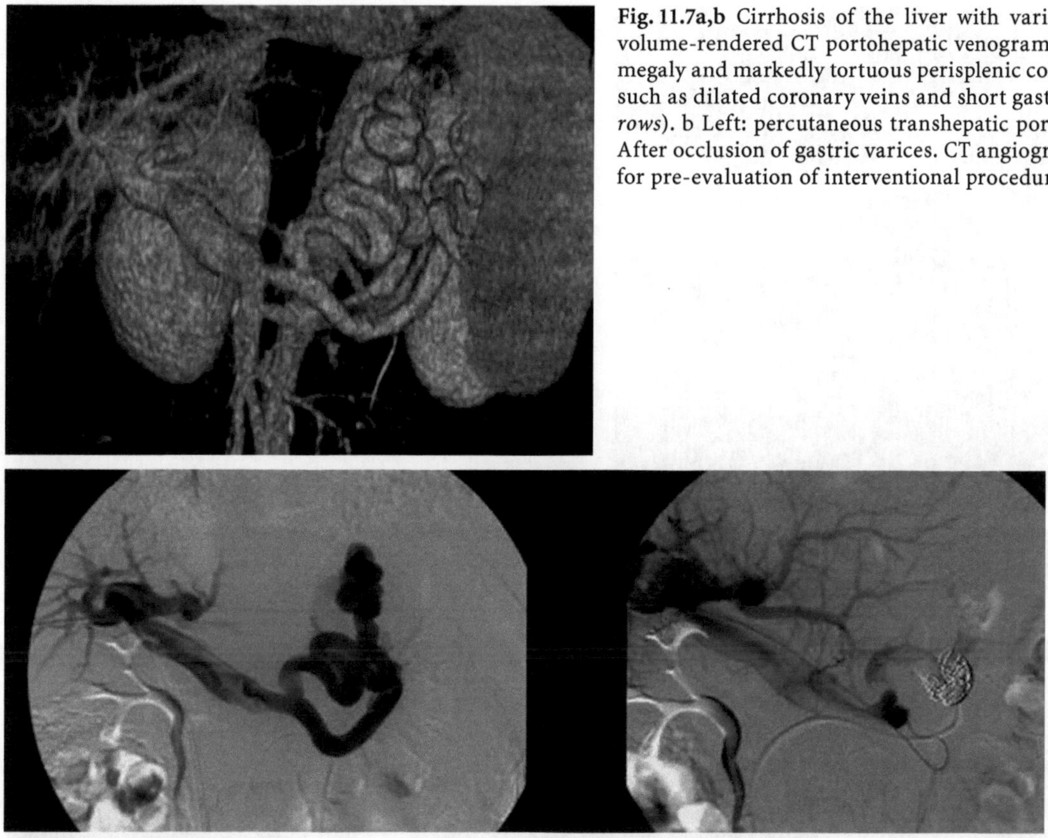

a

b

Fig. 11.7a,b Cirrhosis of the liver with varices. a Coronal volume-rendered CT portohepatic venogram shows splenomegaly and markedly tortuous perisplenic collateral vessels, such as dilated coronary veins and short gastric varices (*arrows*). b Left: percutaneous transhepatic portogram. Right: After occlusion of gastric varices. CT angiography is helpful for pre-evaluation of interventional procedures.

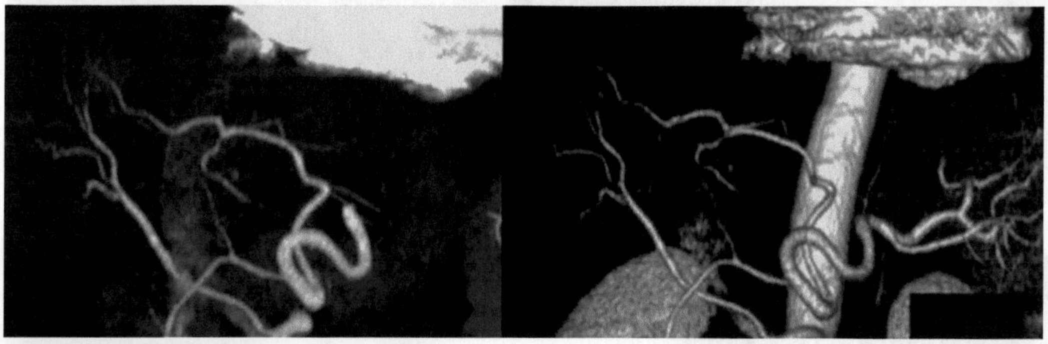

a

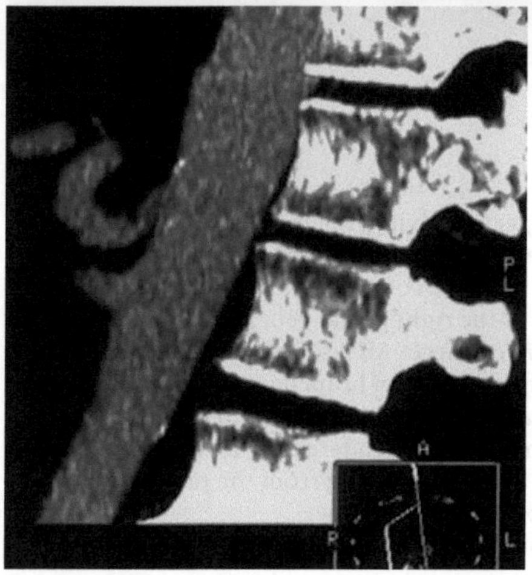

b

Fig. 11.8a,b A case with normal variation of hepatic artery. **a** *Left*: CT arteriogram with target MIP. *Right*: Volume-rendered image. The replaced right hepatic artery arising from the superior mesenteric artery and the replaced left hepatic artery arising from left gastric artery are clearly seen. **b** CT arteriogram with target MIP shows the celiac axis stenosis (*arrow*).

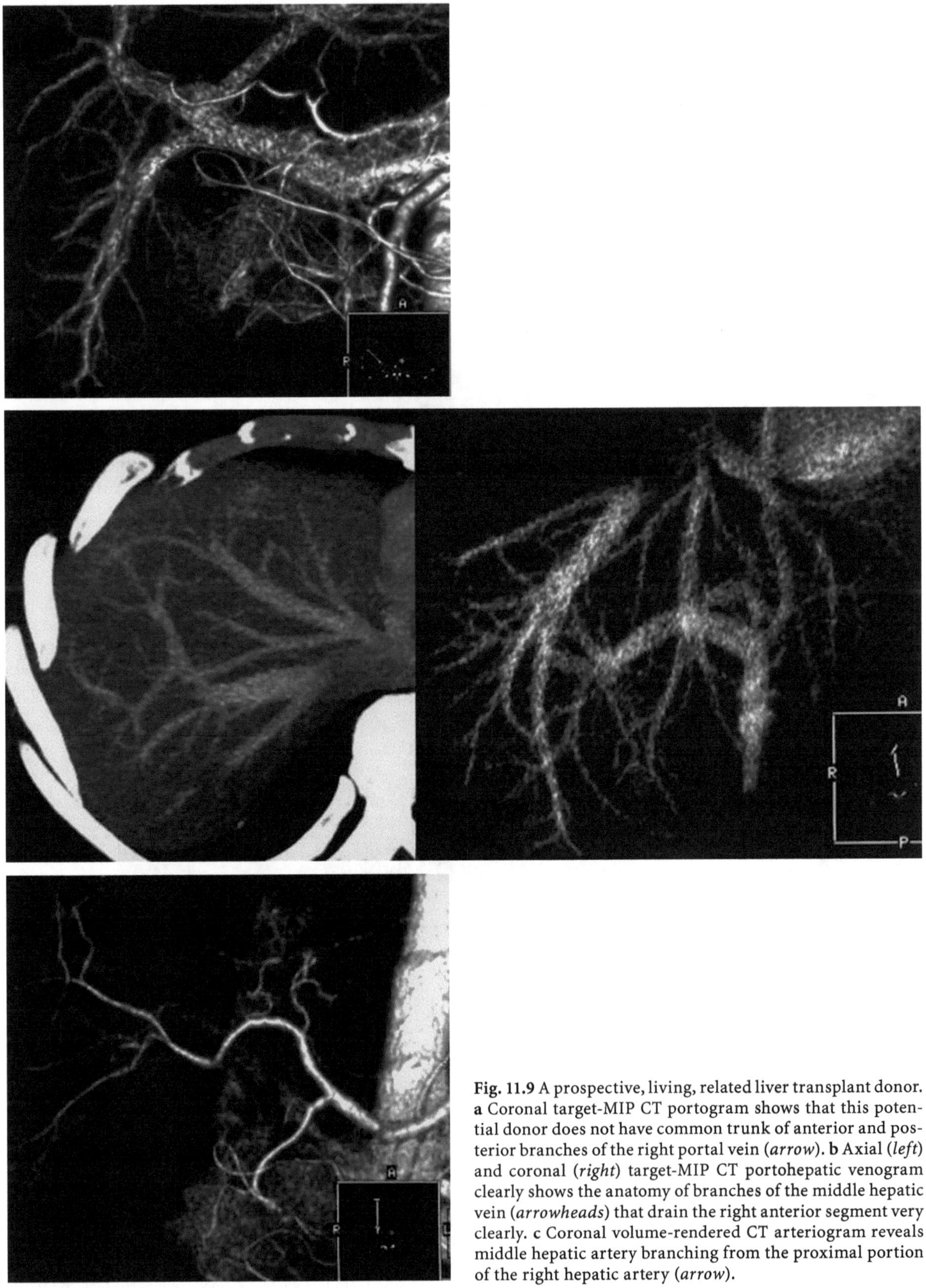

a

b

c

Fig. 11.9 A prospective, living, related liver transplant donor. **a** Coronal target-MIP CT portogram shows that this potential donor does not have common trunk of anterior and posterior branches of the right portal vein (*arrow*). **b** Axial (*left*) and coronal (*right*) target-MIP CT portohepatic venogram clearly shows the anatomy of branches of the middle hepatic vein (*arrowheads*) that drain the right anterior segment very clearly. **c** Coronal volume-rendered CT arteriogram reveals middle hepatic artery branching from the proximal portion of the right hepatic artery (*arrow*).

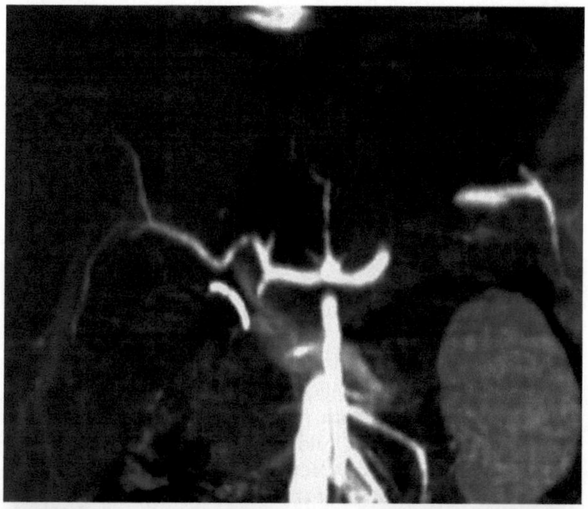
a

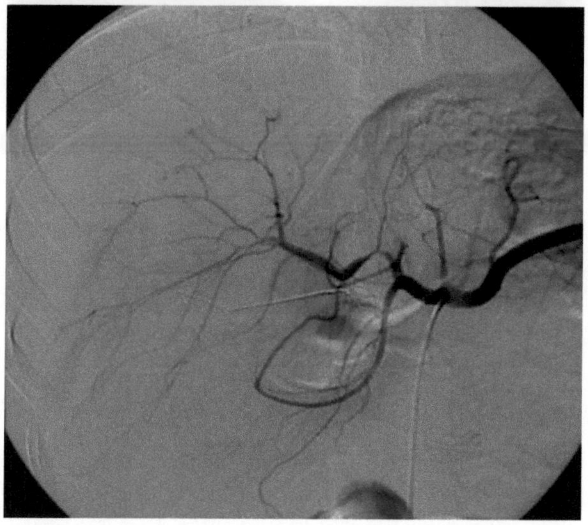
b

Fig. 11.10a,b Complication after transplantation. **a** CT arteriogram with target MIP shows hepatic arterial stenosis (*arrow*) at the point of anastomosis. **b** DSA confirms hepatic arterial stenosis at the same point (*arrow*).

used to successfully detect common and potentially lethal vascular complications, including hepatic artery stenosis, hepatic artery thrombosis, and portal vein stenosis [11] (Fig. 11.10).

11.7 Conclusion

Dynamic MDCT images of liver with the early and late arterial phases and the portal venous phase that are useful for detection of liver tumor, i.e., hepatocellular carcinoma, can also provide CT angiography of hepatic artery, portal vein, and hepatic vein. CT angiography is very beneficial for preoperative or preinterventional radiological assessment or follow-up evaluation of liver disease.

Acknowledgements: We sincerely thank Dr. Shuji Kawata, Mr. Masayuki Kudo, R.T., and Prof. Dr. Hironobu Nakamura for their important help in completing this article.

References

1. Oliver JH 3rd, Baron RL, Federle MP, Jones BC, Sheng R (1997) Hypervascular liver metastases: do unenhanced and hepatic arterial phase CT images effect tumor detection? Radiology 205:709–715
2. Oliver JH 3rd, Baron RL, Federle MP Jr, Rockette HE Jr (1996) Detecting hepatocellular carcinoma: value of unenhanced or arterial phase CT imaging or both used in conjunction with conventional portal venous phase contrast-enhanced CT imaging. Am J Roentogenol 167:71–77
3. Baron RL, Oliver JH 3rd, Dodd GD III, et al. (1996) Hepatocellular carcinoma: evaluation with biphasic contrast enhanced helical CT. Radiology 199:505–511
4. Raptopoulos V, Steer ML, Sheiman RG, et al. (1997) The use of helical CT and CT angiography to predict vascular involvement freom pancreatic cancer: Correlation wtih findings at surgery. Am J Roentgenol 168:971–977
5. Chong M, Freeny PC, Schmiedl UP (1998) Pancreatic arterial anatomy: depiction with dual-phase helical CT. Radiology 208:537–542
6. Nghiem HV, Dimas CT, McVicar JP et al. (1999) Impact of double helical CT and three-dimensional CT arteriography on surgical planning for hepatic transplantation. Abdom Imag 24:278–284
7. Winter TC 3rd, Freeny PC, Nghiem HV et al. (1995) Hepatic arterial anatomy in transplantation candidates: evaluation with three-dimensional CT arteriography. Radiology 195:363–370
8. Lim JH, Kim CK, Lee WJ et al. (2000) Detection of hepatocellular carcinomas and dysplastic nodules in cirrhotic livers: accuracy of helical CT in transplant patients. AJR Am J Roentgenol 175:693–698
9. Bluemke DA, Chambers TP (1995) Spiral CT angiography: an alternative to conventional angiography. Radiology 195:317–319
10. Raptopoulos V, Prassopoulos P, Chuttani R, et al. (1998) Multiplanar CT pancreatography and distal cholangiography with minimum intensity projections. Radiology 207:317–324
11. Katyal S, Oliver JH 3rd, Buck DG, Federle MP (2000) Detection of vascular complications after liver transplantation: early experience in multislice CT angiography with volume rendering. AJR Am J Roentgenol 175:1735–1739
12. Smith PA, Klein AS, Heath DG, Chavin K, Fishman EK (1998) Dual-phase spiral CT angiography with volu-

metric 3D rendering for preoperative liver transplant evaluation: preliminary observations. J Comput Assist Tomogr 22:868–874
13. Uchida M, Ishibashi M, Abe T, Nishimura H, Hayabuchi N (1999) Three-dimensional imaging of liver tumors using helical CT during intravenous injection of contrast medium. J Comput Assist Tomogr 23:435–440
14. Hu H, He HD, Foley WD, SH F (2000) Four multidetector-row helical CT: image quality and volume coverage speed. Radiology 215:55–62
15. Kim T, Murakami T, Takahashi S, et al. (1998) Effects of injection rates of contrast material on arterial phase hepatic CT imaging. AJR Am J Roentgenol 171:429–432
16. Bae KT, Heiken JP, Brink JA (1998) Aortic and hepatic peak enhancement at CT: effect of contrast medium injection rate-pharmacokinetic analysis and experimental porcine model. Radiology 206:455–464
17. Awai K, Takeda K, Onishi H, Hori S (2002) Aortic and hepatic enhancement and tumor-to-liver contrast: analysis of the effect of different concentrations of contrast material at multi-detector row helical CT. Radiology 224:757–763
18. Yamashita Y, Komohara Y, Takahashi M et al. (2000) Abdominal helical CT: evaluation of optimal doses of intravenous contrast material - a prospective randomized study. Radiology 216:718–723
19. Hollett MD, Jeffrey RB, Nino-Murcia M, Jorgensen MJ, Harris DP (1995) Dual-phase helical CT of the liver: value of arterial phase scans in the detection of small (≤1.5 cm) malignant hepatic neoplasms. AJR 164:879–884
20. Murakami T, Kim T, Takamura M, et al. (2001) Hypervascular hepatocellular carcinoma: detection with double arterial phase multidetector row helical CT. Radiology 218:763–767
21. Kim T, Murakami T, Hori M, et al. (2002) Small hypervascular hepatocellular carcinoma revealed by double arterial phase CT performed with single breath-hold scanning and automatic bolus tracking. AJR Am J Roentgenol 178:899–904
22. Rieker O, Duber C, Pitton M, Schweden F, Thelen M (1997) CT angiography versus intraarterial digital subtraction angiography for assessment of aortoiliac occlusive disease. AJR Am J Roentgenol 169:1133–1138
23. Drebin RA, Carpenter L, Hanrahan P (1988) Volume rendering. Comput Graph 22:65–74
24. Ney DR, Drebin RA, Fishman EK, Magid D (1990) Volumetric rendering of computed tomographic data: principles and techniques. IEEE Comput Graph Appl 10:24–32
25. Takahashi S, Murakami T, Takamura M, et al. (2002) Multidetector row helical CT angiography of hepatic vessels: depiction with dual-arterial phase acquisition during single breath hold. Radiology 222:81–88
26. Fishman EK, Magid D, Ney DR et al. (1991) Three-dimensional imaging: state of the art. Radiology 181:321–337
27. Heath DG, Soyer PA, Kuszyk BS et al. (1995) Three-dimensional spiral CT during arterial portography: comparison of 3D rendering techniques. Radiographics 15:1001–1011
28. Kawata S, Murakami T, Kim T, et al. (2002) Multidetector CT angiography of upper abdominal arteries using an eight-detector row CT scanner. Radiology 225:353
29. Ralls PW (1990) Color Doppler sonography of the hepatic artery and portal venous system. AJR Am J Roentgenol 155:522–526
30. Kamel IR, Raptopoulos V, Pomfret EA et al. (2000) Living adult right lobe liver transplantation: imaging before surgery with multidetector multiphase CT. AJR Am J Roentgenol 175:1141–1143
31. Kamel IR, Kruskal JB, Pomfret EA, et al. (2001) Impact of multidetector CT on donor selection and surgical planning before living adult right lobe liver transplantation. AJR Am J Roentgenol 176:193–200

12 Multislice CT Angiography of the Splanchnic Vessels

Andrea Laghi, Riccardo Iannaccone, Riccardo Ferrari, Daniele Marin, and Roberto Passariello

CONTENTS

12.1 Introduction

Computed tomographic angiography (CTA) is a powerful imaging technique for evaluation of the vascular system. It now has the potential to be a diagnostic alternative to conventional angiography, since it is a minimally invasive, safe, relatively comfortable, and low-cost examination. Further reduction of dose exposure can be obtained using dedicated low-dose acquisition protocols [15].

The development of multislice spiral CT (MSCT) technology is a significant advance in CTA [26, 27], particularly in the evaluation of splanchnic vessels [3, 4, 8, 20]. In fact, MSCT allows for acquisition times up to eight times faster than conventional single-slice spiral CT scanners; this feature enables larger anatomical coverage and diminishes misregistration as well as respiratory motion artifacts [23, 30]. Thin-slice collimation protocols can be routinely implemented with greatly enhanced spatial resolution along the longitudinal axis, which provides virtually isotropic 3D voxels; consequently, image quality is improved with better diagnostic capabilities [13, 14]. In addition, contrast-medium administration is optimized, with better vessel enhancement, due to more accurate timing and better separation between the arterial and venous phases.

However, in order to fully exploit the benefits derived from the use of multislice CT, it is of paramount importance not only to improve volumetric acquisition, but also image display. Three-dimensional data sets are reconstructed and interactively evaluated on dedicated workstations using axial and two-dimensional (2D) multiplanar images, as well as more complex rendering techniques such as maximum intensity projections (MIP), surface-shaded displays (SSD), and volume rendering [6, 16, 19].

12.2 Imaging Technique

The choice of an appropriate study technique to evaluate the splanchnic vasculature is mandatory in order to acquire three-dimensional (3D) data sets of high diagnostic quality. Scanning parameters and optimization of contrast-medium administration have to be considered [8, 21].

With regard to scanning parameters, slice collimation, effective slice thickness, pitch, and image reconstruction are the major determinants of a good examination [29]. Parameters need to be optimized on different scanners (in Table 12.1, general guidelines are provided); however, in general, the thinner the collimation and the lower the pitch, the better the slice-sensitivity profile and the higher the longitudinal spatial resolution and consequently the quality of reconstructed images. Image reconstruction is another important factor affecting the quality of 3D images. In principle, in order to obtain an optimal image quality, 20–40% slice overlap should be implemented. However, since the use of a 1-mm-slice collimation protocol produces a considerable number of images (300–400 images per scan per patient), it is sometimes more useful, to reduce the workload

A. Laghi, MD; R. Iannaccone, MD; R. Ferrari, MD;
D. Marin, MD; R. Passariello, MD, Professor
Department of Radiology, University of Rome "La Sapienza", Policlinico Umberto I, Viale Regina Elena n. 324, 00161 Rome, Italy

Table 12.1 Scanning parameters

Field of examination	From the diaphragm to the pelvis (35 –45 cm)
Acquisition	Arterial phase: craniocaudal Venous phase: caudocranial
Kilovoltage	120 kVp
Milliampere seconds	120-165 mAs (depending on tube heat capacity)
Collimation	4-slice scanner: 4 x 1 – 1.25 (HR); 4 x 2.5 (fast) 16-slice scanner: 16 x 0.625 - 0.75 (HR)/16 x 1.5 (fast)
Pitch	1.5 (to be adjusted according to different scanners)
Reconstruction interval	0.8-1.0 mm (4-slice scanners) 0.4-0.8 mm (16-slice scanners)
Acquisition time	30-35 s (4-slice scanners) 15-20 s (16-slice scanners)

Table 12.2 Contrast-medium injection

Injection volume	2 ml/kg of patient body weight
Flow rate	3.5- 5 ml/s
Acquisition delay	Arterial phase: based on bolus test Portal venous phase: around 60 s
Bolus test	Sequential dynamic slices at the level of the celiac trunk following injection of 20 ml of contrast medium

on the workstation, to limit the image reconstruction interval to 1 mm, with no image overlap.

Administration of contrast medium needs to be optimized with regard to timing, volume, and flow rate [29] (see Table 12.2). Due to the fact that each patient has a different circulatory time, there is a substantial risk of scanning the patient too early (with an insufficient amount of contrast material in the vessels) or too late (with opacification of venous vessels during the arterial phase) when a fixed delay time is used (usually 25 or 30 s as start time for the arterial phase). Therefore, we usually utilize the test-bolus technique in which a minibolus (20 ml) of contrast material is injected and a series of single-level CT scans at low dose are acquired every 2 s at the level of the hepatic hilum. The time of maximal opacification of the abdominal aorta is used as the start time for the arterial phase (usually between 18 and 24 s). After the acquisition of the arterial phase, a portal venous phase is also acquired with a 60- to 70-s delay time from the start of contrast-material infusion [1].

Another variable that impacts on contrast-material administration is patient's body weight. Indeed, if a fixed amount of contrast material is used, some patients will receive an insufficient dose of contrast material (with inadequate opacification of the vessels), whereas others will receive an excessive dose of contrast material (which can be spared to reduce the cost of the CT examination). Therefore, to minimize the influence of differences in patient body weight, we usually administer 2 ml of contrast material/kg of patient body weight (e.g., 140 ml for a patient of 70 kg).

A further variable that has to be considered for contrast-material administration is the flow rate. Although excellent vascular studies can be obtained with a contrast-material infusion of 3 ml/s, there is now evidence from the literature that the conspicuity for the analysis of the vascular structures is increased when using higher flow rates, up to 9.6 ml/s [17]. However, in our everyday clinical practice, we try to use a flow rate of 5 ml/s according to patient clinical conditions and availability of an adequate venous access.

Before the study, patients receive 500-800 ml of water as an oral contrast agent in order to produce negative contrast in the stomach and small bowel. The use of a positive oral contrast agent, although very common in the past, is a source of potential difficulties when 3D images need to be reconstructed; indeed, the high density of small-bowel lumen, similar to contrast-enhanced vessels, limits the use of automatic thresholding as well as the possibility of viewing "through the bowel" with volume rendering.

12.3 Image Analysis

Once acquired, images are downloaded to an offline dedicated workstation in order to generate 3D reconstructions. 3D data sets can be examined using different reconstruction techniques, starting with multiplanar reformations along three orthogonal axes and on oblique planes. 3D reconstructions can be obtained by using either maximum-intensity projection (MIP) (Fig. 12.1), or surface-rendering or volume-rendering algorithms [2, 6, 7] (see Table 12.3).

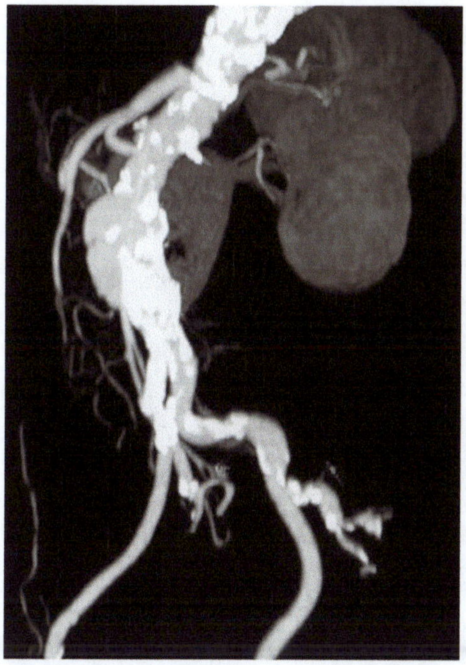

Fig. 12.1 Maximum-intensity projection (MIP). Oblique view of an abdominal aortic aneurysm with diffuse parietal calcifications. MIP algorithm provides optimal evaluation of size and morphology of the aneurysm, but poor assessment of three-dimensional spatial relationships.

Volume rendering is the preferred reconstruction algorithm for better anatomical representation and evaluation of spatial relationships, as well as for faster and easier interaction with 3D data sets, although the diagnosis comes from a combined evaluation of source and reconstructed images.

With volume rendering, selective vessel representation is obtained using different rendering curves (Fig. 12.2a,b) [2]. A panoramic overview of the entire main abdominal branches can be ob-

Table 12.3 Imaging reconstruction technique

Multiplanar reformation	Initial analysis of the data set (usually coronal and sagittal planes). Curvilinear planes: hepatic & splenic arteries
Maximum intensity projection (MIP)	Panoramic evaluation of the entire vascular district (better if bone is removed)
Shaded surface display (SSD)	Usually not necessary
Perspective volume-rendering (pVR)	Surface representations of major vessels; Interactive multiplanar cut planes useful for smaller vessels

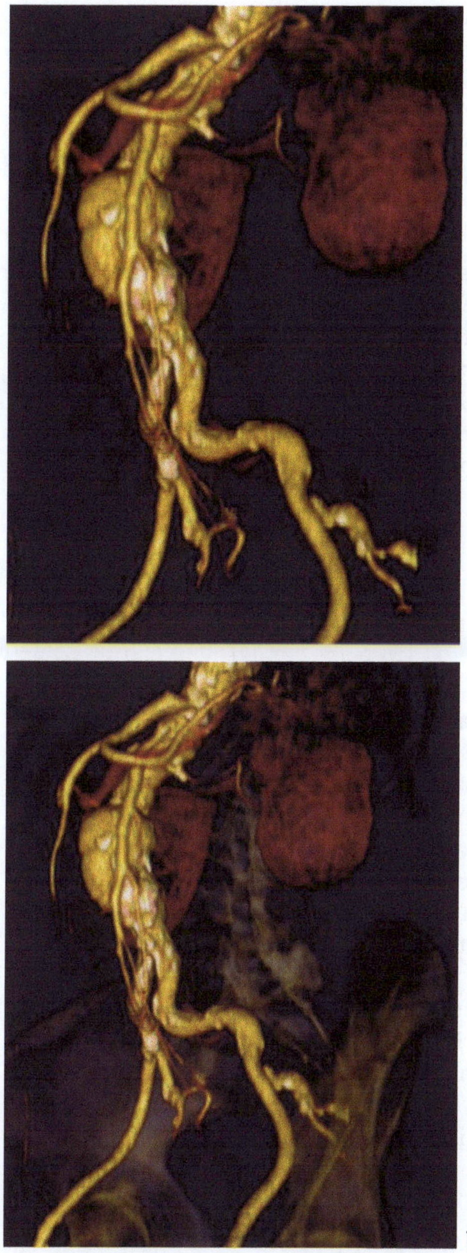

a

b

Fig. 12.2a,b Volume-rendering algorithm. **a** A well-defined 3D image is generated by volume-rendering algorithm thanks to the use of virtual light source. The presence of light and shadows provides an optimal evaluation of spatial relationships among vessels. **b** Modulation of the opacity of different anatomical structures allows to see "through" organs. In the present case, bones are rendered as semi-transparent in order to provide anatomical bony references for the vascular surgeon.

tained using a preset opacity curve showing only the vascular surface. The evaluation of minor vessels (i.e., second, third, and more distal orders of collateral branches) requires the analysis of 3D data sets by using interactive multiplanar cut planes ("oblique trim") and by modulating the opacity of the anatomical structures under evaluation and window/level parameters in order to see vessels "through" abdominal organs. Image analysis requires direct operator interpretation at the workstation, where 2D axial and multiplanar reconstructions and 3D images are simultaneously available. A complete analysis of arterial and venous vessels is obtained within a mean interpretation time of 20 min.

12.4 Normal Anatomy

12.4.1 Arterial Vascular System

The superior mesenteric artery (SMA) usually arises from the abdominal aorta, at the level of L1, less than 1.5 cm below the origin of the celiac trunk. The SMA supplies blood to the duodenum (via the pancreaticoduodenal arcade), jejunum, ileum, right colon, and, usually, transverse colon (Fig. 12.3) [12, 18, 22]. The SMA mostly originates on the left side of the superior mesenteric vein (SMV) as it crosses over the third portion of the duodenum. As it enters the mesentery, the SMA is usually posterior to the SMV. This anatomical relationship has important implications, since the right colic artery and the ileocolic artery cross the SMV as a consequence. However, a recent study [31]et al.] was able to demonstrate that in several cases (67%) the ileocolic artery and the right colic artery may pass on either side of the SMV. The surgeon must dissect the arteries with the SMV, being aware of both possibilities (Fig. 12.4).

Major collateral branches are: the inferior pancreaticoduodenal artery, which has an oblique course, anastomosing superiorly with the superior pancreaticoduodenal artery, a branch of the gastroduodenal artery; the right and middle colic arteries, with the latter absent in up to 80% of normal individuals, supplying blood to the right colon; the jejunal branches, arising from the left side of the SMA above the level of the middle colic artery; and the ileal branches, arising from the left side of the SMA below the level of the middle colic artery and the terminal ileocolic artery, supplying blood to the distal ileum and cecum.

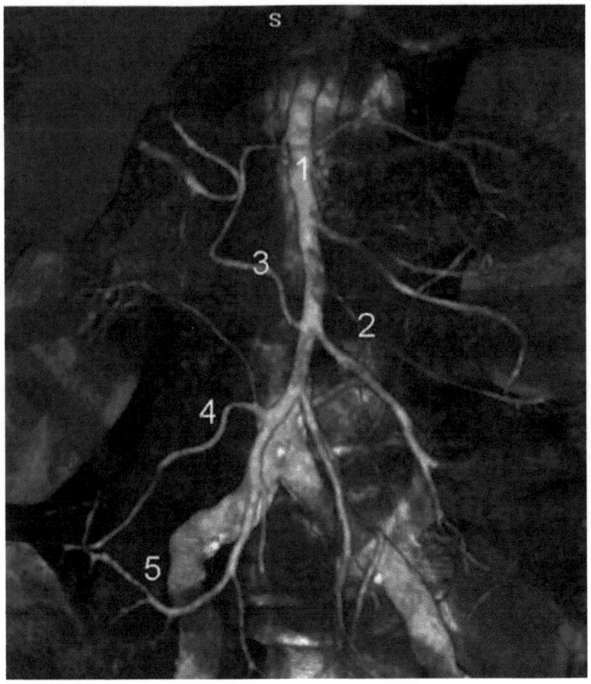

Fig. 12.3 Normal anatomy of the superior mesenteric artery. *1*, SMA; *2*, jejunal branches; *3*, middle colic artery; *4*, right colic artery; *5*, ileocolic artery

Aberrant arteries arising from the SMA are a relatively common finding and include hepatic artery, right hepatic artery, cystic artery, celiac trunk, splenic artery, gastroduodenal artery, right gastroepiploic artery, and left gastric artery [10] (Fig. 12.5).

The inferior mesenteric artery (IMA) arises from the aorta about 7 cm below the origin of the SMA. The IMA divides into the left colic artery, which has a straight superior course, supplying the transverse and descending colon; the sigmoid arteries, two to four vessels supplying the sigmoid colon; and the superior hemorrhoidal artery, a terminal branch that supplies the upper rectum (Fig. 12.6).

The high spatial resolution of multislice CTA allows detailed evaluation of small distal vessels, including the anastomotic arcades along the mesenteric and mesocolic sides of small and large bowel as well as the vasa recta (Fig. 12.7).

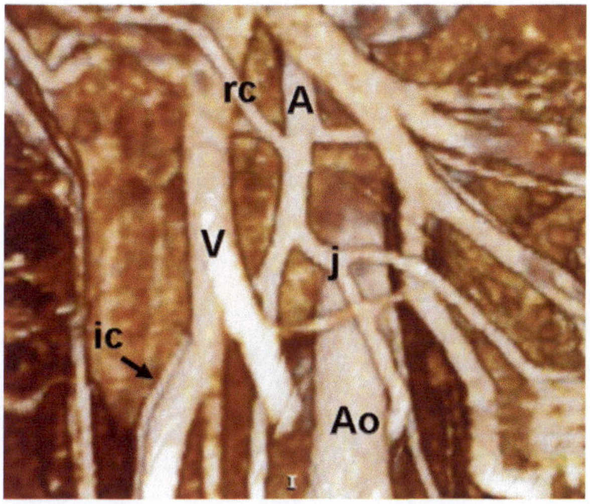

Fig. 12.4 Anatomical relationship between superior mesenteric artery (SMA) and superior mesenteric vein (SMV). The SMA (*A*) is posterior to the SMV (*V*) and the right colic artery (*rc*) crosses the SMV anteriorly. The ileocolic artery (*ic*) passes posterior to the SMV. *Ao*, aorta; *J*, jejunal branches

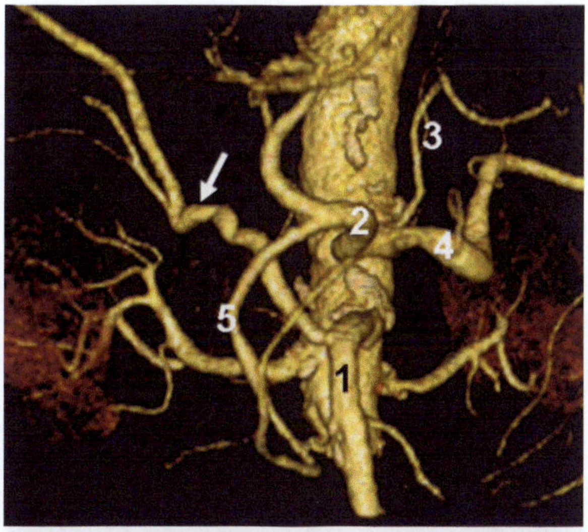

b

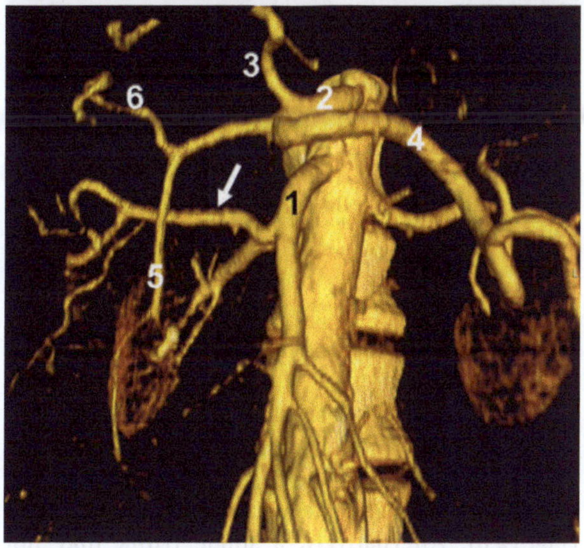

b

Fig. 12.5a,b Anatomical variants represented by anomalous origin (**a**) of the hepatic artery (*arrows*) from superior mesenteric artery and (**b**) right hepatic artery (*arrow*) from superior mesenteric artery. Superior mesenteric artery (*1*), celiac trunk (*2*), left gastric artery (*3*), splenic artery (*4*), and gastroduodenal artery (*5*), left hepatic artery (*6*)

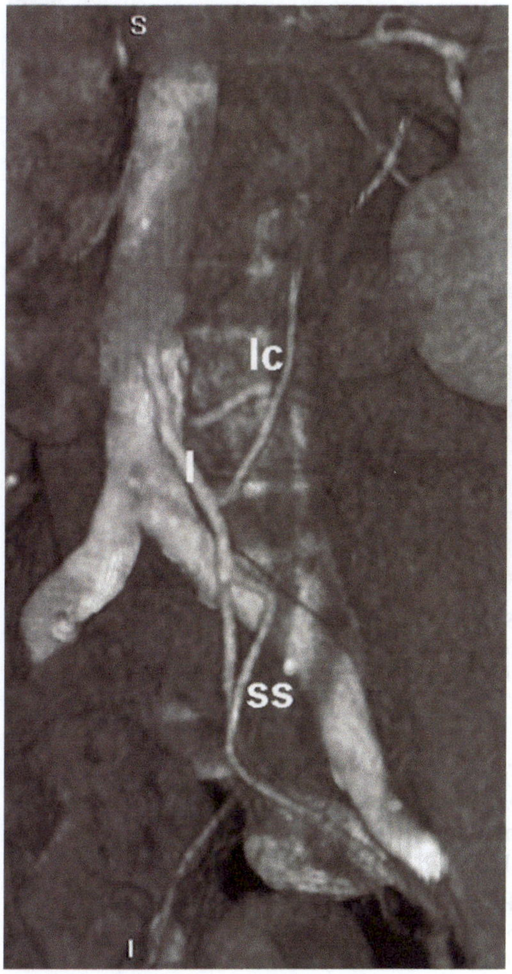

Fig. 12.6 Normal anatomy of the inferior mesenteric artery (*I*) with collaterals: left colic artery (*lc*), which has a straight superior course, supplying the transverse and descending colon, and sigmoid arteries (*SS*), supplying the sigmoid colon.

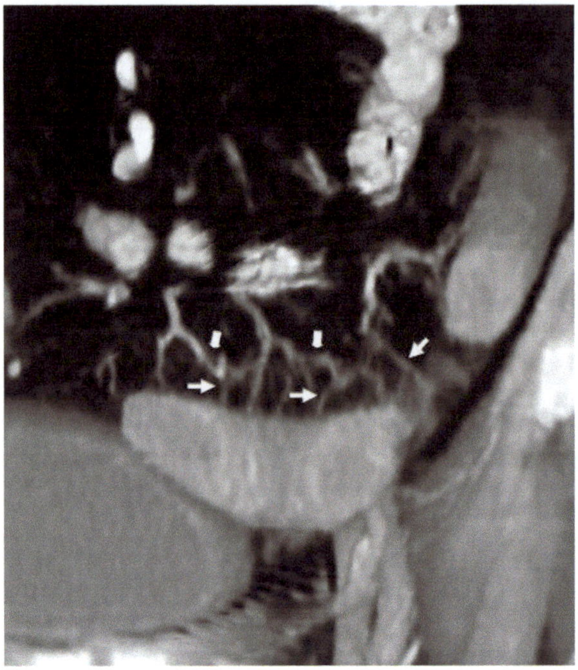

Fig. 12.7 Arterial vascular arcade (*arrowheads*) of the sigmoid colon with vasa recta (*small arrows*) feeding the bowel wall.

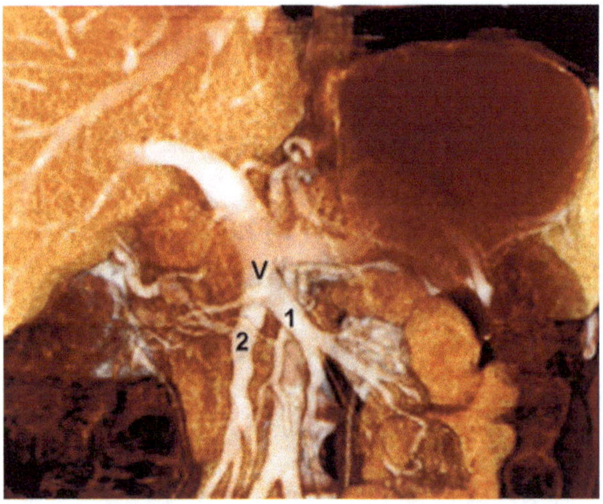

Fig. 12.8 The superior mesenteric vein (*V*) is usually formed by two branches receiving blood from the middle (*1*) and right (*2*) colic veins.

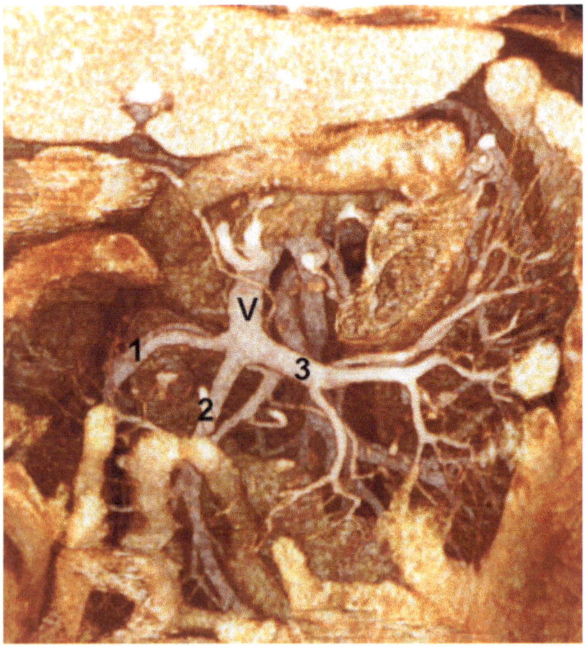

Fig. 12.9 Anatomical variant of the superior mesenteric vein (*V*), which originates from three separate branches. *1*, right colic vein; *2*, ileocolic vein; *3*, jejunal veins

12.4.2 Venous Vascular System

The SMV is usually a single trunk, formed by two branches (right and left), receiving blood from the middle and right colic veins, the ileocolic vein, the gastrocolic vein, and the jejunal and ileal branches (Fig. 12.8). Alternatively, a single trunk may not be present, and the two right and left mesenteric branches may join the splenic vein to form the portal vein [5, 25] (Fig. 12.9). The SMV lies to the right of the SMA as it crosses over the third portion of the duodenum. When the SMA and SMV enter the mesentery, the SMV usually lies anterior to the SMA.

The inferior mesenteric vein (IMV) receives blood from the left colic vein, the sigmoid veins, and the superior hemorrhoidal vein and it may drain into the splenic vein, at the splenoportal angle, or into the SMV (Fig. 12.10).

12.5 Pathological Conditions

There are several clinical applications for MSCT angiography of the mesenteric vessels [4]. In particular, this technique has been demonstrated to be valuable in cases of pancreatic cancer, mesenteric ischemia, and inflammatory bowel disease.

With regard to pancreatic cancer, MSCT angiography plays an important role in the evaluation of the vessels adjacent to the tumor [10, 11, 24]. Infiltration of SMA is a known contraindication to pancreatic

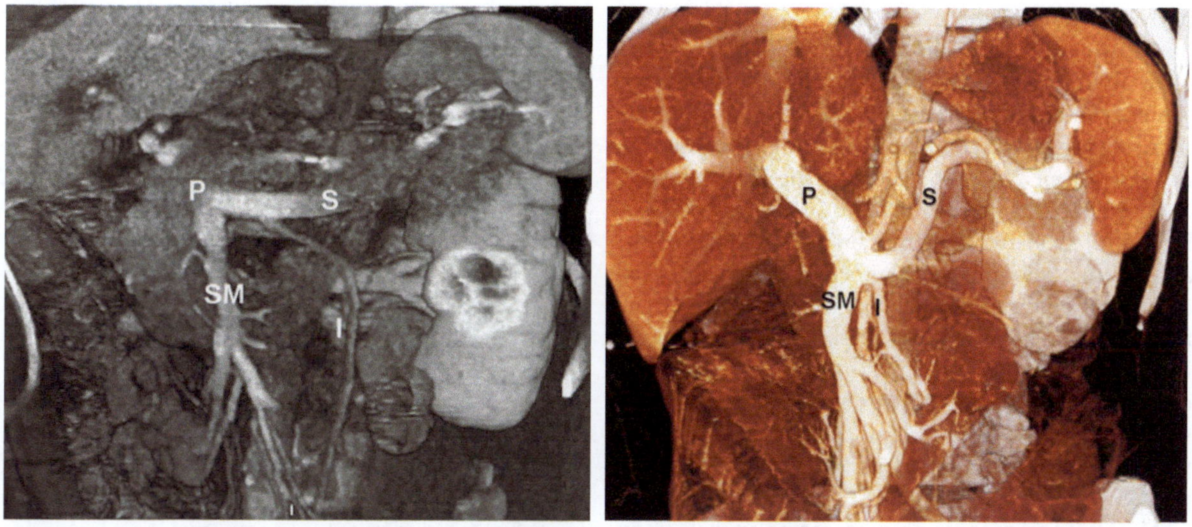

a b

Fig. 12.10a,b Inferior mesenteric vein (*I*) draining into the splenic vein (**a**) and the splenoportal angle (**b**). *P*, portal vein; *S*, splenic vein; *SM*, superior mesenteric vein

surgery. It has been demonstrated that simultaneous evaluation of axial and multiplanar reformatted planes is useful for assessing vascular invasion, and in particular sagittal planes provide excellent evaluation of the posterior fat plane between the SMA and the abdominal aorta, especially useful to rule out vascular encasement. A more precise evaluation of the SMV and the portal vein is also extremely important, since a vessel infiltration of less than 2 cm is considered a criterion for performing pancreatic surgery together with a vascular graft. Again multiplanar reformatted images, in this case along the coronal or coronal oblique planes, provide excellent evaluation of possible vascular infiltration (Fig. 12.11).

Small-bowel ischemia is another important application of MSCT angiography of mesenteric vessels [9]. This disorder occurs when blood flow (arterial or venous) is reduced to the intestines. Mesenteric ischemia can be classified as acute or chronic, and it is usually related to SMA-narrowing or occlusion due to atherosclerotic plaque, thrombosis, or tumoral encasement; other common causes include SMV thrombosis or tumoral encasement; or hypo-

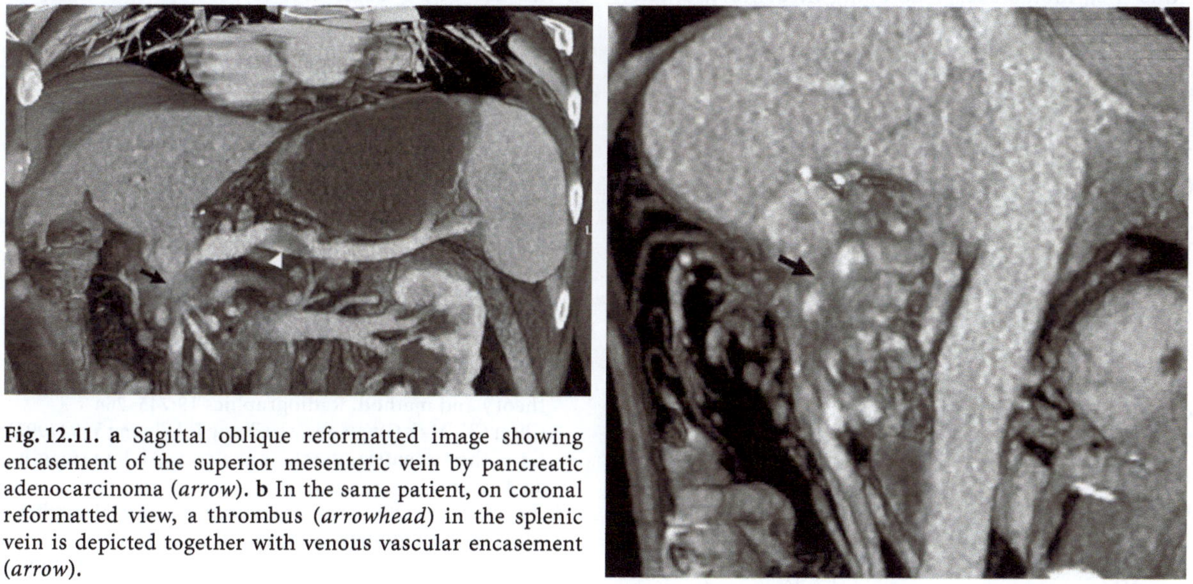

a b

Fig. 12.11. a Sagittal oblique reformatted image showing encasement of the superior mesenteric vein by pancreatic adenocarcinoma (*arrow*). **b** In the same patient, on coronal reformatted view, a thrombus (*arrowhead*) in the splenic vein is depicted together with venous vascular encasement (*arrow*).

perfusion due to atherosclerosis or low cardiac output [6, 18]. At present, conventional angiography has been almost completely replaced by MSCT angiography as imaging modality of choice for the diagnosis of mesenteric ischemia. MSCT angiography can not only often depict the cause of the ischemia, but can also detect ischemic changes in the small-bowel loops and mesentery (such as bowel wall thickening and edema, submucosal hemorrhage, increased or decreased enhancement of the bowel wall, mesenteric stranding or fluid, and pneumatosis). Axial CT images can easily depict narrowing or thrombosis of a major vessel (e.g., SMA or SMV), and 3D reconstructions provide excellent display of collateral vessels, thus providing a road map for the surgical procedure (Fig. 12).

MSCT angiography of mesenteric vessels may also play a role in the assessment of inflammatory disease of the small bowel [12]. Patients with inflammatory bowel disease have changes in mesenteric blood flow that can be detected at MSCT. In particular, patients with Crohn's disease with active bowel inflammation have increased blood flow, whereas patients with quiescent disease have no increased blood flow. Such hemodynamic changes can be identified at MSCT with excellent detail. Specifically, thickening and contrast enhancement of diseased small-bowel loops and engorgement of the vessels feeding the diseased loops can be well demonstrated.

Finally, MSCT angiography might provide diagnostic images in the assessment of vascular changes in the case of small-bowel tumors (i.e., carcinoid, lymphoma) and less frequent pathological conditions (i.e., metastases, sclerosing mesenteritis, etc.) [4].

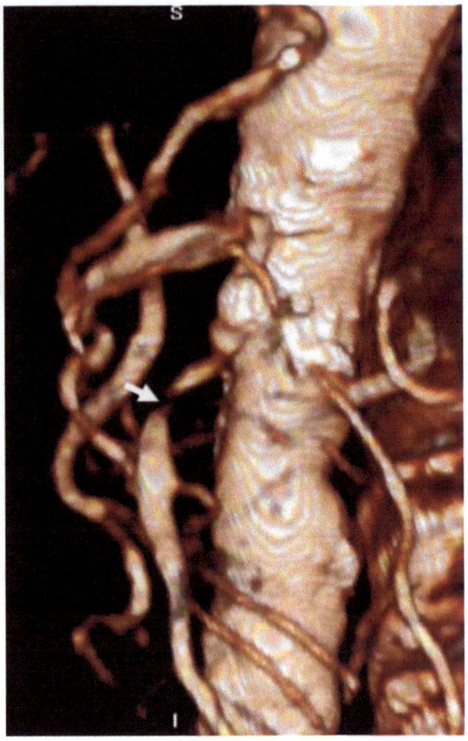

Fig. 12.12 Atherosclerotic stricture of superior mesenteric artery (*arrow*) causing chronic mesenteric ischemia, as shown in this oblique view of volume-rendered CT angiogram of the abdominal vessels.

12.6 Conclusions

With its greatly enhanced image resolution, MSCT angiography seems able to overcome the technical challenge of depicting small mesenteric vessels, providing a detailed anatomical view similar to that of conventional angiography but with the possibility of examination from innumerable viewing angles. Technical requirements include interactive evaluation on a workstation using dedicated reconstruction algorithms, whereas volume-rendering, due to its ability to display the 3D spatial relationships among vessels and surrounding organs, represents the most suitable technique. Widespread applications for these techniques can be expected in the near future, with the greater availability of MSCT equipment, improvement in workstation design and performance, and specific education of radiologists in the use of 3D software. A cost-benefit analysis needs to be performed in order to better understand the impact of this new imaging modality on patient outcomes.

References

1. Bae KT (2003) Peak contrast enhancement in CT and MR angiography: when does it occur and why? Pharmacokinetic study in a porcine model. Radiology 227:809–816
2. Calhoun PS, Kuszyk BS, Heath DG, Carley JC, Fishman EK (1999) 3D volume-rendering of spiral CT data: theory and method. Radiographics 19:745–764
3. Chou CK, Mak CW, Hou CC, Chang JM, Tzeng WS (1997) CT of the mesenteric vascular anatomy. Abdom Imaging 22:477–482
4. Fishman EK (2001) CT angiography: clinical applications in the abdomen. Radiographics 21:3–16
5. Graf O, Boland GW, Kaufman JA, et al. (1997) Anatomic

variants of mesenteric veins: depiction with helical CT venography. Am J Roentgenol 168:1209–1213
6. Heath DG, Soyer PA, Kuszyk BS et al. (1995) 3D spiral CT during arterial portography: comparison of 3D rendering techniques. Radiographics 15:1001–1011
7. Hong KC, Freeny PC (1999) Pancreaticoduodenal arcades and dorsal pancreatic artery: comparison of CT angiography with three-dimensional volume rendering, maximum intensity projection, and shaded-surface display. AJR Am J Roentgenol 172:925–931
8. Horton KM, Fishman EK (2000) 3D CT angiography of the celiac and superior mesenteric arteries with multidetector CT data sets: preliminary observations. Abdom Imaging 25:523–525
9. Horton KM, Fishman EK (2001) Multi-detector row CT of mesenteric ischemia: can it be done? Radiographics 21:1463–1473
10. Horton KM, Fishman EK (2002a) Multidetector CT angiography of pancreatic carcinoma. I. Evaluation of arterial involvement. AJR Am J Roentgenol 178:827–831
11. Horton KM, Fishman EK (2002b) Multidetector CT angiography of pancreatic carcinoma. 2. Evaluation of venous involvement. AJR Am J Roentgenol 178:833–836
12. Horton KM, Fishman EK (2002c) Volume-rendered 3D CT of the mesenteric vasculature: normal anatomy, anatomic variants and pathologic conditions. Radiographics 22:161–172
13. Hu H (1999) Multi slice helical CT: scan and reconstruction. Med Phys 26:5–18
14. Hu H, He HD, Foley WD, Fox SH (2000) Four multidetector-row helical CT: image quality and volume coverage speed. Radiology 215:55–62
15. Jakobs TF, Becker CR, Ohnesorge B et al. (2002) Multislice helical CT of the heart with retrospective ECG gating: reduction of radiation exposure by ECG-controlled tube current modulation. Eur Radiol 12:1081–1086
16. Johnson PT, Heath DG, Kuszyk BS, Fishman EK (1996) CT angiography with volume rendering: advantages and applications in splanchnic vascular imaging. Radiology 200:564–568
17. Kimura M, Shioyama Y, Okumura T, et al. (2003) Very-high-flow injection rate for upper abdominal CT angiography. J Gastroenterol 37 [Suppl 13]:106–111
18. Kornblith PL, Boley SJ, Whitehouse BS (1992) Anatomy of the splanchnic circulation. Surg Clin North Am 72:1–30
19. Kuszyk BS, Heath DG, Ney DR et al. (1995) CT angiography with volume rendering: imaging findings. Am J Roentgenol 165:445–448
20. Laghi A, Iannaccone R, Catalano C, Passariello R (2001) Multislice spiral computed tomography angiography of mesenteric arteries. Lancet 358:638–639
21. Laghi A, Catalano C, Iannaccone R et al. (2001) Multislice spiral CT angiography in the evaluation of the anatomy of splanchnic vessels: preliminary experience. Radiol Med 102:127–131
22. Lin PH, Chaikof EL (2000) Embryology, anatomy and surgical exposure of the great abdominal vessels. Surg Clin North Am 80:417–433
23. McCollough CH, Zink FE (1999) Performance evaluation of a multi-slice CT system. Med Phys 26:2223–2230
24. Raptopoulos V, Steer ML, Sheiman RG, Vrachliotas CA, Movson JS (1997) The use of helical CT and CT angiography to predict vascular involvement from pancreatic cancer: correlation with findings at surgery. Am J Roentgenol 168:971–977
25. Rosenblum JD, Boyle CM, Schwartz LB (1997) The mesenteric circulation: anatomy and physiology. Surg Clin North Am 77:289–306
26. Rubin GD, Shiau MA, Schmidt AJ et al. (1999) Computed tomographic angiography: historical perspective and new state-of-the-art using multi detector-row helical computed tomography. J Comput Assist Tomogr 23: S83–S90
27. Rubin GD, Shiau MC, Kee ST, Logan LJ, Sofilos MC (2000) Aorta and iliac arteries: single versus multiple detector-row helical CT angiography. Radiology 215:670–676
28. Rubin GD (2000) Data explosion: the challenge of multi detector-row CT. Eur J Radiol 36:74–80
29. Rubin GD (2001) Techniques for performing multidetector-row computed tomographic angiography. Tech Vasc Interv Radiol 4:2–14
30. Rydberg J, Buckwalter KA, Caldemeyer KS et al. (2000) Multisection CT: scanning techniques and clinical applications. Radiographics 20:1787–1806
31. Shatary T, Fujita M, Nozawa K, et al. (2003) Vascular anatomy for right colon lymphadenectomy. Surg Radiol Anat 25:86–88

13 Multidetector-Row CT of Renal Arteries

Francesco Fraioli, Carlo Catalano, Linda Bertoletti, and Piergiorgio Nardis

CONTENTS

13.1 Introduction

Multidetector-row spiral CT (MDCT) represents an important clinical tool that is replacing, in many institutions, catheter-based angiography in the evaluation of renal vasculature [1]. For this purpose, MDCT provides a fast, accurate, and noninvasive imaging modality with diverse clinical indications, such as establishing a normal anatomy in transplant donors, delineating the anatomy before partial nephrectomy, screening for stenosis in patients with hypertension, and assessing the status of the renal arteries in aortic disease.

Familiarity with proper MDCT protocols are crucial for an accurate diagnosis. We will review the clinical and technical aspects of renal MDCT angiography (MDCTA) in terms of image acquisition and the reconstruction parameters, contrast-medium application, three-dimensional (3D) visualization, and major clinical disorders.

Multiple vascular diseases affect the renal vasculature and, among these diseases, renal artery stenosis, which is the most common cause of renal hypertension, represents one of the most important pathologies, and its detection is essential, because it is potentially treatable [2, 3], either surgically or by stenting. Therefore, the evaluation of the number and course of renal arteries and the presence and number of accessory arteries appears particularly useful in different situations, such as in the preoperative evaluation of patients with renal tumors, in whom nephron-sparing surgery can be performed [4], in patient candidates for renal transplantation, in donors, and in the follow-up of recipients [5].

Digital subtraction angiography (DSA) has been considered the gold standard for the identification of renal arteries; nevertheless, this procedure may carry some complications which should also be considered for patients with secondary hypertension. A noninvasive screening imaging technique is therefore desirable.

Angiotensin-converting enzyme (ACE) inhibitor scintigraphy, Doppler ultrasonography (US), magnetic resonance angiography (MRA), and CT are used to achieve adequate screening in most patients as a noninvasive modality for renal vasculature disease. Unfortunately, at least before the introduction of MDCT, all these techniques presented some limitations, such as renal scintigraphy, which, although it has been reported to be sensitive to detect renal hypertension, it accounts for some problems in the setting of bilateral renal artery stenosis and renal failure [6].

Doppler ultrasound is an important tool for the evaluation of renal artery stenosis, but it is very often limited by the habitus of the patient and operator dependency; therefore, this limits the possibility to evaluate the presence, number and stenosis of both main and accessory renal arteries [7].

F. Fraioli, MD; L. Bertoletti, MD; P. Nardis, MD
Department of Radiological Sciences, University of Rome "La Sapienza", Policlinico Umberto I, Viale Regina Elena n. 324, 00161 Rome, Italy
C. Catalano, MD
Associate Professor, Department of Radiological Sciences, University of Rome "La Sapienza", Policlinico Umberto I, Viale Regina Elena n. 324, 00161 Rome, Italy

Magnetic resonance angiography turned out to be a valid technique also, because it has shown excellent results in the evaluation of different renal vascular pathologies. Because of the high cost of the examination and the limited spatial resolution that impairs the visualization of segmental branches, its use is restricted to high field-strength magnets and to high-resolution protocols, which are not available everywhere.

The introduction of single-slice spiral CT angiography allowed the assessment of renal arterial disorders; the acquisition of volumetric scans with thin collimations in short times has enabled examination of the entire pathway of the main renal arteries. However, the trade-off between scan volume and spatial resolution along the *z*-axis did not allow, in many cases, visualization of the origin of both main and accessory renal arteries; furthermore, the long acquisition time is often the cause of the opacification of the renal vein with superimposition of arteries. The limited spatial resolution impairs the quality of 3D reconstructions, which have become routine in the clinical evaluation of vascular diseases for radiologists and clinicians.

The recent introduction of MDCT into clinical practice, with the simultaneous acquisition of multiple channels, has had a substantial effect on CT angiography, since it provides the acquisition of large volumes at high resolution with excellent visualization of small branches, including distal collaterals of the main renal and accessory renal arteries. One of the most important promises of multiple-row detector technology is that of a true isotropic spatial resolution. This capability is reasonably achieved with multiple sections of 1-mm thickness or less. Ideally, the true 3D radiograph would have cubic voxels of less than 1 mm acquired over large volumes with very short times, at least within a reasonable breath-hold [8]. For MDCT an exact acquisition protocol must be explained because of the importance, clinically and therapeutically, of depicting both main and accessory arteries.

13.2 Scanning Protocol

Patients are positioned supine with their head first. After a 512-mm initial topogram, the acquisition volume is placed in such a way to comprise all arterial structures from the thoracoabdominal aorta down to the aortic bifurcation.

The *z*-axis (longitudinal) resolution is critical for an adequate visualization of renovascular abnormalities and for further image postprocessing, due to the size and course of the renal arteries. The parameter selection is weighted in order to have an optimal spatial resolution. Acquisition parameters for various types of MDCT scanners are shown in Table 13.1.

13.3 Contrast-Agent Administration

The recent improvement of CT scanners have substantially modified contrast-media administration parameters, such as the delay time, flow rate, volume, and concentration of the contrast-medium injected. Because of high blood flow and short cir-

Table 13.1

MDCT system rotation scanning time (s)	Scanning time (s)	Collimation (mm)	Slice thickness	Reconstruction interval	Feed rotation	Number of slices
4-channel MDCT *0.8 s*	27 s	4×1 4×2.5[a]	1.25 3	0.8	9.3	312
0.5 s	21 s	4×1 4×2.5[a]	1.25 3	0.7	12	357
8-channel 0.5 s	7.5	8×1.25	1.25	0.8	33.5	312
16-channel 0.5 s	7	16×0.75	1	0.5	36	500

[a] A thicker collimation (but always with thinner reconstruction) may be utilized with 4-channel MDCT, both in patients with severe atherosclerotic disease, for whom it gives information on the aorta and its branches and on run off vessels, and in patients with severe respiratory disease, unable to hold their breath for a sufficient time

culation time in the kidneys, the choice of the correct delay time is particularly important to avoid venous superimposition and provide optimal and homogeneous opacification of the arteries. Ideally, scanning occurs during maximal arterial enhancement, before the veins or renal parenchyma pick up the contrast agent.

It is remarkable that, with 4-channel scanners, the injection duration is usually equal to the acquisition time. With faster scanners, such as 8- and 16-channel MDCT, it becomes even more critical to synchronize the arterial enhancement with CT data acquisition, because the time window is substantially shorter. In MDCT systems with acquisition times shorter than 20 s, it is highly recommended to individualize the scan delay. This can either be done with a test bolus injection, to determine the contrast-medium transit time, or with an automated bolus-triggering technique which detects the arrival of the contrast material in the artery of interest and automatically initiates the MDCTA series.

The test-bolus technique consists of an injection of 16 ml of contrast material followed by several serial transverse scans with 1-s interscan delay, in the region that corresponds to the starting point of the acquisition. Usually, to reduce the dose adsorbed by patients, we perform a series of scans with 8-s delays and we stop the acquisition after four or five images after the complete filling of the vessel. By doing this, we usually notice, in the first or second scan, a complete absence of contrast material inside the aorta and consequently a filling and increase in the concentration inside the vessel. A region of interest (ROI) inside the vessel of interest should be used to determine the exact density value before starting the acquisition.

This technique is utilized with a multiple-row CT scanner and provides optimal results in terms of scan delay and adequate filling of renal arteries; nevertheless one of the possible limitations is due to the urographic filling of the caliceal structure just as the start delay is calculated. In our experience this filling does not prevent the visualization of both main and peripheral renal branches but, because of the high contrast density of caliceal and ureteral structures, the 3D visualization could be impaired.

Many CT scanners have an automated detection system for the maximum contrast density built into the software; a ROI is positioned into the target vessel on a nonenhanced image. Consequently, a predefined enhancement threshold value is established. While injecting the contrast medium, a series of low-dose scans are performed and, when the predefined threshold value is reached, the sequence starts automatically after a trigger rate depending on the scanning model.

13.3.1 Bolus Injection

In order to obtain a good renal arterial enhancement, correct intravenous administration of the iodinated contrast agent is crucial. An 18-gauge intravenous cannula must be positioned, generally, in an antecubital vein to allow the injection. Because we believe that an optimal CT angiogram is acquired with the administration of an intravenous contrast-medium bolus for a duration equivalent to the scanning, a shorter scanning time obtained with MDCT allows the use of less contrast medium.

To reach this objective, many different physiological and pharmacological principles have been analyzed to obtain higher and longer concentrations of contrast media during the entire acquisition. One common practical approach to a rational contrast-medium administration is to adopt injection regimens included in the acquisition time.

In our experience, to image the entire renal vasculature, the dose of contrast medium can vary from 80 to 110 ml. A means to reduce the contrast volume, routinely used in our institution, is to flush the contrast agent administered with saline solution. This pushes up the contrast-medium column from the vein to the circulation, prolonging and compacting the column.

13.4 3D Reconstruction and Image Evaluation

It is important that patients do not receive any positive oral contrast agent before the renal MDCTA, because this could severely compromise the 3D image processing. If necessary, negative oral contrast agents such as tap water can be used before imaging.

For the purpose of optimal 3D reconstruction imaging, thin-collimation acquisition and reconstruction parameters (1 mm) allow excellent visualization of the arterial anatomy and pathological involvement. The large volume of data acquired by using such protocols requires evaluation on a dedicated workstation through 3D interaction between axial and 3D reconstruction techniques that simulate conventional angiograms. 3D techniques include maximum-intensity projection (MIP), thin MIP, multiplanar reformation (MPR), and volume rendering.

MIP represents one of the most common reconstruction algorithms commonly employed in examinations. In the MIP technique, each voxel is evaluated from the viewer's eye through the data set, but only maximal voxel values are selected and displayed. The image produced lacks in-depth orientation, but a 3D effect can be produced with rotational viewing of multiple projections. MIP images are very useful to provide information regarding atherosclerotic plaques with the possibility of evaluating the presence of calcifications; on the other hand, sometimes calcium can obscure the visualization of the lumen in relation to the strong hyperdensity.

Since it eliminates the need for preliminary editing, a cumbersome step that in the past hampered the clinical utility of the other 3D reconstruction algorithms, volume rendering is an extremely user-friendly technique. The user actively interacts with the image, editing and modifying the position, orientation, opacity, and brightness of structures.

Our experiences with 3D evaluation proved that images should be evaluated on axial images and only after this reconstructed with different 3D algorithms to better delineate the entire pathway of vessels. Multiplanar (MPR) and curved multiplanar (cMPR) reconstruction are extremely important, because they allow the evaluation of the entire course of vessels along a unique plane and therefore enable performance of a multiplanar view of the entire structure of the abdomen, either vascular or parenchymal.

13.5 Clinical Applications

13.5.1 Normal Anatomy and Variants

Renal arteries in most individuals arise from the abdominal aorta, at the level of L1-L2. Both renal arteries usually course posterior, in relation to the posterior position of the kidneys. More than 30% of the population have accessory arteries, 15% of which are bilateral [9].

MDCT has been proved to be an accurate modality for the depiction of both main and accessory renal arteries, even for arteries of small caliber (less than 2 mm), especially when thin collimations are used; particularly, thin-slice collimations allow determination of the entire course of renal arteries both at the level of the origin (with, for instance, the possibility to differentiate an early bifurcation of the renal artery or the presence of two separate origins from the abdominal aorta) or at the level of the intraparenchymal branches.

Examples of some normal main renal arteries, variants, and accessory vessels are shown in Figs. 13.1; 13.2, 13.3.

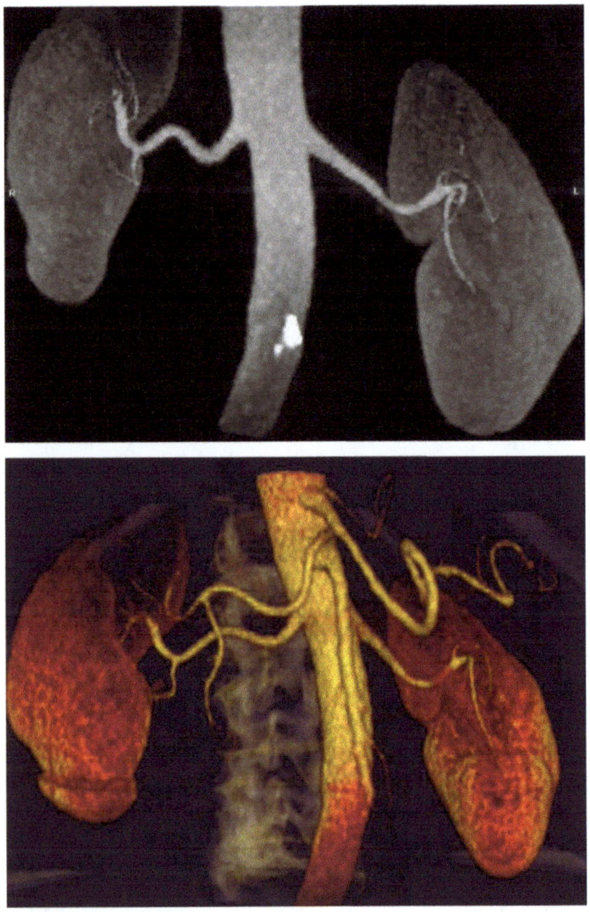

a

b

Fig. 13.1a,b Normal multidetector-row CT angiogram of a 50-year-old man with suspected renovascular hypertension. Acquisition parameters were 4×1-mm detector configuration, 1.25-mm section thickness, 1-mm reconstruction interval. Example of normal main renal artery with maximum-intensity projection (**a**) and volume-rendered (**b**) reconstruction.

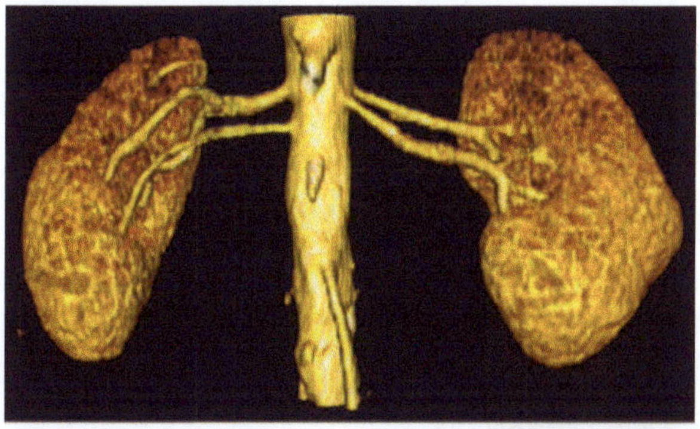

Fig. 13.2 Bilateral accessory arteries with a perfect depiction of the origin and distal intraparenchymal branches.

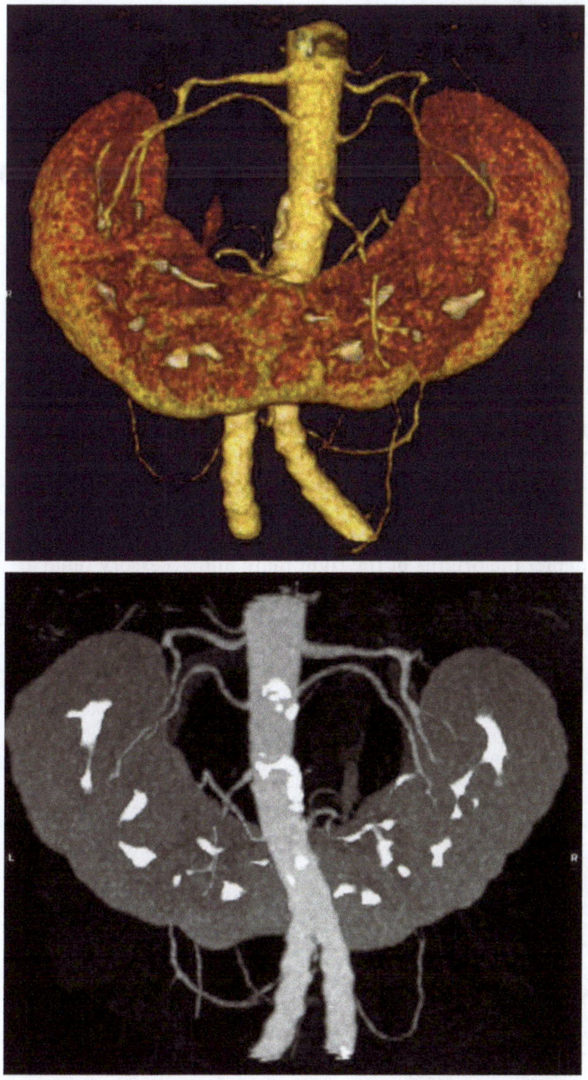

a

b

Fig. 13.3a,b Horseshoe kidney in a 59-year-old male. Three-dimensional coronal reconstruction with volume rendering (**a**) and maximum-intensity projection (**b**) shows the horseshoe kidney with multiple renal arteries.

13.5.2 Renal Artery Stenosis

Although renal hypertension affects less than 5% of the general population, its detection appears particularly useful, since it is potentially treatable, either surgically or with stenting [10]. Catheter-based angiography has been considered, for many years, the gold standard in the evaluation of renal arterial stenosis. Nevertheless, because an important clinical tool not only determines patients with hemodynamically significant stenosis, but performs screening in patients suspected with a renal vascular hypertension, catheter-based angiography cannot be considered as the primary technique for screening because of its invasiveness; for this reason a noninvasive imaging modality is desirable.

The grade of stenosis represents an important parameter that should be considered in the assessment of renal hypertension; in fact, stenoses greater in diameter than 50% are hemodynamically significant and usually treatable (surgically or by stenting), whereas stenoses less than 50% can be treated with antihypertensive drugs.

As reported by previous studies, slices thinner than 2 mm are necessary for an optimal detection and grading of renal artery stenosis [11]. Therefore, particularly in the evaluation of renal arteries, the use of 3D reconstructions, possible only with thinner slices, is helpful to visualize the entire course of the vessels. One-millimeter slice can be routinely performed with MDCT with perfect isotropy of the voxels and a conspicuous increase in the diagnostic performance of 3D reconstructions.

A recent meta-analysis has shown that CTA and MRA are the most accurate, noninvasive techniques for the depiction of renal artery stenosis [12]. Although MRA has the advantages of using a nonionizing radiation and nonnephrotoxic contrast agents, its main limitation is related to lower spatial resolution compared with MDCTA. In fact MRA, in many cases, does not allow the visualization of intraparenchymal branches and especially the visualization of accessory arteries where stenosis (even if in a limited number of cases) can also be responsible of clinical renal hypertension.

Another important advantage of MDCTA over MRA is related to the shorter examination time, especially when multiple sequences are acquired with an MRA examination, with consequently a better acceptance from patients.

Examples of MDCT angiography scans of renal artery plaques and stenosis are shown in Figs. 13.4, 13.5, 13.6.

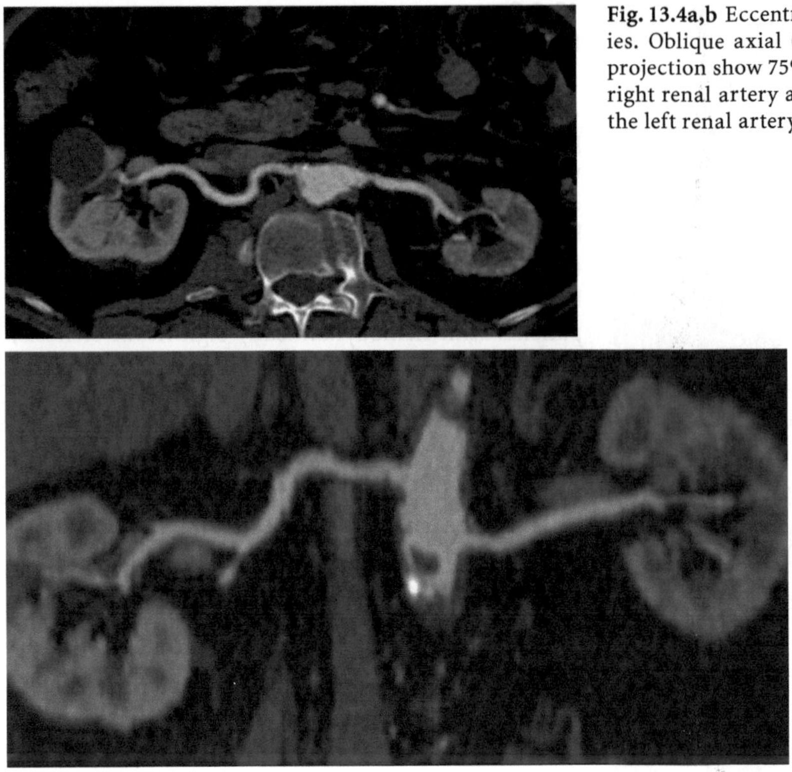

a

b

Fig. 13.4a,b Eccentric stenosis of right and left renal arteries. Oblique axial (**a**) and coronal (**b**) maximum-intensity projection show 75% stenosis of the proximal portion of the right renal artery and 50% stenosis of the proximal part of the left renal artery.

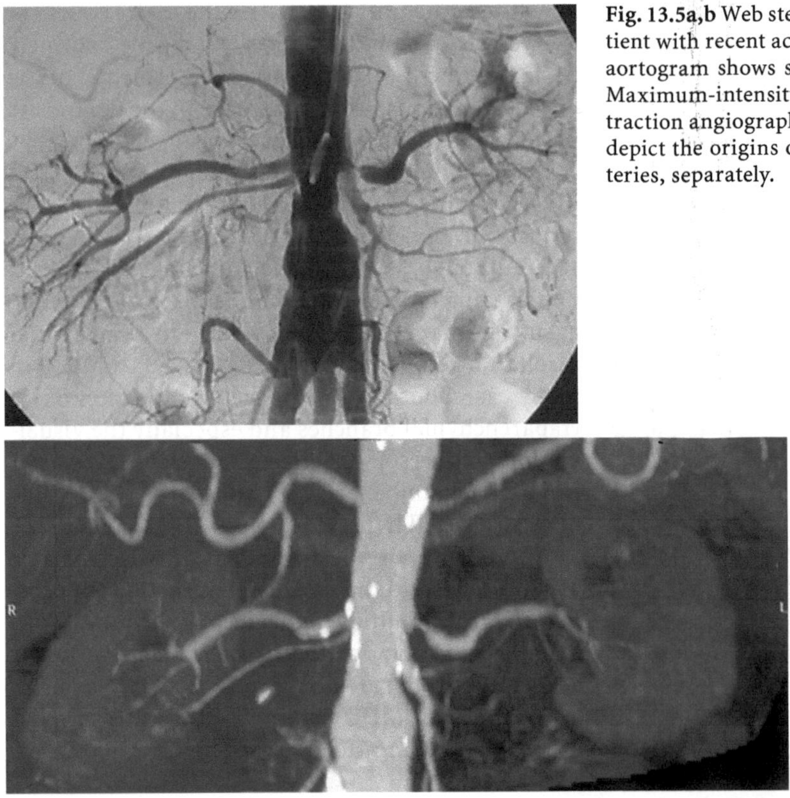

a

b

Fig. 13.5a,b Web stenosis of the main left renal artery in a patient with recent acceleration of hypertension. **a** Abdominal aortogram shows severe stenosis of the left renal artery. **b** Maximum-intensity projection confirms the digital subtraction angiography findings. Both examinations correctly depict the origins of the right main and accessory renal arteries, separately.

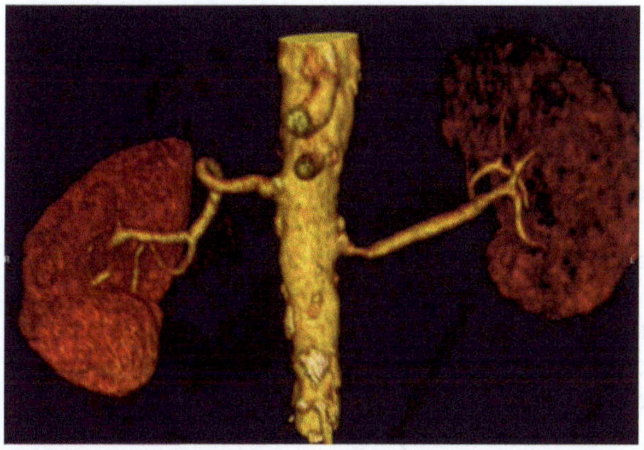

Fig. 13.6 Volume-rendering technique shows a severe stenosis of the left and right renal arteries in 74 patients with renal hypertension.

13.5.3 Fibromuscular Dysplasia

Fibromuscular dysplasia is the second most common cause of renal artery stenosis and accounts for a significant number of patients with renovascular hypertension, the majority of whom are young or middle-aged women. The disease is bilateral in two-thirds of patients [13]. Lesions typically develop in the mid or distal main renal artery, in contrast to the more proximal involvement of atherosclerotic disease.

MDCT angiography, because of its high spatial resolution, represents a reliable, noninvasive screening examination for the detection of fibromuscular dysplasia (Fig. 13.7). The CT findings include arterial stenosis, a string-of-pearls appearance, and focal aneurysms. Aneurysms associated with medial fibrosis are usually fusiform.

Especially in the assessment of mid or distal stenosis of the main renal arteries, MDCT appears more sensitive than other modalities such as MRA, which is impaired by a lower spatial resolution. Selective arteriography with pressure-gradient measurement remains necessary to assess the physiological significance of medial fibroplasias and for the interventional procedure.

13.5.4 Atherosclerotic Disease

CTA has been considered more accurate than DSA in the evaluation of aortic atherosclerosis, and for both dilatative or stenosing diseases; it can evaluate, for instance, mural thrombus in abdominal aneu-

a 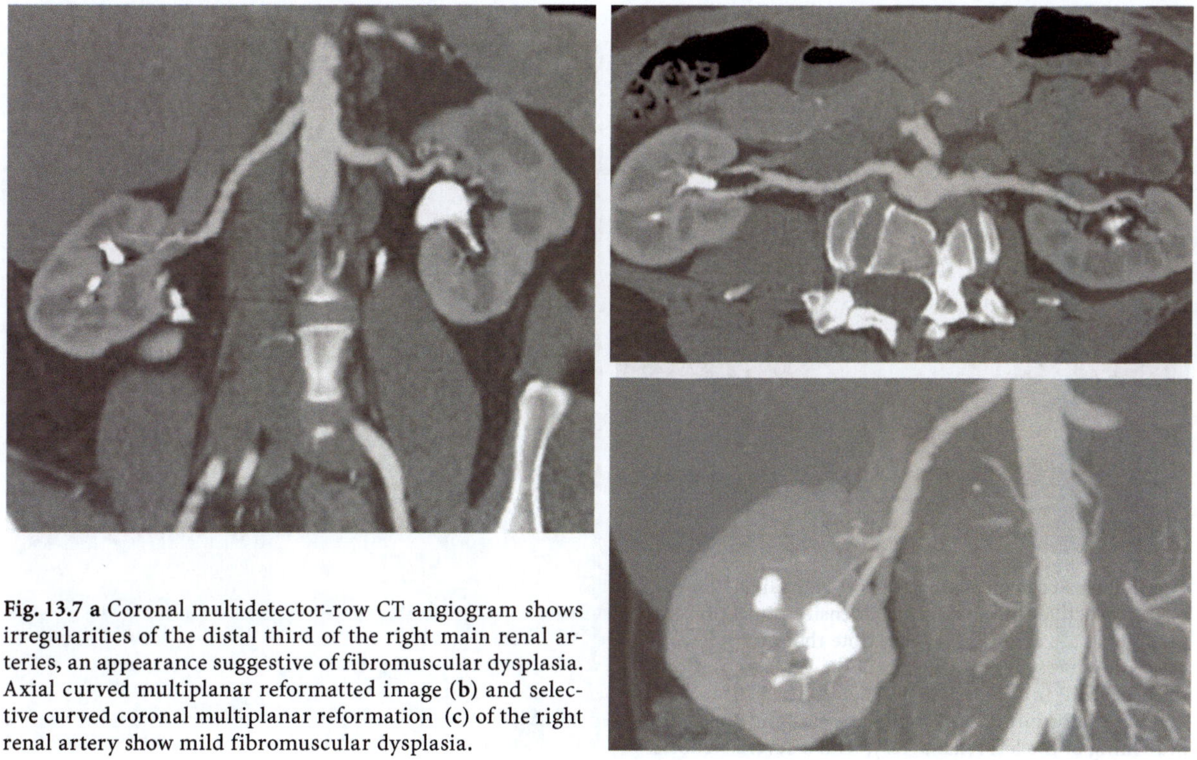 b c

Fig. 13.7 a Coronal multidetector-row CT angiogram shows irregularities of the distal third of the right main renal arteries, an appearance suggestive of fibromuscular dysplasia. Axial curved multiplanar reformatted image (**b**) and selective curved coronal multiplanar reformation (**c**) of the right renal artery show mild fibromuscular dysplasia.

rysms more accurately than DSA. In a variable percentage of patients, renal arteries can be involved in the aneurismal disease of the aorta. In such a situation one of the main problems is related to demonstrating the origin of renal arteries and the presence of supernumerary vessels, because the relation of renal arteries with the aneurysms is critical to optimize a surgical or an endovascular approach. MDCT enables an accurate depiction of the aneurysm neck relative to aortic branch vessels, as well as the relationship between the proximal aspect of the aneurysm and renal artery branches.

Examples of MDCT angiography scans of aortic stenosis involving renal arteries plaques are shown in Fig. 13.8. The aspect that should be stressed is related to the utilization of multiple different reconstruction algorithms; in particular, in our experience, a rapid scrolling of axial images is always performed for an initial view and to measure the maximum diameter of the aneurysm.

In addition, the volume-rendering technique enables the visualization of the relationship between the aortic aneurysm and renal arteries with a spatial and a 3D view. MIP enables demonstration of the presence of ostial calcification but does not allow the evaluation of thrombus; MPR and cMPR reconstruction appear, in our experience, to be the best reconstruction algorithm able to visualize the aortic aneurysm and its relationship with renal arteries, including the presence of calcifications and mural thrombus. The ability of MDCTA to identify renal artery stenosis in the presence of abdominal aortic aneurysms has been recently assessed by Willmann et al. through multidetector-row spiral CT with 3D rendering; the sensitivity and specificity for stenosis greater than 50% were very high for all readers [14].

One of the main problems that usually occurs in the presence of abdominal aortic aneurisms, and often in all arteriosclerotic patients, is the partial obscuration of lumen by calcium; in fact, very often, patients with aneurysms or arteriosclerotic diseases have heavy parietal aortic calcifications responsible for stenosis at the ostium of renal arteries. In our experience, to minimize this effect, a bone window setting is used, both on axial and MIP images.

13.5.5 Renal Artery Aneurysms

Aneurysms of the renal arteries are detected approximately in the 4th and 5th decades of life and represent often isolated cases discovered during examinations performed for other reasons. The most common causes of renal artery aneurysms are represented by atherosclerosis, followed by polyarteri-

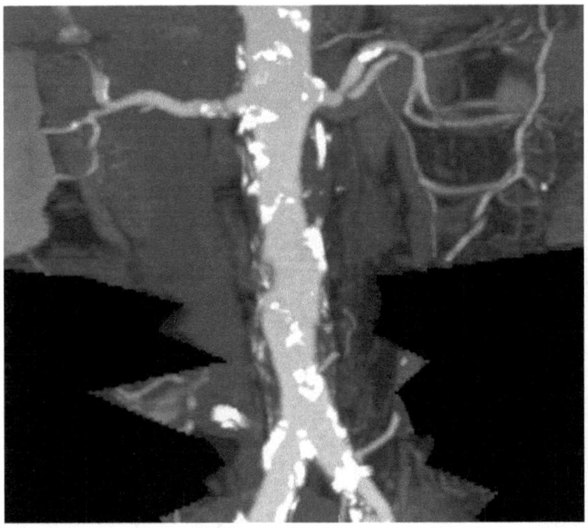

a

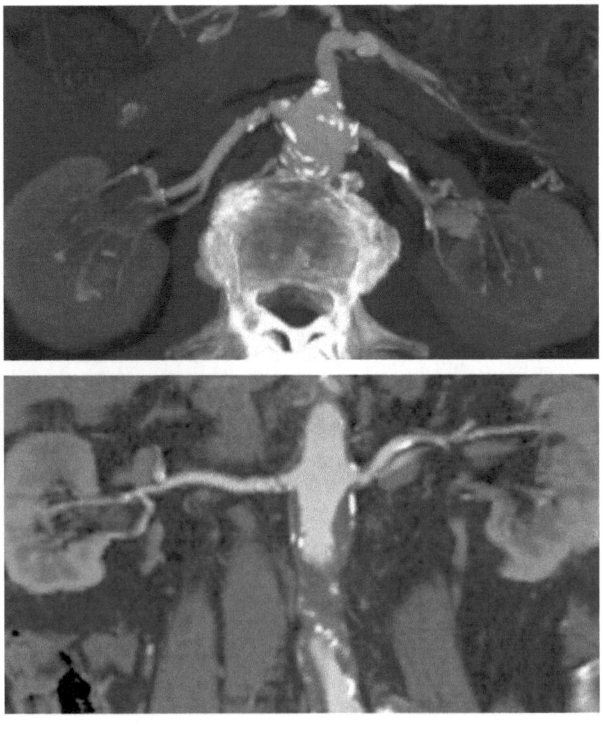

b

c

Fig. 13.8a–c Eccentric stenosis of both right and left renal arteries. Selective thin maximum-intensity projection (MIP) (**a**) shows 75% stenosis (*arrow*). Note that multiple calcifications are present at the origin of the vessels (**b**). Coronal selective MIP (**c**) shows a partially calcified thrombus involving the origin of both renal arteries and the prehilar branching of the left renal artery, with a severe stenosis.

tis nodosa, fibromuscular dysplasia, and trauma [15].

In some cases aneurysms can become quite large and they often develop rim calcifications (Fig. 13.9).

MDCTA represents, at this moment, the gold standard in the evaluation of renal aneurysms, with the potential to define the vascular lumen, the peripheral thrombus, and parietal calcification. In this respect, especially for what concerns polyarteritis nodosa and fibromuscular dysplasia, where the site of aneurysms are often located at the distal branches, MDCT allows better depiction of the presence and the site of aneurisms in relation to the high spatial resolution of the technique than MRA and US.

3D-reconstruction techniques therefore permit a better visualization of the entire length of the vessel, the diameter, and the neck of aneurysms, which may be helpful during interventional or even surgical procedures.

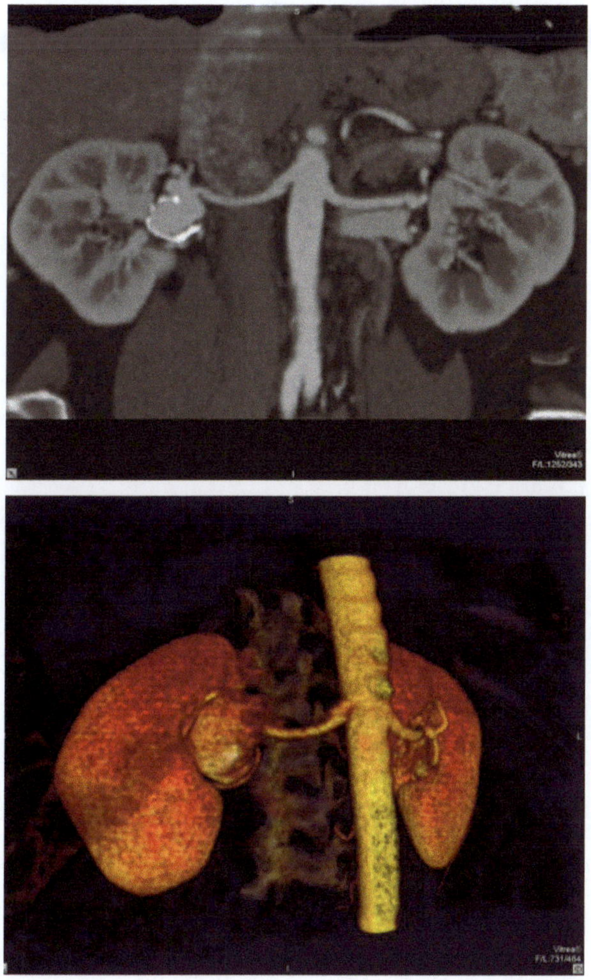

a

a

Fig. 13.9a,b Right renal artery aneurysm in a 59-year-old man. Coronal MIP (**a**) and volume-rendered (**b**) images show a partially calcified, 3-cm renal artery aneurysm.

13.6 Conclusion

Multidetector technology has allowed study of the vascular district with high-resolution protocols at the rate of very low acquisition times: the advantages are image quality, isotropy of the voxels that permit multiplanar and volume-rendering reconstructions, better administration of contrast agent, no superimposition of venous system, and reduction of movement artifacts.

This is a highly reliable technique to depict vascular and parenchymal information and to detect renal artery stenosis, as well as various renal disorders. New scanners will be soon available to reduce time-consuming, ionizing radiation and the amount of contrast-medium administered.

References

1. Platt J, Ellis J, Korobkin M, Reige K (1997) Helical CT evaluation of potential kidney donors: findings in 154 subjects. AJR Am J Roentgenol 169:1325–1330
2. Hillmann BJ (1989) Imaging advances in the diagnosis of renovascular hypertension. AJR Am J Roentgenol 153:5–14
3. National High Blood Pressure Educational Programme Working Group (1996) Update of working group reports on chronic renal failure and renovascular hypertension. Arch Intern Med 156:1938–1947
4. Coll DM, Uzzo RG, Hertz BR et al. (1999) 3-Dimensional volume rendered computed tomography for preoperative evaluation and intraoperative treatment of patients undergoing nephron sparing surgery. J Urol 161:1097–1102
5. Tran T, Heneghan JP, Paulson EK (2002) Preoperative evaluation of potential renal donors using multidetector CT. Abdom Imaging 27:620–625
6. Krijnen P, Oei HY, Claessen RA et al. (2002) Interobserver agreement on captopril renography for assessing renal vascular disease. J Nucl Med 43:330–337
7. Miralles M, Cairols M, Cotillas J et al. (1996) Value of Doppler parameters in the diagnosis of renal artery stenosis. J Vasc Surg 23:428–435
8. Hu H, He HD, Foley WD (2000) Four multidetector-row helical CT: image quality and volume coverage speed. Radiology 215:55–62
9. Abrams HL (1983) Angiography of the kidneys. In: Abrams HL (ed) Abrams' angiography: vascular and interventional radiology, 3rd edn. Medical Education and Research/Little Brown and Co, Boston, pp 445–495

10. Smith PA, Fishman EK (1998) Three-dimensional CT angiography: renal applications. Semin Ultrasound CT MR 19:413–424
11. Brink JA, Lim JT, Wang G et al. (1995) Technical optimization of spiral CT for depiction of renal artery stenosis: in vitro analysis. Radiology 194:157–163
12. Vasbinder GB, Nielmans PJ, Kessels AG et al. (2001) Diagnostic tests for renal artery stenosis in patients suspected of having renovascular hypertension: a meta analysis. Ann Intern Med 135:401–411
13. Harrison EG Jr, Hunt JC, Bernatz PE (1967) Morphology of fibromuscular dysplasia of the renal arteryin renovascular hypertension. Am J Med 43:97–112
14. Willmann JK, Wildermuth S, Pfammatter T et al. (2003) Aortoiliac and renal arteries: prospective intraindividual comparison of contrast-enhanced 3D MR angiography and multi-detector row CT. Angiogr Radiol 226:798–811
15. Kadir S (1986) Angiography of the kidneys. In: Kadir S (ed) Diagnostic angiography. Saunders, Philadelphia, pp 445–495

14 Multidetector-Row CT Angiography of Peripheral Arteries: Imaging Upper-Extremity and Lower-Extremity Vascular Disease

Dominik Fleischmann, Jeffrey C. Hellinger, and Alessandro Napoli

CONTENTS

14.1 Introduction

Since its first clinical implementation in the early 1990s, computed tomography angiography (CTA) has had a substantial impact on diagnostic vascular imaging. During this time, spiral CT has evolved technologically, with improvements in X-ray tubes' capabilities, gantry rotation, and interpolation algorithm performances. The greatest advance, though, has been the introduction of multidetector-row computed tomography (MDCT). Currently capable of acquiring 16 channels of helical data simultaneously, MDCT scanners have substantially improved the quality and ease of performing angiographic studies. As a result, CTA has become a robust method of diagnostic angiographic imaging, challenging digital subtraction angiography (DSA) in most vascular systems. As CTA for extremity vascular disease has become a common examination in many radiology departments, a discussion of MDCT angiography (MDCTA) technique is required. A clinical overview of extremity vascular disease is first presented, with the focus on peripheral atherosclerotic arterial disease (PAD). Next, the chapter addresses the MDCT principles, which optimize peripheral vascular imaging. A discussion of contrast-medium (CM) administration strategies proceeds, with attention toward injection protocol and bolus timing. Finally, an outline of 3-dimensional (3D) visualization techniques is presented.

D. Fleischmann, MD
Assistant Professor of Radiology, Department of Radiology, Division of Cardiovascular Imaging, Stanford University Medical Center, 300 Pasteur Drive, Room S-068B, Stanford, CA 94305-5105, USA
J. C. Hellinger, MD
Department of Radiology, Division of Cardiovascular Imaging, Stanford University Medical Center, 300 Pasteur Drive, Room S-068B, Stanford, CA 94305-5105, USA
A. Napoli, MD
Department of Radiology, University of Rome "La Sapienza", Policlinico Umberto I, Viale Regina Elena n. 324, 00161 Rome, Italy

14.2 Upper- and Lower-Extremity Vascular Disease

Indications for upper-extremity (UE) and lower-extremity (LE) vascular imaging include PAD, vasculitis, venous occlusive disease, vascular masses, trauma, and preoperative vascular mapping. PAD more commonly affects the LE, and therefore the other indications will be more frequently encountered for UE CTA referrals, in particular vasculitis. One additional indication for UE vascular imaging is assessment of failing hemodialysis access.

14.2.1 Infrarenal Aortic and Extremity Atherosclerotic Arterial Disease

14.2.1.1 Clinical Overview

Twenty-seven million people in Europe and North America (16% of the population 55 years and older) have PAD, most involving the LE [1]. The secondary arterial narrowing or obstruction reduces blood flow to the affected limb during exercise or at rest. A spectrum of symptoms results, the severity of which depends on the extent of the involvement and the available collateral circulation. These symptoms may range from intermittent claudication to limb-threatening ischemia (i.e., rest pain, tissue loss). Patients may not recognize the symptoms and therefore patients frequently present with advanced disease. Even once patients present to a primary-care physician, PAD is often underdiagnosed. As referrals to a vascular surgeon are not required, since the CTA is noninvasive, MDCTA offers primary-care physicians the potential to noninvasively screen more patients before limbs are nonsalvageable.

14.2.1.2 Evaluating PAD

For patients with PAD, treatment options include medical management or endovascular (angioplasty/stent) and/or surgical revascularization. In claudicant patients, treatment aims at improving flow to the buttocks, thigh, and/or calf muscles. For patients in danger of losing their limbs, treatment goals are similar; however, foremost is the aim to prevent development of or progression of tissue loss and the need for extremity amputation. For patients suspected of having PAD therefore, the principle goal of CTA is to evaluate the extent of disease and characterize vessel morphology such that CTA can offer a means to address treatment planning. For patients with lesions amenable to intervention, CTA also provides a road map, in particular target vessels for potential distal surgical anastomoses (Fig. 14.1). To ensure clinical decision-making needs are answered, clinical data is reviewed, beginning with a patient's history and physical examination. If previously obtained, inquiry is also made as to segmental blood pressure measurements (i.e., ankle-brachial index, ABI), ultrasound with Doppler flow, and/or plethysmography. Knowledge of the patient data will ensure

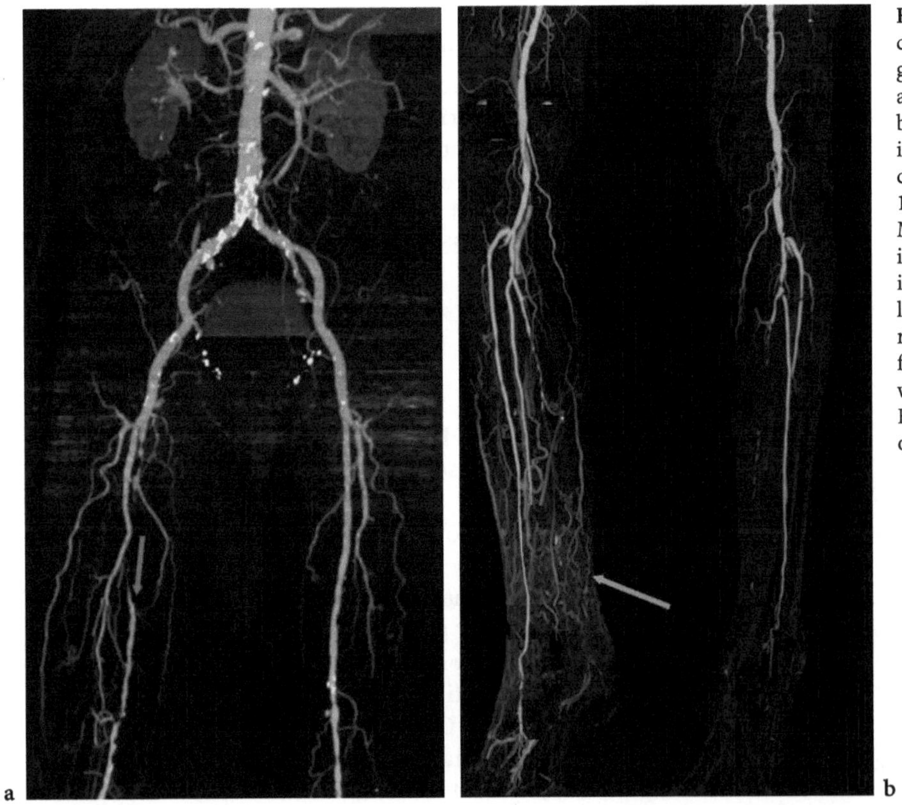

Fig. 14.1 a,b Multidetector-row computed tomography angiography was performed on a 70-year-old male with one block bilateral lower-extremity claudication and a right-calf nonhealing ulcer, utilizing 16×1.25 detector collimation. Maximum-intensity projection images demonstrate bilateral infrainguinal and infrapopliteal outflow disease. **a** On the right there is proximal superficial femoral artery occlusion with distal reconstitution. **b** Hyperemia is noted at the site of the nonhealing ulcer.

and also facilitate planning the examination protocol. Most importantly, this clinical background will afford that the study is interpreted in context to the patient as, regardless of the pathology, only symptomatic lesions will warrant intervention.

Lesions can be distinguished by type (i.e., atheromatous vs thromboembolic); chronicity (i.e., acute vs chronic); severity [i.e., mild stenosis (<50% narrowing), moderate stenosis (50-75% stenosis), severe stenosis (75-99% narrowing), occlusion]; length (i.e., focal, short segment, long segment); vessel-wall location (i.e., circumferential vs eccentric); and vascular territory distribution (i.e., inflow vs outflow). Regarding lesion type and chronicity, atheromatous lesions are treated by endovascular (i.e., angioplasty and/or stent) or surgical means (i.e., graft bypass). Patients may present in a subacute to chronic state, with the degree of collateral vessels serving as a marker for distinction. Acute thromboembolic lesions are usually first amenable to pharmacological and/or mechanical thrombectomy, followed by definitive endovascular or surgical repair. No collateral vessels will be present in the acute setting, unless the event occurs in a previously diseased region. Regarding severity, it is important to keep in mind that such descriptions broadly categorize PAD, but in general lesions with more than 50% narrowing of a vessel are most often hemodynamically significant. Regarding lesion length and vessel wall location, traditionally, focal, noneccentric to short-segment (<10 cm) lesions are most amenable to successful endovascular repair in contrast to long-segment (>10 cm in length) and/or eccentric lesions. The latter type lesions traditionally are reserved for surgical bypass. Regarding territory distribution, it is important to evaluate disease as aorto-iliac inflow, femoral-popliteal and tibioperoneal outflow, or combined pathology. Inflow and outflow pathology offer different strategies. Endovascular therapy for inflow disease has greater long-term patency than infrainguinal and infrapoliteal outflow (Fig. 14.2). Although drug-eluding stents offer promising initial endovascular results for outflow disease, at present surgical revascularization remains the current treatment recommendation. When combined inflow and outflow lesions are present, proximal in-flow lesions are treated first.

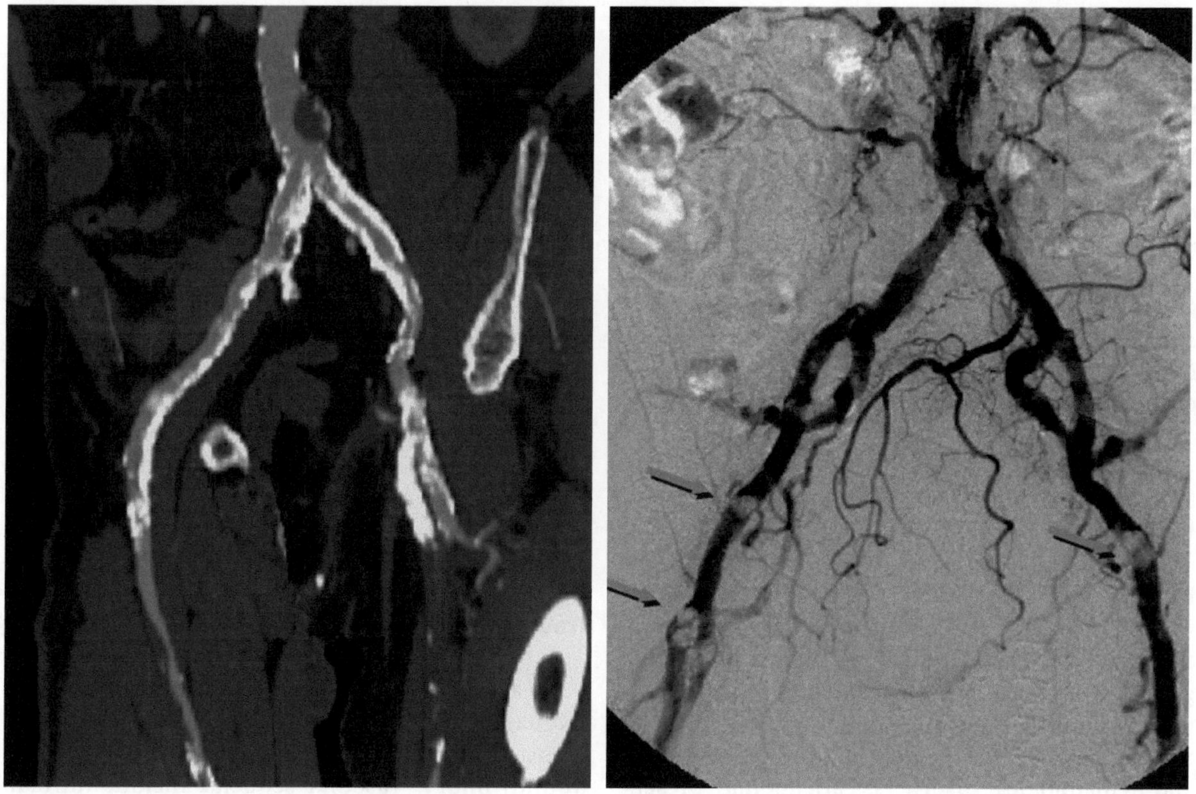

a b

Fig. 14.2a,b Computed tomographic angiography was carried out on a patient with bilateral proximal lower-extremity claudication. Left anterior oblique maximum-intensity projection image (**a**) demonstrates tandem, hemodynamically significant inflow disease, confirmed on digital subtraction angiography (**b**).

14.2.1.3 Diagnostic Value of Lower-Extremity CTA for PAD

CTA should be considered as the first-line imaging modality for diagnostic evaluation of suspected PAD [2]. It is an accurate and reliable examination, at reduced cost and time, compared with DSA. Furthermore it eliminates the inherent risks of DSA and is more convenient for patients. Most importantly, by imaging the entire blood pool without dependence on arterial flow, CTA provides a robust means to depict collateral networks on a single injection and acquisition. This is particularly the case for patients with aortic occlusion and/or severe disease involving inflow and/or outflow territories.

Regarding CTA accuracy, to evaluate the performance of 4-channel MDCT (4-MDCT) angiography in the assessment of the *infrarenal* aorta and lower-extremity arterial system, we studied 50 patients with suspected peripheral arterial occlusive disease [3]. Patients underwent both 4-MDCTA and DSA. Arterial anatomy was divided into 23 anatomic segments (infrarenal aorta, right and left common iliac artery, internal iliac artery, external iliac artery, common femoral artery, superficial femoral artery, deep femoral artery, popliteal artery, anterior tibial artery, tibioperoneal trunk, posterior tibial artery, and peroneal artery). Findings were classified as normal, moderate disease (<50% stenosis), focal severe stenosis (>50% stenosis), diffuse disease (multiple severe stenoses), and occlusion. At consensus reading, the sensitivity, specificity, and accuracy of MDCTA as compared to DSA were, respectively, 96%, 93%, and 94%, with a κ-value of 0.812 (almost perfect agreement). The results of this study confirm that MDCTA is accurate for assessing PAD, independent of the grade of ischemia.

14.2.2 Vasculitis

Extremity vasculitis targets both large and small vessels, with UE vascular territories most commonly affected. The arteritides include Takayasu arteritis, giant cell arteritis, and thromboangitis obliterans, while common small-vessel vasculitides include Systemic lupus erythema nodosa, scleroderma, and hematological disorders. Patients may present with a combination of claudication, rest ischemia, and/or Raynaud's phenomenon, depending on the disease burden, level of involvement, and collateral flow [4]. Systemic symptoms are not uncommon. In our experience, CTA has been performed to assess proximal disease in patients clinically presenting with vasculitis symptoms (Fig. 14.3). However, if evaluation is to primarily assess distal outflow and digital anatomy, DSA rather than UE CTA, may be the study of choice, as this assessment may require intra-arterial vasodilators.

14.2.3 Veno-occlusive Disease

Venous occlusive disease may result from in-situ stasis (i.e., systemic diseases, hypercoaguable state), instrumentation (i.e., catheters), trauma, and extrinsic compression [5, 6]. Diagnosis can be made noninvasively by ultrasound. In some instances, venography may be required. CT venography is an alternative to conventional venography for evaluating suspected UE or LE venous thrombosis (Fig. 14.4). Similar to imaging for arterial disease, CT venography affords the opportunity to evaluate nonvascular structures, which may be the cause for venous thrombosis (i.e., Paget–Schroetter syndrome).

14.2.4 Vascular Masses

Common vascular masses include aneurysms, hemangiomas, and arteriovenous malformations. Aneurysms may be atherosclerotic, poststenotic (i.e., thoracic outlet syndrome), posttraumatic (pseudoaneurysm), mycotic, or secondary to a connective tissue disorder (i.e., Ehlers-Danlos syndrome). Similar to DSA, extremity CTA for aneurysms should always include distally to the digits for assessment of downstream embolization (Fig. 14.5). CTA for hemangiomas and arteriovenous malformations, however, can be limited in volume coverage.

14.2.5 Trauma

Both acute and chronic vascular trauma can be evaluated with CTA. Acute trauma results from blunt (i.e., crush) or penetrating (i.e., gunshot wound) injury. Vascular sequelae include intimal tears with or without transection, pseudoaneurysms, and occlusion (Fig. 14.6). Chronic trauma is secondary to repeated intimal and/or media in-

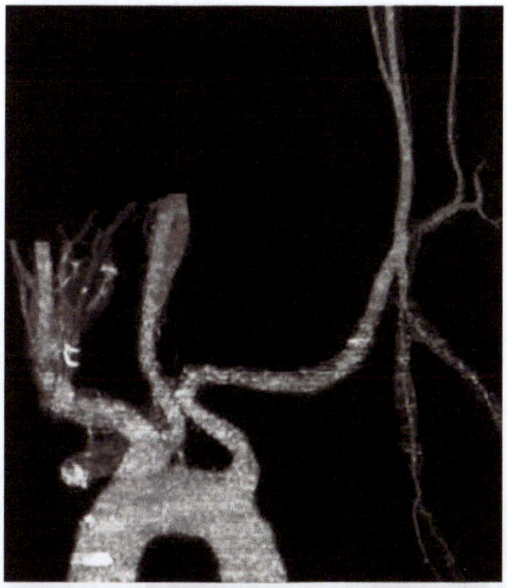

a

Fig. 14.3a-c A 45-year-old woman with known scleroderma vasculitis involving both hands presented with a new, subacute left second-digit ulcer. Upper-extremity computed tomographic angiography was requested to exclude proximal pathology which may have been contributing to the changes. Acquired at 1.25 mm nominal section thickness on a 16-channel multidetector-row computed tomography scanner, maximum-intensity projection (**a**) and volume-rendered images (**b, c**) of the inflow and proximal outflow vessels show normal proximal vessels without a source for thromboembolism. Palmar and digital vessels were poorly opacified, related to the known vasculitis (not shown). Incidental note is made of normal variant radial artery off the brachial artery (*arrow*).

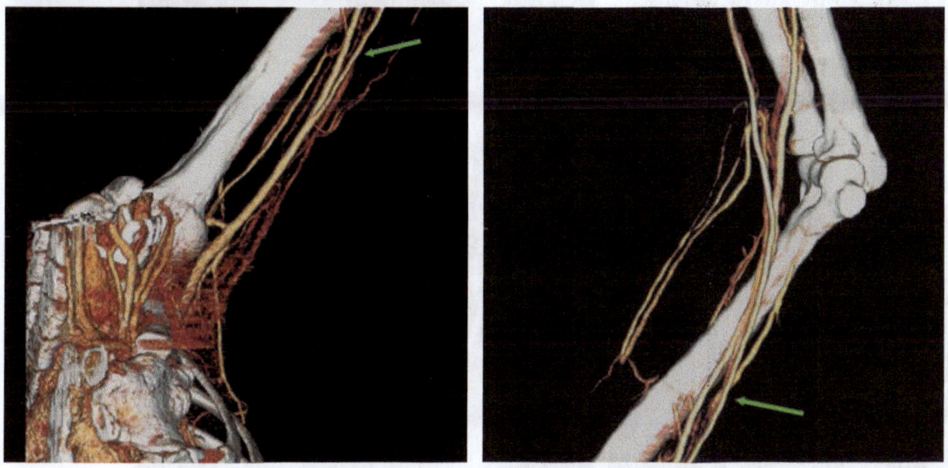

b c

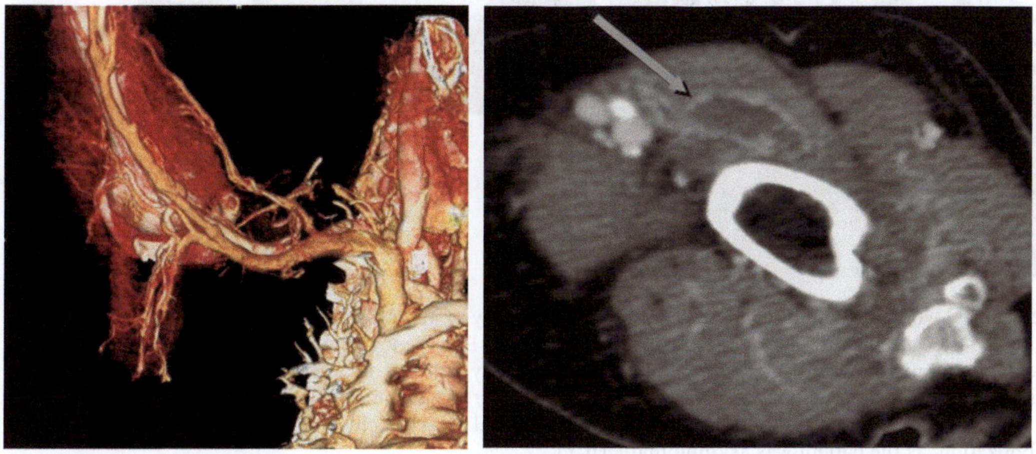

a b

Fig. 14.4a,b A 76-year-old woman with acquired hemophilia presented with a swollen, erythematous right upper arm. Initial ultrasound was suboptimal, but suggested subclavian and peripheral right upper-arm venous thrombosis. As anticoagulation was contraindicated, upper-extremity CT venography was performed. From the antecubital fossa through to the cavoatrial junction, 1.25-mm images were acquired on a 16-row multidetector-row computed tomography scanner. A volume-rendered image (**a**) confirms patency of peripheral and central veins, without thrombus. Axial images provided a correct alternative diagnosis, intramuscular hematoma (**b**).

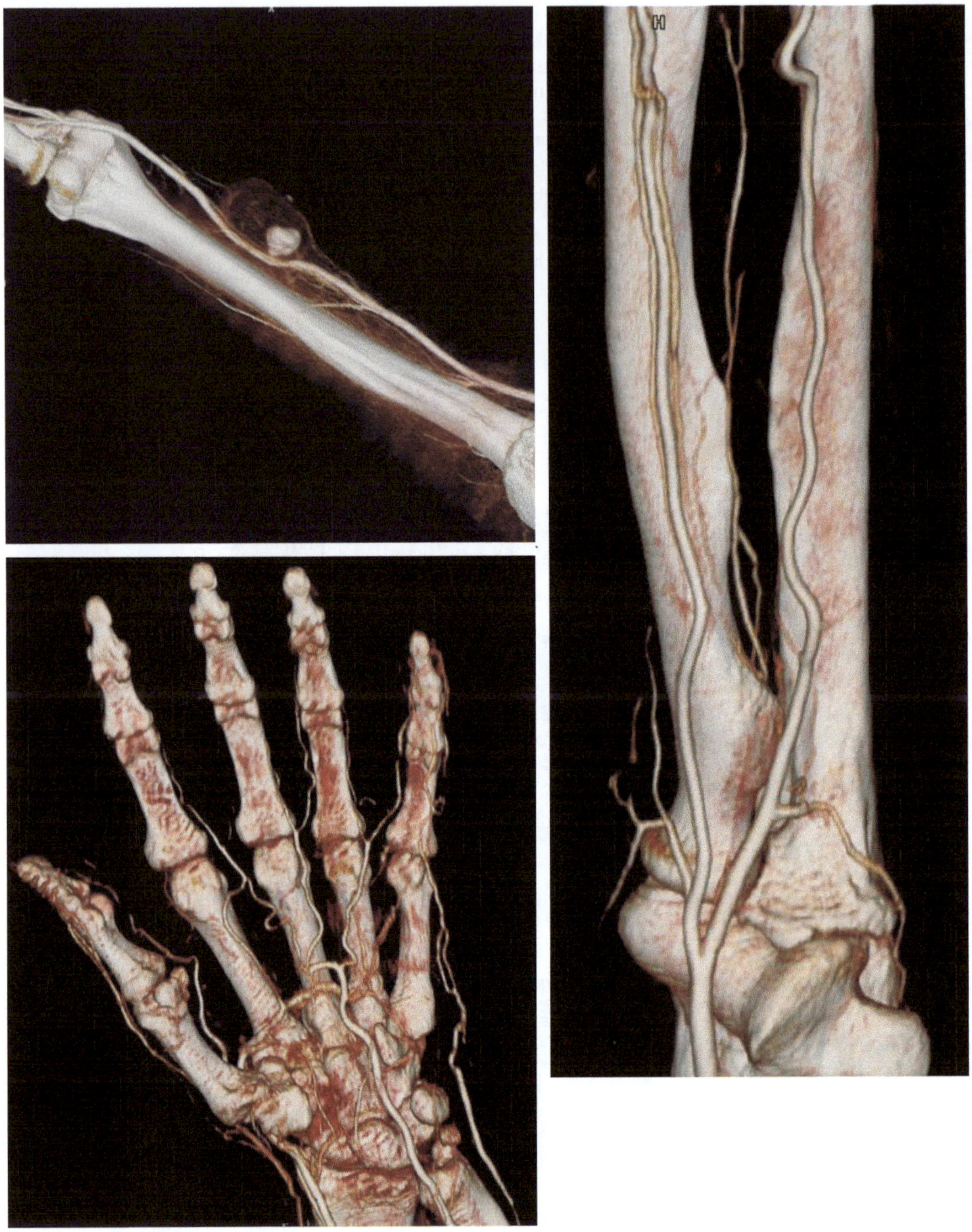

a b c

Fig. 14.5a-c A 62-year-old woman in the intensive care unit, with a history of atherosclerotic disease, developed a left arm pulsatile mass shortly after attempted placement of an arterial catheter. Emergency computed tomographic angiography was performed on a 16-channel multidetector-row computed tomography scanner. Scan coverage was from the shoulder through to the digits. Volume-rendered image in **a** identifies a brachial artery saccular pseudoaneurysm. Distal runoff to the hand shows proximal interosseous and radial second and third digital artery occlusions, indeterminate if reflective of downstream embolization, as the patient was asymptomatic (**b, c**).

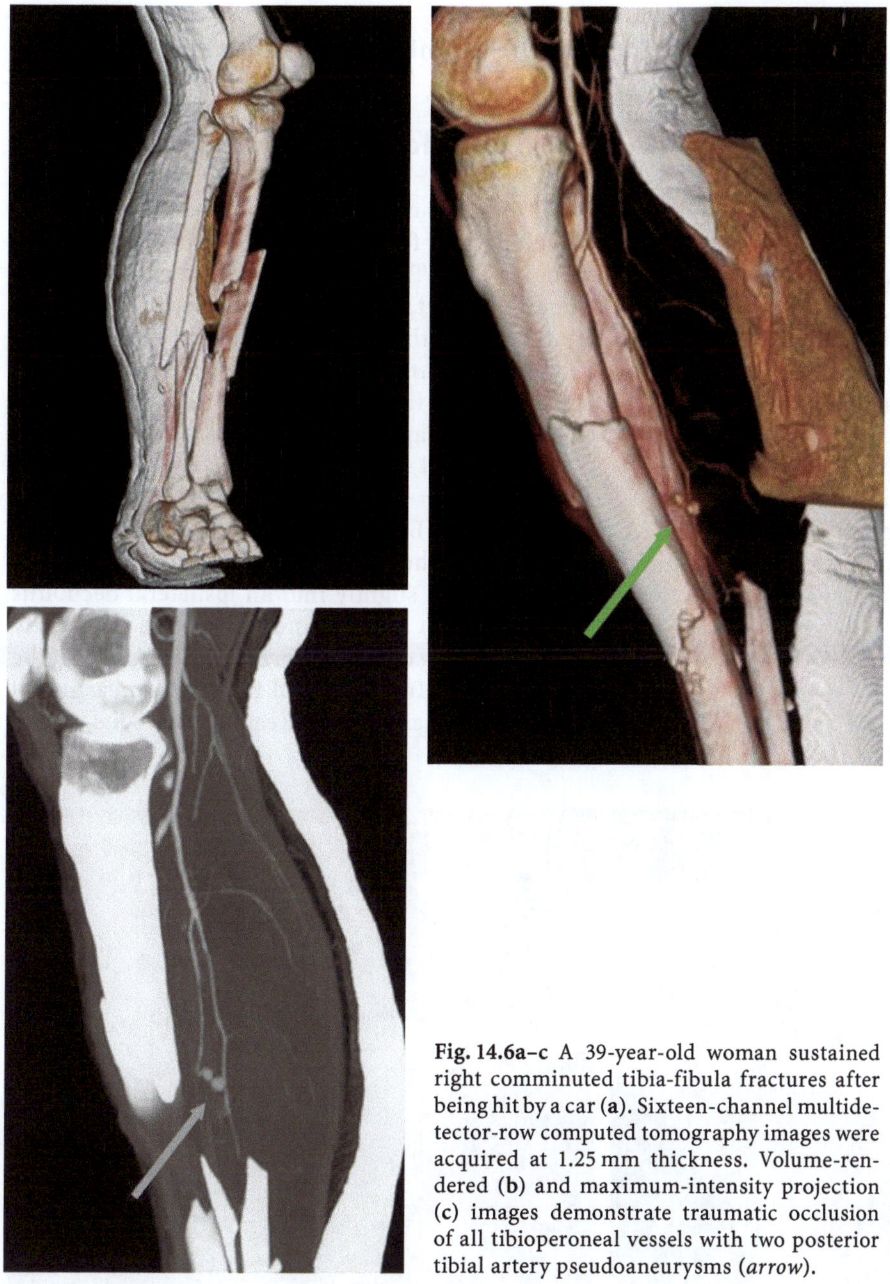

Fig. 14.6a–c A 39-year-old woman sustained right comminuted tibia-fibula fractures after being hit by a car (**a**). Sixteen-channel multidetector-row computed tomography images were acquired at 1.25 mm thickness. Volume-rendered (**b**) and maximum-intensity projection (**c**) images demonstrate traumatic occlusion of all tibioperoneal vessels with two posterior tibial artery pseudoaneurysms (*arrow*).

jury, often related to repetitive use with normal (i.e., hypothenar hammer syndrome) or abnormal bony/soft tissue structure (i.e., thoracic outlet syndrome). This results in intimal irregularity, stenosis, and thrombosis, and aneurysms may result. In both acute and chronic settings, a search should be made for distal embolization, collateral networks should be defined, and vascular injuries should be interpreted in the context of relevant musculoskeletal findings.

14.2.6 Vascular Mapping: Tissue Reconstruction

Wounds may require reconstruction by transferring tissue with an intact vascular supply. Conventional flap repair involves local or distant tissue continuity between the donor and recipient sites. Free flaps employ microsurgical techniques to transfer tissue from one region of the body to a distant recipient site. Preoperative knowledge of recipient and/or donor vessel patency and caliber, in addition to perivascular soft tissues (i.e., fibrosis), can facilitate surgical planning. CTA offers a noninvasive means to comprehensively obtain this information (Fig. 14.7).

14.2.7 Hemodialysis Access

Surgically created arteriovenous fistulae (AVF) and polytetrafluoroethylene (PTFE) bridge grafts (AVG) are means for permanent hemodialysis access. Functional AVF and AVG success begins with patient selection. While duplex ultrasonography and less often DSA are performed to assess continuous vessel patency and suitable caliber, CTA is an alternative for arterial and venous mapping. CTA also has a role in assessment of dysfunctioning AVF and AVG (i.e., low flow/venous pressures; elevated venous pressures/urea recirculation time; Fig. 14.8).

14.3 MDCTA Technique: Extremity Vasculature

14.3.1 Patient Preparation and Positioning

An 18- to 20-gauge IV catheter is placed into an antecubital fossa, forearm, or dorsum hand superficial vein. For UE-CTA this should be in the contralateral extremity. Next, patients are positioned on the CT gantry table with the affected extremity(s) in the isocenter of the scanner. For LE-CTA, patients are placed supine and feet first. Legs are stabilized with cushions and adhesive tape. To facilitate infrapopliteal postprocessing and distinction of tibioperoneal vessels from bone, feet can be secured with slight internal rotation. For UE-CTA, the symptomatic extremity is raised above the patient's head. If needed, the patient is rotated slightly into an ipsilateral decubitus position. When the extremity cannot be adequately raised, imaging can be performed with the arm at the patient's side. Tape is useful to secure forearm and hand position, as well as spreading the digits.

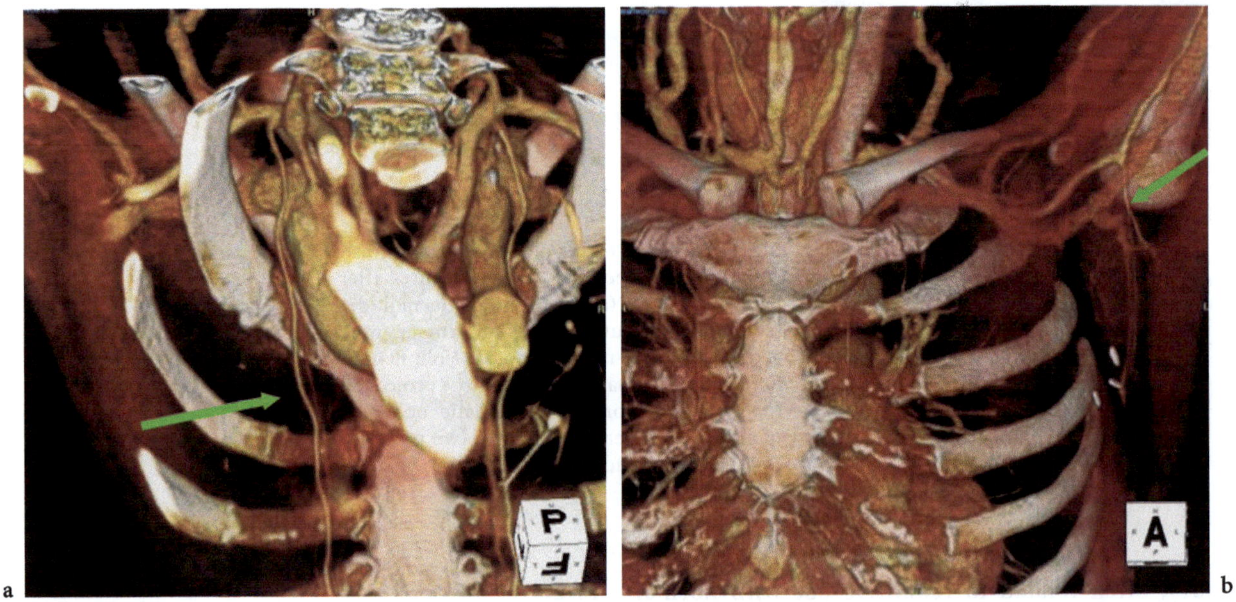

Fig. 14.7a,b A 57-year-old woman, status post bilateral mastectomy, was under consideration for possible bilateral TRAM reconstruction. CTA was requested to evaluate patency and caliber of internal mammary and thoracodorsal arteries. 1.25 mm images were acquired on 16-channel multidetector-row computed tomography from the mid arms through the chest. Left internal mammary artery is shown on the posterior view to have normal caliber throughout its course (**a**). The left thoracodorsal artery is patent, but diminutive (**b**). Note adjacent left axillary surgical clips.

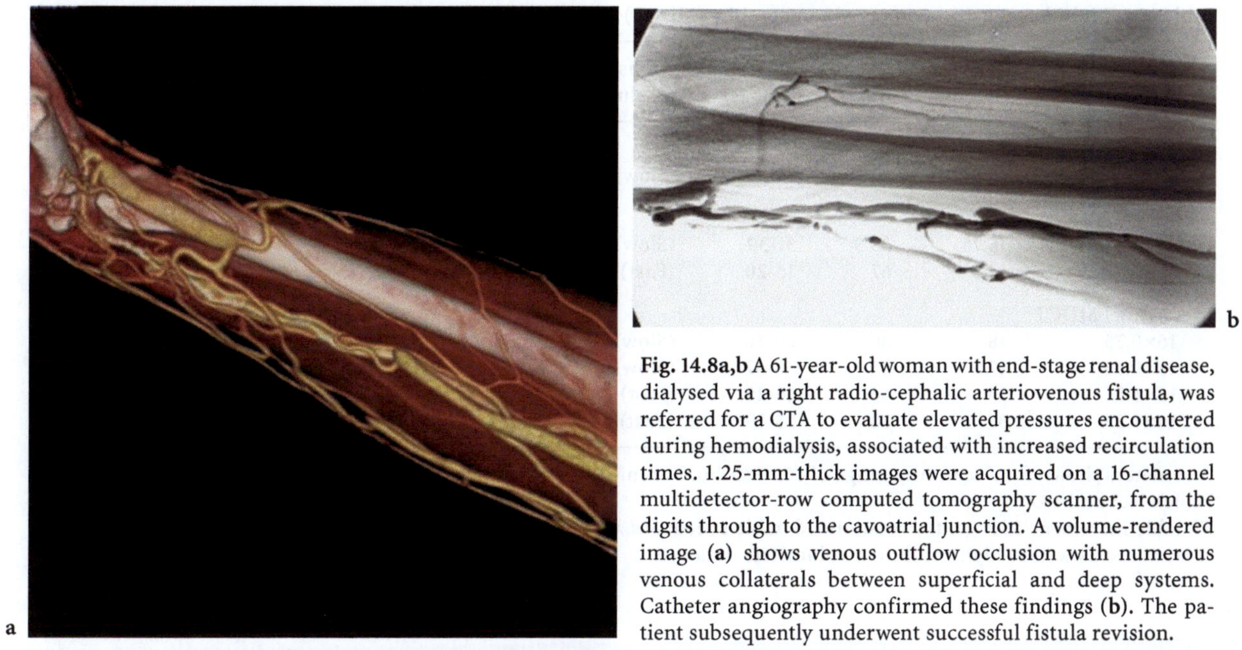

Fig. 14.8a,b A 61-year-old woman with end-stage renal disease, dialysed via a right radio-cephalic arteriovenous fistula, was referred for a CTA to evaluate elevated pressures encountered during hemodialysis, associated with increased recirculation times. 1.25-mm-thick images were acquired on a 16-channel multidetector-row computed tomography scanner, from the digits through to the cavoatrial junction. A volume-rendered image (**a**) shows venous outflow occlusion with numerous venous collaterals between superficial and deep systems. Catheter angiography confirmed these findings (**b**). The patient subsequently underwent successful fistula revision.

14.3.2 Scan Coverage

Determining the scan coverage for both UE- and LE-CTA will reflect the patient's presentation and indications for the examination. In general, coverage can either be targeted to the region of clinical interest or include complete inflow and outflow anatomy. For LE-CTA, complete anatomical coverage should include from the supraceliac aorta proximally to the pedal arteries distally. The average distance for LE-CTA varies between 1,200 and 1,400 mm, depending on the patient's height. For UE-CTA, complete arterial coverage includes from the aortic arch proximally, through to the digital vessels distally, while complete venous coverage includes from the digits through to the cavoatrial junction. Complete UE-CTA varies between 800 and 1,000 mm, depending on arm length. Two clinical scenarios warrant modification of complete UE and LE coverage. When thromboembolism is a consideration, scan coverage should include the heart, to assess for a cardiogenic source. When vascular compression is a consideration (i.e., thoracic outlet syndrome, popliteal entrapment syndrome), symptomatic extremities are first scanned in the neutral position with limited thin-section acquisition. Patients are then repositioned with a challenged maneuver and scanned with complete arterial coverage.

14.3.3 CTA Acquisition Parameters

Detector configuration and table speed determine the acquisition time. Acquisition duration in turn impacts CM-injection techniques. When a 4-MDCT scanner with a gantry rotation time of 0.5 s is used, the following protocol has been proved successful [3]: 4×2.5- mm collimation, with a 2.5-mm-section thickness and a table feed of 15 mm/gantry rotation (30 mm/s), resulting in scan times between 35 and 45 s, depending on the patient length. Thin-section acquisition (~1.25 mm) improves 3D postprocessing and depiction of small vessels (i.e., pedal). When acquiring with 4-MDCT, scan durations will approach 60–70 s, resulting in more venous contamination.

Compared with 4-MDCT, 8-channel MDCT (8-MDCT) affords greater temporal resolution, while 16-channel MDCT (16-MDCT) affords both greater temporal and spatial resolution. When compared with 4-MDCT, for the same volume coverage, collimation, gantry rotation, and nominal section thickness, scan times are twice as fast with 8-MDCT and 4 times faster with 16-MDCT. When progressing to the 16-MDCT, thinner sections can be obtained (0.625 mm) with still twice the scan time of 4-MDCT. The thinner acquisition (≤1.25 mm) provides high-resolution isotropic datasets, which improves image quality and 3D postprocessing. Acquisition parameters for 4-, 8-, and 16-channel systems are given in Table 14.1.

Table 14.1. Multidetector-row computed tomography (MDCT) acquisition parameters

Collimation (mm)	TI (mm/360°)	TS (mm/s)	Scanning time (s)	z-axis resolution	Scanning protocol	Injection protocol
4-Channel MDCT						
4×2.5	15	30	35-45	(Slow)	Standard	A
8-Channel MDCT						
8×1.25	16.75	33.5	31-39	(Slow)	Std/high-res.	A
8×2.5	33.5	67	16-20	(Fast)	Standard	B
16-Channel MDCT						
16×0.75	18	36	29-36	(Slow)	Std./high-res.	A
16×0.63	17.5	35	30-37	(Slow)	Std./high-res.	A
16×1.5	33	66	16-20	(Fast)	Standard	B
16×1.25	35	70	15-19	(Fast)	Standard	B

Parameters shown for a scanning range of 105-130 cm. For injection protocols A and B see Tables 14.3 and 14.4
TI, table increment/360° gantry rotation; *TS*, table speed; *Std./high-res.*, allows reconstruction of standard as well as high-resolution volumetric data sets

14.3.4 Image Reconstruction

Standard-resolution CTA data sets can be obtained from 2.5- to 3- mm MDCT acquisitions, whereby overlapping images are reconstructed every 1- to 1.5- mm increment. High-resolution isotropic data sets can be obtained from thin-collimation (≤1.25 mm) acquisitions, whereby overlapping images are reconstructed at 0.5- to 0.8- mm increments. Thinner reconstructions produce higher image quality for depicting small vessels (i.e., crural), but require greater processing speed and archival storage to handle the larger amount of data (Table 14.2). Furthermore, the thin-section data sets are limited by increased image noise in the abdomen, requiring increased milliamperes.

Table 14.2. MDCT image reconstruction

	Standard resolution	High resolution
Section thickness	2.5–3 mm	1–1.25 mm
Reconstruction interval	1–1.5 mm	0.5–0.8 mm
Advantage	Sufficient for most indications	Optimal resolution for small vessels
Limitations	z-axis blurring (crural arteries)	Increase image noise (abdomen) and large number of images

14.4 Contrast-Medium Delivery for Extremity CTA

Synchronizing CM injection with spiral acquisition is the limiting factor to achieve optimal vascular enhancement. As technology progresses to faster MDCT scanners, CM administration will become more challenging, requiring continuous modifications of CM protocols. Regardless of the MDCT, three issues have to be taken into consideration:

1. The CM transit time from the IV injection site to the beginning of the scan volume varies for individual patients. For instance, in 95% of patients, the contrast arrival time between the injection site and the abdominal aorta ranges between 14 and 28 s. To account for this variability, scan delays should be individualized. This can be accomplished either using test-bolus or automated bolus-triggering techniques. Most vendors now have automated bolus triggering and, in our experience, we have found this to be most efficient and practical. For an abdominal aortogram with LE runoff CTA, bolus triggering is performed in the infrarenal abdominal aorta, while for an arch aortogram with UE runoff CTA, a level in the mid- to distal brachial artery is selected
2. Because many patients have coexisting cardiovascular disease with reduced cardiac output, initial enhancement profiles may be shallow. Thus, for a LE runoff, if the CT acquisition is initiated shortly after bolus arrival, opacification may not

yet have reached adequate enhancement levels. An increase in the initial injection flow rate (e.g., 5-6 ml/s for the first 5 s of the injection), use of high-concentration contrast medium (≥350-400 mg I/ml), or an increased scanning delay relative to the contrast arrival in the aorta (i.e., 8 s) are options to eliminate this problem

3. In a patient with PAD, flow-limiting arterial stenoses and occlusions may be present anywhere in the inflow and outflow territories. For example, in a patient presenting with LE claudication, lesions may occur between the infrarenal aorta and the pedal arteries. This will result in variable contrast arrival time to the outflow vessels. In a study examining CM LE-CTA administration in a group of 20 patients with PAD, bolus transit times from the aorta to the popliteal arteries ranged from 4 to 24 s (average 10 s). Clinical stage of disease (intermittent claudication vs limb threatening ischemia) was no predictor of aortopopliteal bolus transit time. Extrapolated for the entire peripheral arterial tree and across all individuals, an injection duration of 35 s was necessary to guarantee optimal opacification of the aorta down to the pedal branches in all (>97.5%) patients. With 4-channel MDCT, this is not a relevant problem, because acquisition times (and injection times) are usually longer than 35 s. With 8- and 16-MDCT, however, acquisitions may outrun the bolus, if the scanning protocol does not account for possible slow arterial filling.

14.4.1 Practical Approach to Contrast-Medium Injection for Extremity CTA

Strategies for optimal CM delivery can be divided into two groups, according to the acquisition speed. For slow acquisitions (scan times ≥35 s), biphasic injections yield optimal arterial opacification [7]. For fast acquisitions, i.e., 8- and 16-MDCT, an increased scanning delay relative to the CM transit time is optimal. The protocols for these strategies are provided in Tables 14.3 and 14.4.

14.5 Visualization

In daily clinical practice, the large extremity-CTA data sets can limit workload efficiency. To manage this "data overload," it is recommended that examinations are viewed on workstations through a combination of 3D and 2D real-time interaction and axial source images. Most information can be interpreted from the real-time postprocessed images, through standard or advanced techniques, using appropriate window settings (Table 14.5). Findings and the extent of disease can be corroborated on the

Table 14.3 Peripheral CTA contrast-medium (CM) delivery for scan-times >35 s

Suitable acquisition protocols	4×2.5 mm 8×1.25 mm 16×0.75 mm 16×0.63 mm	scan-times between 32 and 50 s (or more)
Biphasic Injection	6.0 ml/s for 6 s (36 ml) +3.3 ml/s for (scan-time – 10 s)	
Scanning delay	Determined from test-bolus or bolus triggering	
Example:	for an acquisition time of 40 s: 30 ml@6 ml/s+100 ml @ 3.3 ml/s The total CM volume is 130 ml, the total injection time is 36 s	

Flow rates and volumes refer to 300 mg I/ml CM. Injection rates are smaller for high-concentration
CM:26 ml@5.0 ml/s +
85 ml@2.8 ml/s for 350 mg I/ml agent.
22 ml@4.5 ml/s + 75 ml@2.5 ml/s for 400 mg I/ml agent

Table 14.4 Injection protocol B. Peripheral CTA CM delivery for scan-times ≤35s

Suitable acquisition protocols:	8×2.5 mm 16×1.25 mm 16×1.5 mm	scan times in the range of 20s
Injection duration	35 s	
Injection rates[a]	5 ml/s → 175 ml 4.5 ml/s → 160 ml 4 ml/s → 140 ml	
Scanning delay:	determined by the t_{CMT} plus an additional trigger delay added to the time of contrast arrival. The trigger delay is chosen according to the scan time: trigger delay (s) = 40 s – scan time (s)	
Examples	30 s → t_{CMT} + 10 s 25 s → t_{CMT} + 15 s 20 s → t_{CMT} + 20 s 15 s → t_{CMT} + 25 s	

t_{CMT}, CM transit time, as determined by a test-bolus or automated bolus triggering
[a]Higher-concentration CM and shorter scan times require smaller injection rates and volumes

Table 14.5 Image postprocessing

	Volumetric (3D) overview	Cross-sectional (2D) detail
Purpose	Provides general overview of vessel tree, including collaterals	Allows detailed analysis of flow channel and vessel wall
Techniques	Maximum-intensity projection (MIP) Volume rendering (VR)	Multiplanar reformations (MPR) Curved planar reformations (CPR)
Advantages	Excellent spatial perception Easy display of findings to referring physician	Allows accurate grading of stenoses/ occlusion, even in presence of calcifications and stents
Limitations	Portions of vessel tree may be obscured by bone Vessel lumen is obscured in the presence of stents and calcified plaque	Limited spatial perception

transverse source images. Review of source images is also required for the assessment of vessel-wall pathology and nonvascular disease.

Standard postprocessing techniques include maximum intensity projection (MIP), thin MIP, volume rendering (VR), multiplanar (MPR), and curved planar (CPR) techniques. MIP and VR offer virtual 3D angiographic images that can be manipulated in any plane. They provide a general overview of the normal and abnormal vascular anatomy and offer an easy means to display findings. Interpretation of both, however, can be limited by adjacent bone, calcified atherosclerotic plaque, and metallic stents. In these instances, MPR and CPR, in addition to the source images, should be reviewed. Although MPR and CPR are 2D longitudinal cross-sectional evaluations, they provide detailed analysis of the flow channel along with the vessel wall, leading toward more accurate grading of stenoses and/or occlusions. Compared with MPR, CPR affords vessel display in a single path, eliminating angles and tortuosity, which can hinder MPR interpretation and display.

To increase CTA productivity and limit the time spent on generating postprocessed images, advanced CTA postprocessing techniques for extremity CTA have been developed, including algorithms for (semi-)automated bone removal and vessel tracking. These are available in many commercially available workstations. We have developed a research software program that automatically traces the centerline of the entire peripheral arterial tree – from the aorta down to the crural and pedal arteries. The centerline tree is used to create a "composited" image of multiple CPR through the entire arterial tree in a single view. A set of 21 "multipath CPRs" created over a viewing range of 180° combines the advantages of detailed luminal display while maintaining spatial perception.

14.6 Conclusions

Advancement in MDCT technology and gantry rotation both have substantially impacted CT angiography. Faster acquisitions with improved spatial resolution have broadened the role for CT imaging of the upper and lower extremity vascular systems. With fundamental knowledge of MDCT acquisition technique and CM injection protocols, high-quality, reliable data sets can be obtained, providing robust 2D and 3D images. Visualization techniques are fundamental to interpretation and work efficiency. With advancements in automated algorithms, maneuvering through the large data sets will continue to improve. Such work will facilitate continued CTA acceptance, obviating the need for DSA in most diagnostic vascular algorithms.

References

1. Criqui MH, Coughlin SS, Fronek A (1985) Noninvasively diagnosed peripheral arterial disease as a predictor of mortality: results from a prospective study. Circulation 72:768–773
2. Rubin GD, Schmidt AJ, Logan LJ, Sofilos MC (2001) Multi-detector row CT angiography of lower extremity arterial inflow and runoff: initial experience. Radiology 221(1):146–158
3. Catalano C, Fraioli F, Laghi A, Napoli A et al. (2004) Infrarenal aortic and lower-extremity arterial disease: diagnostic performance of multi-detector row CT angiography. Radiology 231(2):555–563
4. Greenfield LJ, Rajagopalan S, Olin JW (2002) Upper extremity arterial disease. Cardiol Clin 20:623–631
5. Joyce JW (1992) Occlusive arterial disease of the upper extremity. Cardiovasc Clin 22(3):147–160
6. Zimmerman NB (1993) Occlusive vascular disorders of the upper extremity. Hand Clin 9(1):139–150
7. Fleischmann D, Rubin GD, Bankier AA, Hittmair K (2000) Improved uniformity of aortic enhancement with customized contrast medium injection protocols at CT angiography. Radiology 214(2):363–871

15 Three-Dimensional Evaluation of the Venous System in Varicose Limbs by Multidetector Spiral CT

Jean-François Uhl and Alberto Caggiati

CONTENTS

15.1 Introduction

The anatomy of the venous system of the lower extremities is extremely complex and variable, especially in varicose and/or postthrombotic limbs [2]. There is a need for research into even more global and morphologically accurate techniques for examination of the vascular tree.

Traditional venography lost its title of gold standard for the morphofunctional examination of the venous tree of the lower limbs because, in the majority of cases, Duplex ultrasonography (US) furnishes a more accurate imaging and more complete hemodynamic evaluation with a less traumatic, expensive and time-consuming technique.

Recent advances in computer techniques have brought an innovative technique for investigation of venous disease based upon the use of spiral CT (veno-CT or VCT). Veno-CT furnishes an accurate three-dimensional (3D) representation of the whole venous system of the lower limb, demonstrating, in same cases, hemodynamic patterns which are not available from Duplex US.

J-F. Uhl, MD
Varicose Vein Surgical Center, 113 av. Charles De Gaulle, 92200 Neuilly, France; and Laboratoire d'Anatomie, Université Paris V – Necker, 75006 Paris, France
A. Caggiati, MD
Department of Anatomy, University of Rome "La Sapienza", Via Borrelli, 50, 00161 Rome, Italy

15.2 Principles of Spiral CT

The spiral or helical CT scan is the result of two different moves combined: Firstly, the rotation of an X-ray tube attached with detectors rotating around the patient's bed; Secondly, a continuous linear translation of the same bed. This enables the acquisition of volume data, with different results: 3D reconstructed images and slices.

15.2.1 Methods

The three steps of the VCT investigation are data acquisition, reconstruction, and postprocessing.

After treatment, reconstructed images are transmitted by intranet and can be seen on a PC by the angiologist (Fig. 15.1).

15.2.1.1 Data Acquisition

A multislice and multidetector CT scan (Siemens Somatom sensation 16) is used, producing 400–600 slices by series during 25–40 s. The protocol details are shown in Table 15.1, for 8- and 16-detector spiral CT.

The patient lies on his/her back (feet-first into the scanner), with no contact points with the table

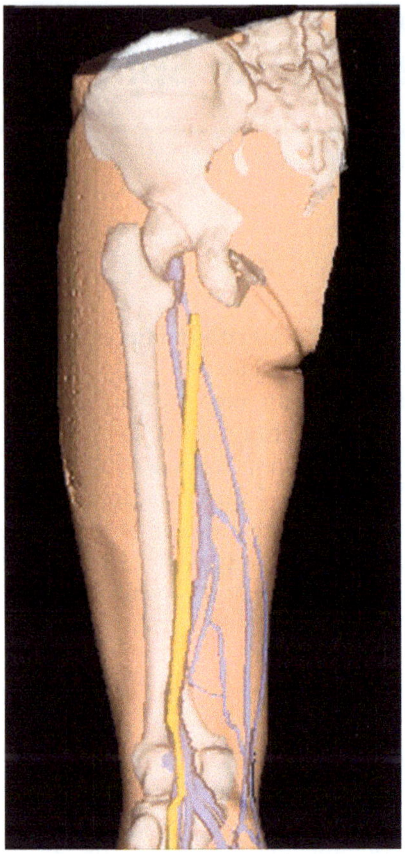

Fig. 15.1 A reconstructed image after data transmission

except for the buttocks and heels: It is important to avoid any compression of the calf and posterior thigh during acquisition time. The patient has to keep perfectly still during this short time and is often asked to make a Valsalva maneuver.

15.2.1.2 Data Reconstruction

Raw data are processed to perform a slice reconstruction. We use a slice width of 2 mm with a slice increment of 1.5 mm, a filter B30, and a zoom factor of 1.7 (Table 15.1)

15.2.1.3 Postprocessing of Data

To obtain 3D reconstruction of the venous system, the data are sent by intranet on a dedicated workstation for postprocessing using dedicated 3D reconstruction software.

Surface-rendering technique. (Also called "surface-shading rendering" – SSR). Huge progress has been made since 1994 in 3D image reconstruction. At the beginning, a manual segmentation of the image was necessary to obtain reconstructed 3D images by a SSR 3D model. A pixel extraction had to be done by the observer using appropriate windowing: the maximal minimal-density threshold was chosen manually in order to select the voxels corresponding to an anatomical structure. Although performed on Sun or Silicon graphics workstations, this technique was time-consuming and used only some of the data. In turn, it is possible to achieve manual reconstruction of some other structure of interest as nerves (Fig. 15.2).

Volume-rendering techniques (VRT). Today, beautiful 3D images of the venous system (Fig. 15.3) are quickly produced by reconstruction with VRT, with easy-to-

Table 15.1 Multislice and multidetector spiral CT protocols

Protocols	Acquisition	Reconstruction	Postprocessing	Contrast injection
8-Detector CT: 400 slices in 30 s	120 kV 130 mAs slice collimation: 8×2.5 mm field 512 rotation time 0.5-s feed/ rotation 15 mm FOV 380 mm	Slice width 3 mm Slice increment 2 mm filter B20 Matrix 512×512 Zoom factor 1.7	1994–1997 Surface-shading rendered (with manual segmentation)	Medrad MCT injector system Uniphasic injection 20 ml of iodine contrast medium in 180 ml of serum Puncture of a vein of the dorsal foot or rarely the varices of the thigh
16-Detector CT: 600 slices in 25 s	120 kV 150 mAs slice collimation: 16×1.5 mm field 512 FOV 380 mm	Slice width 2 mm slice increment 1.5 mm filter B30 matrix 512×512 zoom factor 1.7	1998-2002 Volume rendering Fast & automatic with tissue transparency	

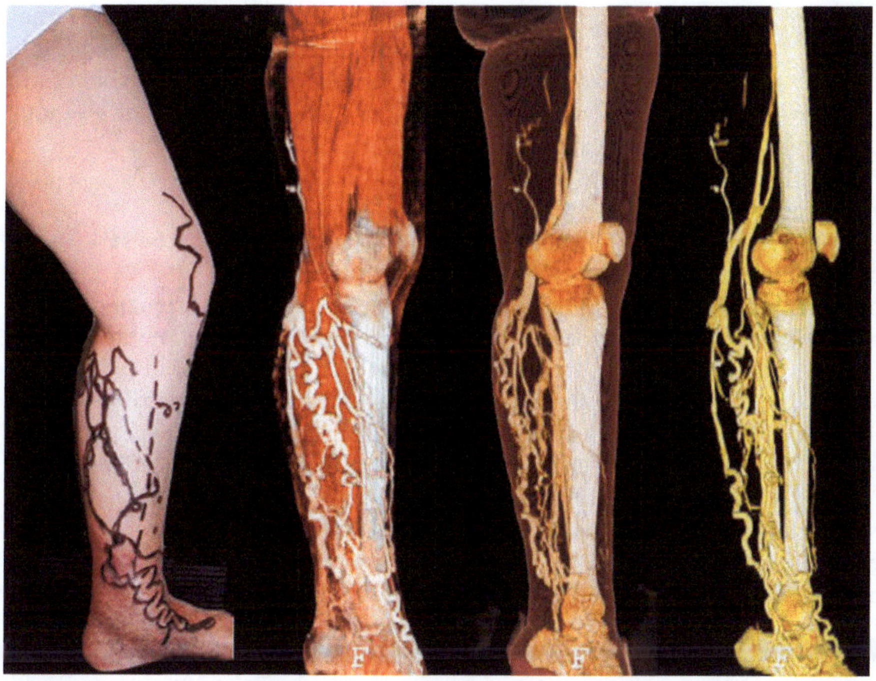

Fig. 15.2 Surface rendering with sciatic nerve reconstruction

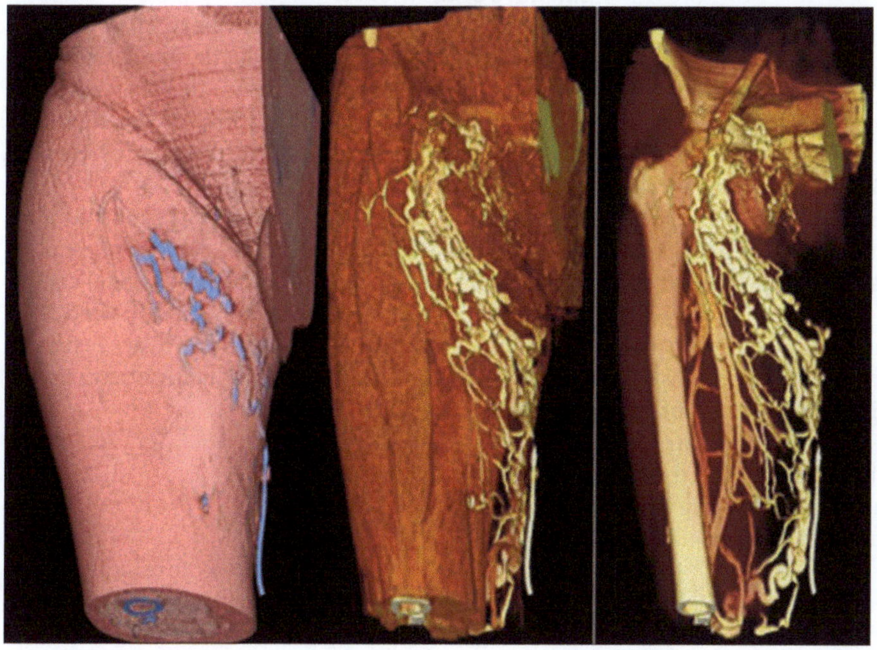

Fig. 15.3 Volume rendering: different transparencies of the tissues

use, built-in protocols. This saves time and takes full advantage of all the 3D information of the dataset. New 3D dedicated software running on a PC with 1 gigabyte of RAM are now available for this purpose.

Main functions of VRT are: rotation, tilt, pan, zoom, and use of different transparencies of the tissues in real time. Automatic presets are available to directly visualize skin, muscles, or vessels. Quick and easy images are captured or animated. Output functions are useful to transmit resulting images to a PC.

The VRT software we use is Plug & View 3D (VOXAR Inc.; Tiani-Medgraph).

15.2.1.4
Contrast-Medium Injection

An injection of diluted contrast is to be preferred in order to enhance the contrast of the venous network, allowing display of it alone, without the surrounding tissues with the VRT software (by using automated preset protocols).This is also true for the perforators: their course and precise connection with the deep veins are to be checked before surgery. Lastly, it is mandatory to investigate the detailed morphology of the deep system.

15.2.1.5
Venous Puncture

A dorsal foot vein puncture is performed in most cases. In particular cases, the cannulation of a varix of the leg or thigh could be necessary, to opacify a varicose network of the root of the limb, a pelvic varix, or a pelvic origin of the reflux, or to show an excluded varicose region.

15.2.1.6
Injection Technique

We use an automated Medrad MCT injector system. A uniphasic injection of 20 ml of iodine contrast medium is done in 180 ml of serum, at the rate of 2-3 ml/s. The duration of injection (usually 1 min) is synchronized with acquisition time, starting 30 s before and lasting until the end of acquisition.

Associated techniques can be used to enhance the contrast: a Valsalva maneuver is frequently asked of the patient. A tourniquet is put at the root of the thigh in case of investigation of the popliteal area. A balloon placed in the suprailiac area is inflated during acquisition for better evaluation of the inguinal veins.

15.2.1.7
Contrast-less 3D Venography

3D imaging of the venous tree can be obtained also without contrast-medium injection [3–5].

Technique. Parameters of acquisition: 125 kVp; 120 mA; collimation 2; pitch 4; 1 reconstruction. Images were reformatted at the CT console and transferred in a DICOM format to a dedicated workstation equipped with dedicated software such as Voxar (www.voxar.com).

Contrast-less veno-CT visualizes the external face of the veins, not their lumen. As a consequence, contrast injection is necessary when the goal of the examination is to evaluate the patency of a venous segment.

15.2.1.8
Transmission of 3D Images to the Specialist

The slices and a selection of 3D reconstructed images can be saved on a CD, but the best way to achieve the data transmission between the radiologist and the angiologist is to export the movie files of a rotating 3D model using different transparencies of the tissues: skin, muscle, vessels. (Fig. 15.3). These dynamic data are easily built and exported by the new VRT software.

One of the best ways is to use the QTVR software (Quicktime virtual reality) from Apple. It achieves a true interaction with a rotation of the 3D model according to the horizontal move of the mouse, and modifies tissue transparency according to the vertical move of the mouse.

In that way, the surgeon can have all of the information about the veno-CT available on his laptop computer in the operating room, together with the data of paper cartography [5] and of the US skin-mapping [6]. They can be used together as a roadmap for surgery.

By an exquisite depiction of the venous course, VCT may avoid the anatomical pitfalls of venous surgery. This makes possible a better surgical choice of technique, and a more accurate and limited skin approach. Accordingly, it improves the aesthetic result as well as the efficacy, reducing the varicose vein recurrence rate.

15.2.1.9
Limits, Pitfalls, and Drawbacks

Technical problems. Venous puncture was rarely impossible (3-4% of the limbs). However, a VCT without injection is possible, providing detailed anatomical information, but restricted to the superficial network [3].

Limits. The main drawback is that VCT provides no hemodynamic data, and it can only be performed in a prone position. It means that the Duplex US examination (in a standing position) is always necessary. It provides a complete map of the superficial venous network and perforators with anatomical and hemodynamic data [7]. In addition, a preoperative skin-mapping is performed [8], to be use as a guideline by the surgeon during surgery.

Pitfalls. The possible lack of injection of some veins means a careful differentiation from a venous thrombosis has to be made. It may be due to competent valves, venous congenital agenesis or hypoplasia, or compression point(s), usually calf, by the table. There is an exclusion area in case of huge and/or high-located varicose veins. The region is not filled by the foot injection: the solution is to make a direct puncture of the varix to obtain good visualization, so there is a case for pelvic varix visualization. A direct puncture of a perineal vein is the best way to get a fine injection of these complex networks. (Fig. 15.4). The main reason is an improper bolus timing of contrast-material injection, usually a too-short injection time: the contrast material had no time to reach the anatomical region of interest. In order to avoid this problem, one can use a tourniquet and/or a Valsalva maneuver. This is particularly true for popliteal fossa investigation: here the tourniquet of the root of the limb increases the quality of contrast and avoids an examination failure. In case of difficulty, we have to keep in mind that 3D reconstructions are not fully reliable. These clever postprocessing routines create images that do not exist. Hence, to avoid a misunderstanding or a false diagnosis by the use of the 3D images, do not hesitate to go back to the original slices and also to compare with other investigations (US).

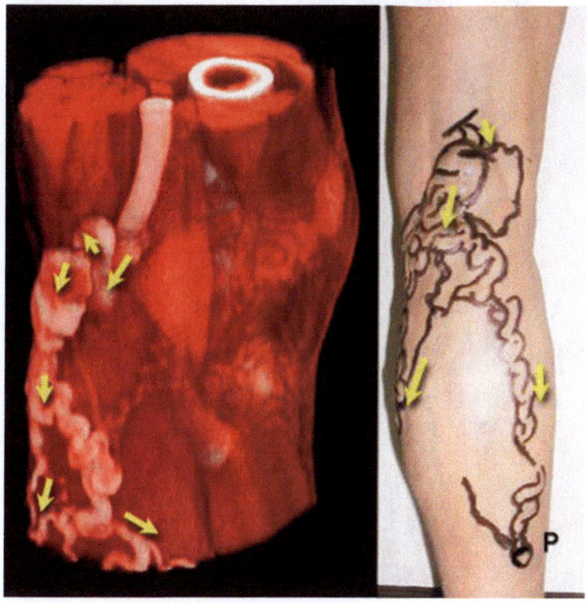

Fig. 15.4 Puncture of the varix of the thigh to enhance contrast

Drawbacks. X-ray exposure is the main criticism of CT venography. A pure venogram can be obtained by other "radiation-free" and less-invasive techniques, but they provide a lower quality of images: MR venography without gadolinium injection using protocols that incorporate 2D time-of-flight acquisition. Recently, Fraser et al. [6] proposed a new MR venography technique called VESPA (venous enhanced subtracted peak arterial) with gadolinium injection, using spatial subtraction which eliminates the need to cannulate a foot vein.

15.2.2 Clinical Applications

15.2.2.1 Preoperative Assessment of CVI on Varicose Patients

On the basis of the experience derived from a large series of investigations, VCT is usefully recommended in about 15% of patients undergoing surgery for varicose veins. [9]. It is particularly useful in the following cases:

- Postoperative recurrences, especially at the popliteal fossa. (Fig. 15.5)
- High termination (Fig. 15.6) or dystrophic termination of the short saphenous vein (Fig. 15.7)
- Duplication of the saphenous popliteal junction (Fig. 15.8)
- Varicose veins of the long saphenous region fed by an ascending flux of the Giacomini vein via a saphenous popliteal reflux (Fig. 15.9)
- Large and complex varicose networks, to improve information furnished by clinical and US mapping (Fig. 15.10; skin mapping, 1; VCT skin level, 2; and VCT muscle level, 3)
- Patients with large perforators of the thigh

In all these cases, the association with color-coded Duplex of the venous network is mandatory, because VCT does not provide hemodynamic data.

15.2.2.2 Investigation of Pelvic Varix

The pelvic origin of varicose veins is not rare, and is responsible for specific symptoms. Color Duplex using a vaginal probe is useful to study hemodynamics.

VCT investigates the reflux route and anatomical connections of the *pelvic* network: a possible cause of reflux is an incompetent lumbo-ovarian vein com-

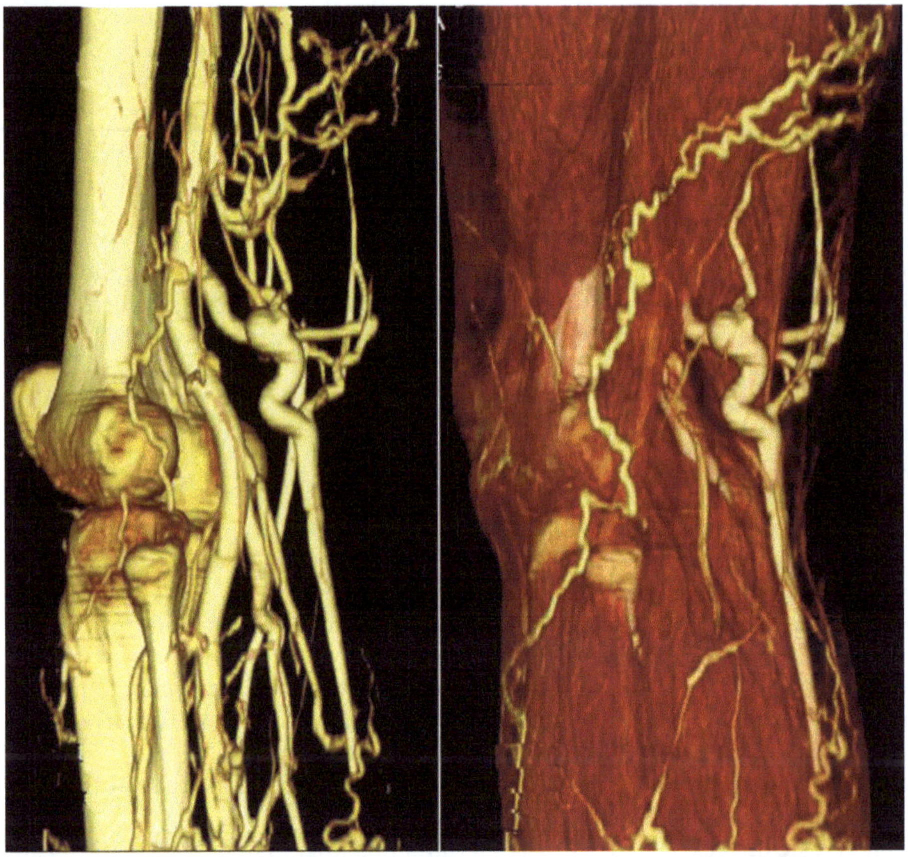

Fig. 15.5 Popliteal fossa cavernoma following short saphenous vein surgery

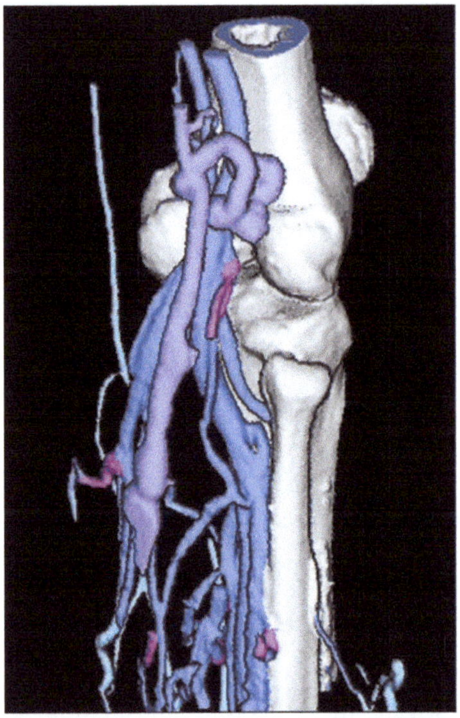

Fig. 15.6 High termination of the short saphenous vein

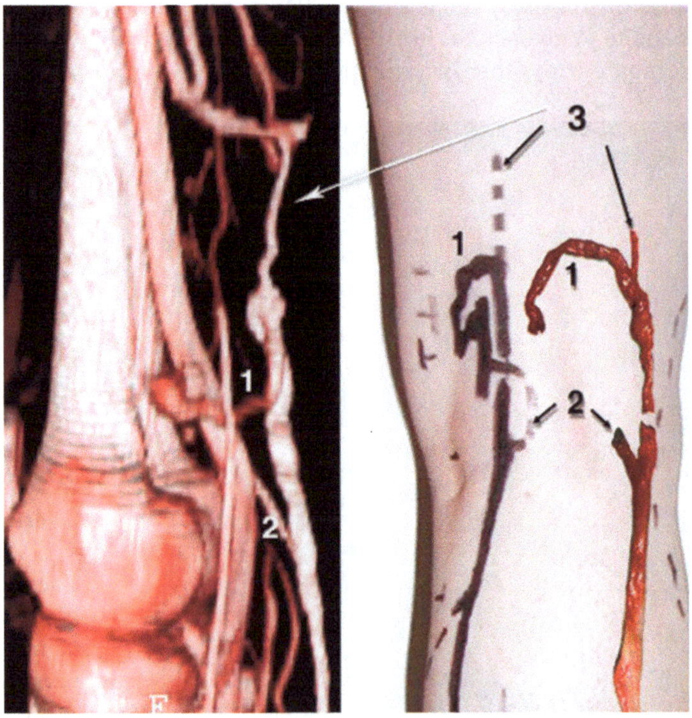

Fig. 15.7 Dystrophic short saphenous vein and saphenous popliteal junction

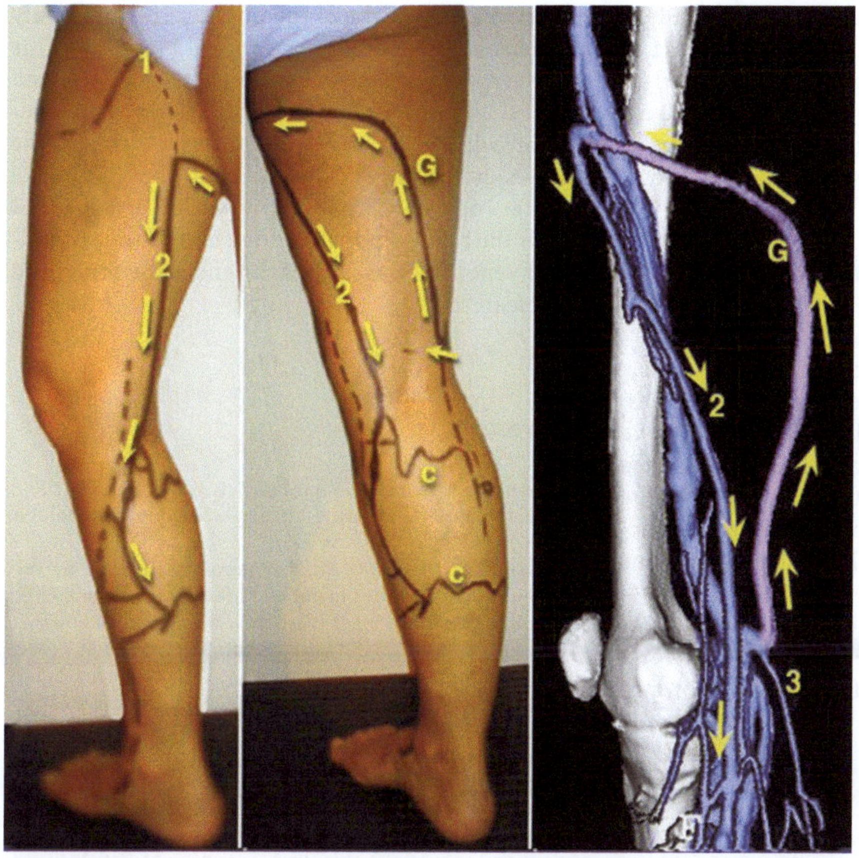

Fig. 15.8 Duplication of the saphenous popliteal junction

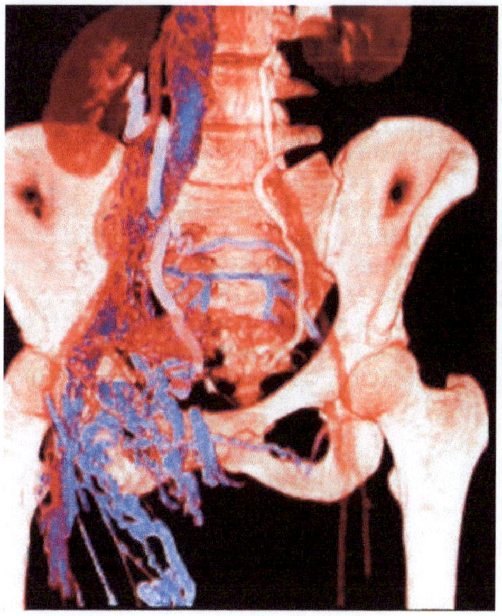

Fig. 15.9 Long saphenous vein varix fed by the Giacomini vein

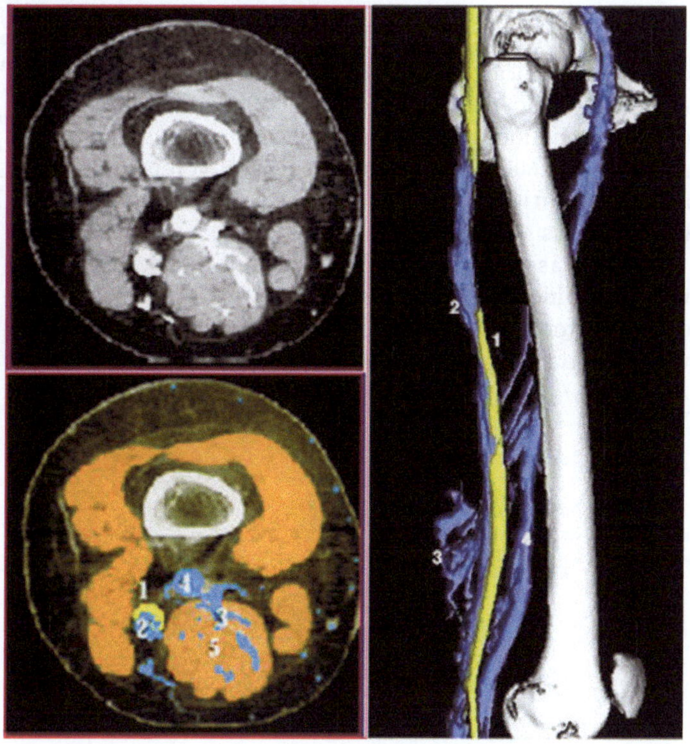

Fig. 15.10 Improved information about complex network

ing from the inferior vena cava, feeding the pudendal network by the inguinal canal. In such a case, interventional radiology using a coil associated to foam with sclerotic agent is the best choice to treat the origin of the reflux, associated with removal of the varix of the limb by phlebectomies.

15.2.2.3 Investigation of a Varix of the Sheath of the Sciatic Nerve

According to neurovenous embryogenesis, varicosis of the sciatic nerve follows the route of the nerves: sciatic nerve at the thigh level, fibular nerve at the knee level, and lateral saphenous nerve below knee level [7]. VCT usually shows the deep route at the thigh along the sciatic nerve: on the 3D reconstructions as well as on the slices, the dystrophic venous network infiltrates the sheath of the nerve. It is associated here with a stasis in the muscular arcades of the semimembranosus muscle (Fig. 15.12; network, 1; femoral vein, 2; dilatation of the semimembranosus arcades, 3).

15.3 Conclusion

The aim of spiral VCT (veno-CT) is to provide a precise 3D anatomical depiction of the venous network. A multislice and multidetector spiral CT acquisition of the lower limb with contrast injection produces about 400 to 600 slices in 30 s. Dedicated volume-rendering software compute interactive 3D images of the venous system.

Always associated with color-coded Duplex, which provides hemodynamic data, VCT is a powerful new tool to investigate patients with varicose veins, particularly in the case of a recurrences or for complex networks of the popliteal fossa; it truly provides a 3D roadmap for surgical planning. This role seems to be extremely important in selected cases, such as in the presence of pelvic venous congestion with reflux transmitted to the veins of the leg. Beside the patient's assessment, the VCT make us enter into the virtual reality world. Hence, it is a tool of the highest potential for a better understanding of venous disease, to learn venous anatomy, and for research.

References

1. Lemasle P, Lefebvre-Vilardebo M, Uhl JF, et al. (2000) La varicose de la gaine du nerf sciatique. Phlébologie 53:363–373
2. Claude Gillot (1998) Atlas anatomique du système veineux superficiel des membres inférieurs. Editions Phlébologiques Françaises (French and English versions)
3. Caggiati A, Ricci S, Lucchichienti G, Pavone P (2000) Visualisation tridimensionnelle de l'arbre veineux superficial par scanner hélicoidal. Phlebologie 53:275–277
4. Caggiati A, Luccichenti G, Pavone P (2000) 3D phlebography of the saphenous venous system. Circulation 102: E33--35
5. Caggiati A, Ricci S, Laghi A, Lucchichenti G, Pavone P (2001) 3D contrastless varicography by spiral computed tomography. Eur J Vasc Endovasc Surg 21:374–376
6. Fraser DGW, Moody AR, Davidson IR, Martel AR, Morgan PS (2003) Deep venous thrombosis: venous enhanced subtracted peak arterial MR venography versus conventionnal venography for diagnosis. Radiology 226:810–820
7. Lemasle P, Lefebvre-Vilardebo M, Uhl JF, et al. (2000) La cartographie veineuse superficielle. Considérations pratiques. Phlébologie 53:363–373
8. Uhl JF, Lefebvre-Vilardebo M, Lemasle P (1995) L'échomarquage pré-opératoire des varices des membres inférieurs: une exploration essentielle pour l'efficacité de la chirurgie d'exérèse. Phlébologie 48:359–365
9. Uhl JF, Verdeille S, Martin-Bouyer Y (2003) Interêt du phléboscan hélicoïdal avec reconstruction 3D dans le bilan pré-opératoire des varices. Phlébologie 56:11–16

Subject Index

List of Contributors

HISASHI ABE, MD
Department of Radiology
Osaka University Graduate School of Medicine D1
2-2 Yamadaoka, Suita-City
Osaka 565-0871
Japan

CARLO BARTOLOZZI, MD
Professor and Chairman
Division of Diagnostic and Interventional Radiology
Department of Oncology, Transplants,
and Advanced Technologies in Medicine
University of Pisa
Via Roma 67
56126 Pisa
Italy

CHRISTOPH R. BECKER, MD
Associate Professor, Department of Clinical Radiology
University Hospital Grosshadern
University Munich
Marchioninistr. 15
81377 Munich
Germany

LINDA BERTOLETTI, MD
Department of Radiological Sciences
University of Rome "La Sapienza"
Policlinico Umberto I
Viale Regina Elena n. 324
00161 Rome
Italy

LORENZO BONOMO, MD
Professor, Department of Radiology
Policlinico Agostino Gemelli
Università Cattolica del Sacro Cuore
L.go F. Vito, 1
00168 Rome
Italy

ALBERTO CAGGIATI, MD
Department of Anatomy
University of Rome "La Sapienza"
Via Borrelli, 50
00161 Rome
Italy

CARLO CATALANO, MD
Associate Professor, Department of Radiological Sciences
University of Rome "La Sapienza"
Policlinico Umberto I
Viale Regina Elena n. 324
00161 Rome
Italy

DAVIDE CARAMELLA, MD
Diagnostic and Interventional Radiology
Department of Oncology, Transplants,
and Advanced Technologies in Medicine
University of Pisa
Via Roma 67
56126 Pisa
Italy

MICHAEL D. DAKE, MD
Department of Radiology
Stanford University Medical Center
300 Pasteur Drive
SHS H3647
Stanford, CA 94305-5642
USA

MASSIMILIANO DANTI, MD
Department of Radiological Sciences
University of Rome "La Sapienza"
Policlinico Umberto I
Viale Regina Elena n. 324
00161 Rome
Italy

RICCARDO FERRARI, MD
Department of Radiological Sciences
University of Rome "La Sapienza"
Policlinico Umberto I
Viale Regina Elena n. 324
00161 Rome
Italy

DOMINIK FLEISCHMANN, MD
Assistant Professor of Radiology
Department of Radiology
Thoracic and Cardiovascular Imaging Sections
Stanford University Medical Center
300 Pasteur Drive, Room S-072
Stanford CA, 94305-5105
USA

Thomas Flohr, PhD
Siemens Medical Solutions, CT Concepts
Siemensstr. 1
91301 Forchheim
Germany

Francesco Fraioli, MD
Department of Radiological Sciences
University of Rome "La Sapienza"
Policlinico Umberto I
Viale Regina Elena n. 324
00161 Rome
Italy

Jeffrey C. Hellinger, MD
Department of Radiology
Division of Cardiovascular Imaging
Stanford University Medical Center
300 Pasteur Drive, Room S-068B
Stanford CA, 94305-5105
USA

Toshinori Hirai, MD
Department of Radiology
Kumamoto University School of Medicine
1-1-1 Honjo
Kumamoto 860-8556
Japan

Man Hon, MD
Attending, Department of Radiology
Winthrop-University Hospital
259 First Street
Mineola, NY 11501
USA
and
Assistant Professor of Clinical Radiology
State University of New York at Stony Brook
Stony Brook, NY
USA

Masatoshi Hori, MD, PhD
Department of Radiology
Osaka University Graduate School of Medicine D1
2-2 Yamadaoka, Suita-City
Osaka 565-0871
Japan

Riccardo Iannaccone, MD
Department of Radiological Sciences
University of Rome "La Sapienza"
Policlinico Umberto I
Viale Regina Elena n. 324
00161 Rome
Italy

Roberto Iezzi, MD
Department of Radiology
University of Chieti
"SS. Annunziata" Hospital
Via dei Vestini
66031 Chieti Scalo
Italy

Douglas S. Katz, MD
Vice Chair and Director of Body CT
Department of Radiology
Winthrop-University Hospital
259 First Street
Mineola, NY 11501
USA
and
Associate Professor of Clinical Radiology
State University of New York at Stony Brook
Stony Brook, NY
USA

Azzam Anwar Khankan, MD
Department of Radiology
Osaka University Graduate School of Medicine D1
2-2 Yamadaoka, Suita-City
Osaka 565-0871
Japan

Tonsok Kim, MD
Department of Radiology
Osaka University Graduate School of Medicine D1
2-2 Yamadaoka, Suita-City
Osaka 565-0871
Japan

Yukunori Korogi, MD
Department of Radiology
Kumamoto University School of Medicine
1-1-1 Honjo
Kumamoto 860-8556
Japan

Masatomo Kuwabara, MD
Department of Radiology
Osaka University Graduate School of Medicine D1
2-2 Yamadaoka, Suita-City
Osaka 565-0871
Japan

Andrea Laghi, MD
Department of Radiological Sciences
University of Rome "La Sapienza"
Policlinico Umberto I
Viale Regina Elena n. 324
00161 Rome
Italy

Jonathan M. Levin, MD
Department of Radiology
Stanford University Medical Center
300 Pasteur Drive
SHS H3647
Stanford, CA 94305-5642
USA

Daniele Marin, MD
Department of Radiological Sciences
University of Rome "La Sapienza"
Policlinico Umberto I
Viale Regina Elena n. 324
00161 Rome
Italy

Biagio Merlino, MD
Department of Radiology
Policlinico Agostino Gemelli
Università Cattolica del Sacro Cuore
L.go F. Vito, 1
00168 Rome
Italy

Takamichi Murakami, MD, PhD
Associate Professor and Vicechairman
Department of Radiology
Osaka University Graduate School of Medicine D1
2-2 Yamadaoka, Suita-City
Osaka 565-0871
Japan

Hironobu Nakamura, MD, PhD
Department of Radiology
Osaka University Graduate School of Medicine D1
2-2 Yamadaoka, Suita-City
Osaka 565-0871
Japan

Alessandro Napoli, MD
Department of Radiology
University of Rome "La Sapienza"
Policlinico Umberto I
Viale Regina Elena n. 324
00161 Rome
Italy

Piergiorgio Nardis, MD
Department of Radiological Sciences
University of Rome "La Sapienza"
Policlinico Umberto I
Viale Regina Elena n. 324
00161 Rome
Italy

Emanuele Neri, MD
Diagnostic and Interventional Radiology
Department of Oncology, Transplants,
and Advanced Technologies in Medicine
University of Pisa
Via Roma 67
56126 Pisa
Italy

Francesco Odoguardi, MD
Diagnostic and Interventional Radiology
Department of Oncology, Transplants,
and Advanced Technologies in Medicine
University of Pisa
Via Roma 67
56126 Pisa
Italy

Roberto Passariello, MD
Professor, Department of Radiological Sciences
University of Rome "La Sapienza"
Policlinico Umberto I
Viale Regina Elena n. 324
00161 Rome
Italy

Federica Pediconi, MD
Department of Radiological Sciences
University of Rome "La Sapienza"
Policlinico Umberto I
Viale Regina Elena n. 324
00161 Rome
Italy

Stefan Schaller, PhD
Siemens Medical Solutions, CT Concepts
Siemensstr. 1
91301 Forchheim
Germany

U. Joseph Schoepf, MD
Department of Radiology
Medical University of South Carolina
169 Ashley Avenue
Charleston, SC 29425
USA

Mutsumasa Takahashi, MD
Kumamoto University
School of Medicine
International Imaging Center
1-2-23 Kuhonji
Kumamoto 862-0976
Japan

Jean-François Uhl, MD
Varicose Vein Surgical Center
113 av. Ch. De Gaulle
92200 Neuilly, France

and

Laboratoire d'Anatomie
Université Paris V – Necker
45 rue des saints pères
75006 Paris, France

Paola Vagli, MD
Diagnostic and Interventional Radiology
Department of Oncology, Transplants,
and Advanced Technologies in Medicine
University of Pisa
Via Roma 67
56126 Pisa
Italy

Yasuyuki Yamashita, MD
Department of Radiology
Kumamoto University School of Medicine
1-1-1 Honjo
Kumamoto 860-8556
Japan

MEDICAL RADIOLOGY Diagnostic Imaging and Radiation Oncology

Titles in the series already published

DIAGNOSTIC IMAGING

Innovations in Diagnostic Imaging
Edited by J. H. Anderson

Radiology of the Upper Urinary Tract
Edited by E. K. Lang

The Thymus - Diagnostic Imaging, Functions, and Pathologic Anatomy
Edited by E. Walter, E. Willich, and W. R. Webb

Interventional Neuroradiology
Edited by A. Valavanis

Radiology of the Pancreas
Edited by A. L. Baert, co-edited by G. Delorme

Radiology of the Lower Urinary Tract
Edited by E. K. Lang

Magnetic Resonance Angiography
Edited by I. P. Arlart, G. M. Bongartz, and G. Marchal

Contrast-Enhanced MRI of the Breast
S. Heywang-Köbrunner and R. Beck

Spiral CT of the Chest
Edited by M. Rémy-Jardin and J. Rémy

Radiological Diagnosis of Breast Diseases
Edited by M. Friedrich and E.A. Sickles

Radiology of the Trauma
Edited by M. Heller and A. Fink

Biliary Tract Radiology
Edited by P. Rossi, co-edited by M. Brezi

Radiological Imaging of Sports Injuries
Edited by C. Masciocchi

Modern Imaging of the Alimentary Tube
Edited by A. R. Margulis

Diagnosis and Therapy of Spinal Tumors
Edited by P. R. Algra, J. Valk, and J. J. Heimans

Interventional Magnetic Resonance Imaging
Edited by J.F. Debatin and G. Adam

Abdominal and Pelvic MRI
Edited by A. Heuck and M. Reiser

Orthopedic Imaging
Techniques and Applications
Edited by A. M. Davies and H. Pettersson

Radiology of the Female Pelvic Organs
Edited by E. K.Lang

Magnetic Resonance of the Heart and Great Vessels
Clinical Applications
Edited by J. Bogaert, A.J. Duerinckx, and F. E. Rademakers

Modern Head and Neck Imaging
Edited by S. K. Mukherji and J. A. Castelijns

Radiological Imaging of Endocrine Diseases
Edited by J. N. Bruneton in collaboration with B. Padovani and M.-Y. Mourou

Trends in Contrast Media
Edited by H. S. Thomsen, R. N. Muller, and R. F. Mattrey

Functional MRI
Edited by C. T. W. Moonen and P. A. Bandettini

Radiology of the Pancreas
2nd Revised Edition
Edited by A. L. Baert
Co-edited by G. Delorme and L. Van Hoe

Emergency Pediatric Radiology
Edited by H. Carty

Spiral CT of the Abdomen
Edited by F. Terrier, M. Grossholz, and C. D. Becker

Liver Malignancies
Diagnostic and Interventional Radiology
Edited by C. Bartolozzi and R. Lencioni

Medical Imaging of the Spleen
Edited by A. M. De Schepper and F. Vanhoenacker

Radiology of Peripheral Vascular Diseases
Edited by E. Zeitler

Diagnostic Nuclear Medicine
Edited by C. Schiepers

Radiology of Blunt Trauma of the Chest
P. Schnyder and M. Wintermark

Portal Hypertension
Diagnostic Imaging-Guided Therapy
Edited by P. Rossi
Co-edited by P. Ricci and L. Broglia

Recent Advances in Diagnostic Neuroradiology
Edited by Ph. Demaerel

Virtual Endoscopy and Related 3D Techniques
Edited by P. Rogalla, J. Terwisscha Van Scheltinga, and B. Hamm

Multislice CT
Edited by M. F. Reiser, M. Takahashi, M. Modic, and R. Bruening

Pediatric Uroradiology
Edited by R. Fotter

Transfontanellar Doppler Imaging in Neonates
A. Couture and C. Veyrac

Radiology of AIDS
A Practical Approach
Edited by J.W.A.J. Reeders and P.C. Goodman

CT of the Peritoneum
Armando Rossi and Giorgio Rossi

Magnetic Resonance Angiography
2nd Revised Edition
Edited by I. P. Arlart, G. M. Bongratz, and G. Marchal

Medical Radiology Diagnostic Imaging and Radiation Oncology

Titles in the series already published

Pediatric Chest Imaging
Edited by Javier Lucaya and Janet L. Strife

Applications of Sonography in Head and Neck Pathology
Edited by J. N. Bruneton in collaboration with C. Raffaelli and O. Dassonville

Imaging of the Larynx
Edited by R. Hermans

3D Image Processing
Techniques and Clinical Applications
Edited by D. Caramella and C. Bartolozzi

Imaging of Orbital and Visual Pathway Pathology
Edited by W. S. Müller-Forell

Pediatric ENT Radiology
Edited by S. J. King and A. E. Boothroyd

Radiological Imaging of the Small Intestine
Edited by N. C. Gourtsoyiannis

Imaging of the Knee
Techniques and Applications
Edited by A. M. Davies and V. N. Cassar-Pullicino

Perinatal Imaging
From Ultrasound to MR Imaging
Edited by Fred E. Avni

Radiological Imaging of the Neonatal Chest
Edited by V. Donoghue

Diagnostic and Interventional Radiology in Liver Transplantation
Edited by E. Bücheler, V. Nicolas, C. E. Broelsch, X. Rogiers, and G. Krupski

Radiology of Osteoporosis
Edited by S. Grampp

Imaging Pelvic Floor Disorders
Edited by C. I. Bartram and J. O. L. DeLancey
Associate Editors: S. Halligan, F. M. Kelvin, and J. Stoker

Imaging of the Pancreas
Cystic and Rare Tumors
Edited by C. Procacci and A. J. Megibow

High Resolution Sonography of the Peripheral Nervous System
Edited by S. Peer and G. Bodner

Imaging of the Foot and Ankle
Techniques and Applications
Edited by A. M. Davies, R. W. Whitehouse, and J. P. R. Jenkins

Radiology Imaging of the Ureter
Edited by F. Joffre, Ph. Otal, and M. Soulie

Imaging of the Shoulder
Techniques and Applications
Edited by A. M. Davies and J. Hodler

Radiology of the Petrous Bone
Edited by M. Lemmerling and S. S. Kollias

Interventional Radiology in Cancer
Edited by A. Adam, R. F. Dondelinger, and P. R. Mueller

Duplex and Color Doppler Imaging of the Venous System
Edited by G. H. Mostbeck

Multidetector-Row CT of the Thorax
Edited by U. J. Schoepf

Functional Imaging of the Chest
Edited by H.-U. Kauczor

Radiology of the Pharynx and the Esophagus
Edited by O. Ekberg

Radiological Imaging in Hematological Malignancies
Edited by A. Guermazi

Imaging and Intervention in Abdominal Trauma
Edited by R. F. Dondelinger

Multislice CT
2nd Revised Edition
Edited by M. F. Reiser, M. Takahashi, M. Modic, and C. R. Becker

Intracranial Vascular Malformations and Aneurysms
From Diagnostic Work-Up to Endovascular Therapy
Edited by M. Forsting

Radiology and Imaing of the Colon
Edited by A. H. Chapman

Coronary Radiology
Edited by M. Oudkerk

Dynamic Contrast-Enhanced Magnetic Resonance Imaging in Oncology
Edited by A. Jackson, D. L. Buckley, and G. J. M. Parker

Imaging in Treatment Planning for Sinonasal Diseases
Edited by R. Maroldi and P. Nicolai

Clinical Cardiac MRI
With Interactive CD-ROM
Edited by J. Bogaert, S. Dymarkowski, and A. M. Taylor

Focal Liver Lesions
Detection, Characterization, Ablation
Edited by R. Lencioni, D. Cioni, and C. Bartolozzi

Multidetector-Row CT Angiography
Edited by C. Catalano and R. Passariello

Medical Radiology Diagnostic Imaging and Radiation Oncology

Titles in the series already published

Radiation Oncology

Lung Cancer
Edited by C.W. Scarantino

Innovations in Radiation Oncology
Edited by H. R. Withers and L. J. Peters

Radiation Therapy of Head and Neck Cancer
Edited by G. E. Laramore

Gastrointestinal Cancer – Radiation Therapy
Edited by R.R. Dobelbower, Jr.

Radiation Exposure and Occupational Risks
Edited by E. Scherer, C. Streffer, and K.-R. Trott

Radiation Therapy of Benign Diseases
A Clinical Guide
S. E. Order and S. S. Donaldson

Interventional Radiation Therapy Techniques – Brachytherapy
Edited by R. Sauer

Radiopathology of Organs and Tissues
Edited by E. Scherer, C. Streffer, and K.-R. Trott

Concomitant Continuous Infusion Chemotherapy and Radiation
Edited by M. Rotman and C. J. Rosenthal

Intraoperative Radiotherapy – Clinical Experiences and Results
Edited by F. A. Calvo, M. Santos, and L.W. Brady

Radiotherapy of Intraocular and Orbital Tumors
Edited by W. E. Alberti and R. H. Sagerman

Interstitial and Intracavitary Thermoradiotherapy
Edited by M. H. Seegenschmiedt and R. Sauer

Non-Disseminated Breast Cancer
Controversial Issues in Management
Edited by G. H. Fletcher and S.H. Levitt

Current Topics in Clinical Radiobiology of Tumors
Edited by H.-P. Beck-Bornholdt

Practical Approaches to Cancer Invasion and Metastases
A Compendium of Radiation Oncologists' Responses to 40 Histories
Edited by A. R. Kagan with the Assistance of R. J. Steckel

Radiation Therapy in Pediatric Oncology
Edited by J. R. Cassady

Radiation Therapy Physics
Edited by A. R. Smith

Late Sequelae in Oncology
Edited by J. Dunst and R. Sauer

Mediastinal Tumors. Update 1995
Edited by D. E. Wood and C. R. Thomas, Jr.

Thermoradiotherapy and Thermochemotherapy

Volume 1:
Biology, Physiology, and Physics

Volume 2:
Clinical Applications

Edited by M.H. Seegenschmiedt, P. Fessenden, and C.C. Vernon

Carcinoma of the Prostate
Innovations in Management
Edited by Z. Petrovich, L. Baert, and L.W. Brady

Radiation Oncology of Gynecological Cancers
Edited by H.W. Vahrson

Carcinoma of the Bladder
Innovations in Management
Edited by Z. Petrovich, L. Baert, and L.W. Brady

Blood Perfusion and Microenvironment of Human Tumors
Implications for Clinical Radiooncology
Edited by M. Molls and P. Vaupel

Radiation Therapy of Benign Diseases
A Clinical Guide
2nd Revised Edition
S. E. Order and S. S. Donaldson

Carcinoma of the Kidney and Testis, and Rare Urologic Malignancies
Innovations in Management
Edited by Z. Petrovich, L. Baert, and L.W. Brady

Progress and Perspectives in the Treatment of Lung Cancer
Edited by P. Van Houtte, J. Klastersky, and P. Rocmans

Combined Modality Therapy of Central Nervous System Tumors
Edited by Z. Petrovich, L. W. Brady, M. L. Apuzzo, and M. Bamberg

Age-Related Macular Degeneration
Current Treatment Concepts
Edited by W. A. Alberti, G. Richard, and R. H. Sagerman

Radiotherapy of Intraocular and Orbital Tumors
2nd Revised Edition
Edited by R. H. Sagerman, and W. E. Alberti

Modification of Radiation Response
Cytokines, Growth Factors, and Other Biolgical Targets
Edited by C. Nieder, L. Milas, and K. K. Ang

Radiation Oncology for Cure and Palliation
R. G. Parker, N. A. Janjan, and M. T. Selch

Clinical Target Volumes in Conformal and Intensity Modulated Radiation Therapy
A Clinical Guide to Cancer Treatment
Edited by V. Grégoire, P. Scalliet, and K. K. Ang

Advances in Radiation Oncology in Lung Cancer
Edited by Branislav Jeremić

Springer

MIX
Papier aus verantwortungsvollen Quellen
Paper from responsible sources
FSC® C105338

If you have any concerns about our products,
you can contact us on
ProductSafety@springernature.com

In case Publisher is established outside the EU,
the EU authorized representative is:
Springer Nature Customer Service Center GmbH
Europaplatz 3, 69115 Heidelberg, Germany

Printed by Libri Plureos GmbH
in Hamburg, Germany